WORLD HEALTH ORGANIZATION

The

WORLD
HEALTH
REPORT
2001

Mental Health:

New Understanding, New Hope

WHO Library Cataloguing in Publication Data

The World health report : 2001 : Mental health : new understanding, new hope.

1. Mental health 2. Mental disorders 3. Community mental health services
4. Cost of illness 5. Forecasting 6.World health – trends
I.Title: Mental health : new understanding, new hope

ISBN 92 4 156201 3   (NLM Classification: WA 540.1)
ISSN 1020-3311

The World Health Organization welcomes requests for permission to reproduce or translate its publications, in part or in full. Applications and enquiries should be addressed to the Office of Publications, World Health Organization, 1211 Geneva 27, Switzerland, which will be glad to provide the latest information on any changes made to the text, plans for new editions, and reprints and translations already available.

The designations employed and the presentation of the material in this publication, including tables and maps, do not imply the expression of any opinion whatsoever on the part of the Secretariat of the World Health Organization concerning the legal status of any country, territory, city or area or of its authorities, or concerning the delimitation of its frontiers or boundaries. Dotted lines on maps represent approximate border lines for which there may not yet be full agreement.

The mention of specific companies or of certain manufacturers' products does not imply that they are endorsed or recommended by the World Health Organization in preference to others of a similar nature that are not mentioned. Errors and omissions excepted, the names of proprietary products are distinguished by initial capital letters.

Information concerning this publication can be obtained from:
World Health Report
World Health Organization
1211 Geneva 27, Switzerland
Fax: (41-22) 791 4870
Email: whr@who.int

Copies of this publication can be ordered from: bookorders@who.int

The principal writers of this report were Rangaswamy Srinivasa Murthy (editor-in-chief), José Manoel Bertolote, JoAnne Epping-Jordan, Michelle Funk, Thomson Prentice, Benedetto Saraceno, and Shekhar Saxena. The report was directed by a steering committee formed by Susan Holck, Christopher Murray (chair), Rangaswamy Srinivasa Murthy, Thomson Prentice, Benedetto Saraceno, and Derek Yach.

Contributions were gratefully received from Gavin Andrews, Sarah Assamagan, Myron Belfer, Tom Bornemann, Meena Cabral de Mello, Somnath Chatterji, Daniel Chisholm, Alex Cohen, Leon Eisenberg, David Goldberg, Steve Hyman, Arthur Kleinmann, Alan Lopez, Doris Ma Fat, Colin Mathers, Maristela Monteiro, Philip Musgrove, Norman Sartorius, Chitra Subramaniam, Naren Wig, and Derek Yach.

Valuable input was received from an internal advisory group and a regional reference group, the members of which are listed in the Acknowledgements. Additional help and advice were appreciated from regional directors, executive directors at WHO headquarters and senior policy advisers to the Director-General.

The report was edited by Angela Haden and Barbara Campanini. The tables and figures were coordinated by Michel Beusenberg. Translation coordination and other administrative support for the World Health Report team was provided by Shelagh Probst, assisted by Pearl Harlley. The index was prepared by Liza Furnival.

The cover incorporates the World Health Day 2001 logo, which was designed by Marc Bizet.

Design by Marilyn Langfeld. Layout by WHO Graphics
Printed in France
2001/13757 – Sadag – 20000

CONTENTS

CHAPTER 5

TABLES

FIGURES

Boxes

MESSAGE FROM THE

DIRECTOR-GENERAL

*M*ental illness is not a personal failure. It doesn't happen only to other people. We all remember a time not too long ago when we couldn't openly speak about cancer. That was a family secret. Today, many of us still do not want to talk about AIDS. These barriers are gradually being broken down.

The theme of World Health Day 2001 was "Stop exclusion – Dare to care". Its message was that there is no justification for excluding people with a mental illness or brain disorder from our communities – there is room for everyone. Yet many of us still shy away from, or feign ignorance of such individuals – as if we do not dare to understand and care. The theme of this report is "New understanding, new hope". It shows how science and sensibility are combining to break down real and perceived barriers to care and cure in mental health. For there is a new understanding that offers real hope to the mentally ill. Understanding how genetic, biological, social and environmental factors come together to cause mental and brain illness. Understanding how inseparable mental and physical health really are, and how their influence on each other is complex and profound. And this is just the beginning. I believe that talking about health without mental health is a little like tuning an instrument and leaving a few discordant notes.

WHO is making a simple statement: mental health – neglected for far too long – is crucial to the overall well-being of individuals, societies and countries and must be universally regarded in a new light.

Our call has been joined by the United Nations General Assembly, which this year marks the 10th anniversary of the rights of the mentally ill to protection and care. I believe *The World Health Report 2001* gives renewed emphasis to the UN principles laid down a decade ago. The first of these principles is that there shall be no discrimination on the grounds of mental illness. Another is that as far as possible, every patient shall have the right to be treated and cared for in his or her own community. And a third is that every patient shall have the right to be treated in the least restrictive environment, with the least restrictive or intrusive treatment.

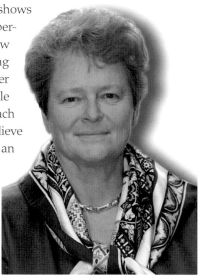

Dr Gro Harlem Brundtland

Throughout the year, our Member States have taken our struggle forward by focusing on various aspects of mental health whether it be medical, social or political. This year WHO is also supporting the development and launching of global campaigns on depression management and suicide prevention, schizophrenia and epilepsy. The World Health Assembly 2001 discussed mental health in all its dimensions. For us at the World Health Organization and in the extended community of health professionals, this heightened and sustained focus is an opportunity and a challenge.

A lot remains to be done. We do not know how many people are not getting the help they need – help that is available, help that can be obtained at no great cost. Initial estimates suggest that about 450 million people alive today suffer from mental or neurological disorders or from psychosocial problems such as those related to alcohol and drug abuse. Many of them suffer silently. Many of them suffer alone. Beyond the suffering and beyond the absence of care lie the frontiers of stigma, shame, exclusion, and more often than we care to know, death.

Major depression is now the leading cause of disability globally and ranks fourth in the ten leading causes of the global burden of disease. If projections are correct, within the next 20 years, depression will have the dubious distinction of becoming the second cause of the global disease burden. Globally, 70 million people suffer from alcohol dependence. About 50 million have epilepsy; another 24 million have schizophrenia. A million people commit suicide every year. Between ten and 20 million people attempt it.

Rare is the family that will be free from an encounter with mental disorders.

One person in every four will be affected by a mental disorder at some stage of life. The risk of some disorders, including Alzheimer's disease, increases with age. The conclusions are obvious for the world's ageing population. The social and economic burden of mental illness is enormous.

Today we know that most illnesses, mental and physical, are influenced by a combination of biological, psychological and social factors. Our understanding of the relationship between mental and physical health is rapidly increasing. We know that mental disorders are the outcome of many factors and have a physical basis in the brain. We know they can affect everyone, everywhere. And we know that more often than not, they can be treated effectively.

This report deals with depressive disorders, schizophrenia, mental retardation, disorders of childhood and adolescence, drug and alcohol dependence, Alzheimer's disease and epilepsy. All of these are common and usually cause severe disability. Epilepsy is not a mental problem, but we have included it because it faces the same kind of stigma, ignorance and fear associated with mental illnesses.

Our report is a comprehensive review of what we know about the current and future burden of all these disorders and their principal contributing factors. It deals with the effectiveness of prevention and the availability of, and barriers to, treatment. We deal in detail with service provision and service planning. And, finally, the report outlines policies needed to ensure that stigma and discrimination are broken down, and that effective prevention and treatment are put in place and adequately funded.

In more ways than one, we make this simple point: we have the means and the scientific knowledge to help people with mental and brain disorders. Governments have been remiss, as has been the public health community. By accident or by design, we are all responsible for this situation. As the world's leading public health agency, WHO has one, and only one option – to ensure that ours will be the last generation that allows shame and stigma to rule over science and reason.

Gro Harlem Brundtland
Geneva
October 2001

OVERVIEW

*T*his landmark World Health Organization publication aims to raise public and professional awareness of the real burden of mental disorders and their costs in human, social and economic terms. At the same time it intends to help dismantle many of those barriers – particularly of stigma, discrimination and inadequate services – which prevent many millions of people worldwide from receiving the treatment they need and deserve.

In many ways, *The World Health Report 2001* provides a new understanding of mental disorders that offers new hope to the mentally ill and their families in all countries and all societies. It is a comprehensive review of what is known about the current and future burden of disorders, and the principal contributing factors. It examines the scope of prevention and the availability of, and obstacles to, treatment. It deals in detail with service provision and planning; and it concludes with a set of far-reaching recommendations that can be adapted by every country according to its needs and its resources.

The ten recommendations for action are as follows.

1. PROVIDE TREATMENT IN PRIMARY CARE

The management and treatment of mental disorders in primary care is a fundamental step which enables the largest number of people to get easier and faster access to services – it needs to be recognized that many are already seeking help at this level. This not only gives better care; it cuts wastage resulting from unnecessary investigations and inappropriate and non-specific treatments. For this to happen, however, general health personnel need to be trained in the essential skills of mental health care. Such training ensures the best use of available knowledge for the largest number of people and makes possible the immediate application of interventions. Mental health should therefore be included in training curricula, with refresher courses to improve the effectiveness of the management of mental disorders in general health services.

2. MAKE PSYCHOTROPIC DRUGS AVAILABLE

Essential psychotropic drugs should be provided and made constantly available at all levels of health care. These medicines should be included in every country's essential drugs list, and the best drugs to treat conditions should be made available whenever possible. In some countries, this may require enabling legislation changes. These drugs can ameliorate symptoms, reduce disability, shorten the course of many disorders, and prevent relapse. They often provide the first-line treatment, especially in situations where psychosocial interventions and highly skilled professionals are unavailable.

3. GIVE CARE IN THE COMMUNITY

Community care has a better effect than institutional treatment on the outcome and quality of life of individuals with chronic mental disorders. Shifting patients from mental hospitals to care in the community is also cost-effective and respects human rights. Mental health services should therefore be provided in the community, with the use of all available resources. Community-based services can lead to early intervention and limit the stigma of taking treatment. Large custodial mental hospitals should be replaced by community care facilities, backed by general hospital psychiatric beds and home care support, which meet all the needs of the ill that were the responsibility of those hospitals. This shift towards community care requires health workers and rehabilitation services to be available at community level, along with the provision of crisis support, protected housing, and sheltered employment.

4. EDUCATE THE PUBLIC

Public education and awareness campaigns on mental health should be launched in all countries. The main goal is to reduce barriers to treatment and care by increasing awareness of the frequency of mental disorders, their treatability, the recovery process and the human rights of people with mental disorders. The care choices available and their benefits should be widely disseminated so that responses from the general population, professionals, media, policy-makers and politicians reflect the best available knowledge. This is already a priority for a number of countries, and national and international organizations. Well-planned public awareness and education campaigns can reduce stigma and discrimination, increase the use of mental health services, and bring mental and physical health care closer to each other.

5. INVOLVE COMMUNITIES, FAMILIES AND CONSUMERS

Communities, families and consumers should be included in the development and decision-making of policies, programmes and services. This should lead to services being better tailored to people's needs and better used. In addition, interventions should take account of age, sex, culture and social conditions, so as to meet the needs of people with mental disorders and their families.

6. ESTABLISH NATIONAL POLICIES, PROGRAMMES AND LEGISLATION

Mental health policy, programmes and legislation are necessary steps for significant and sustained action. These should be based on current knowledge and human rights considerations. Most countries need to increase their budgets for mental health programmes from existing low levels. Some countries that have recently developed or revised their policy and legislation have made progress in implementing their mental health care programmes. Mental health reforms should be part of the larger health system reforms. Health insurance schemes should not discriminate against persons with mental disorders, in order to give wider access to treatment and to reduce burdens of care.

7. DEVELOP HUMAN RESOURCES

Most developing countries need to increase and improve training of mental health professionals, who will provide specialized care as well as support the primary health care programmes. Most developing countries lack an adequate number of such specialists to staff mental health services. Once trained, these professionals should be encouraged to remain in their country in positions that make the best use of their skills. This human resource development is especially necessary for countries with few resources at present. Though primary care provides the most useful setting for initial care, specialists are needed to provide a wider range of services. Specialist mental health care teams ideally should include medical and non-medical professionals, such as psychiatrists, clinical psychologists, psychiatric nurses, psychiatric social workers and occupational therapists, who can work together towards the total care and integration of patients in the community.

8. LINK WITH OTHER SECTORS

Sectors other than health, such as education, labour, welfare, and law, and nongovernmental organizations should be involved in improving the mental health of communities. Nongovernmental organizations should be much more proactive, with better-defined roles, and should be encouraged to give greater support to local initiatives.

9. MONITOR COMMUNITY MENTAL HEALTH

The mental health of communities should be monitored by including mental health indicators in health information and reporting systems. The indices should include both the numbers of individuals with mental disorders and the quality of their care, as well as some more general measures of the mental health of communities. Such monitoring helps to determine trends and to detect mental health changes resulting from external events, such as disasters. Monitoring is necessary to assess the effectiveness of mental health prevention and treatment programmes, and it also strengthens arguments for the provision of more resources. New indicators for the mental health of communities are necessary.

10. SUPPORT MORE RESEARCH

More research into biological and psychosocial aspects of mental health is needed in order to increase the understanding of mental disorders and to develop more effective interventions. Such research should be carried out on a wide international basis to understand variations across communities and to learn more about factors that influence the cause, course and outcome of mental disorders. Building research capacity in developing countries is an urgent need.

THREE SCENARIOS FOR ACTION

International action is critical if these recommendations are to be implemented effectively, because many countries lack the necessary resources. United Nations technical and developmental agencies and others can assist countries with mental health infrastructure development, manpower training, and research capacity building.

To help guide countries, the report in its concluding section provides three "scenarios for action" according to the varying levels of national mental health resources around the world. Scenario A, for example, applies to economically poorer countries where such resources are completely absent or very limited. Even in such cases, specific actions such as training of all personnel, making essential drugs available at all health facilities, and moving the mentally ill out of prisons, can be applied. For countries with modest levels of resources, Scenario B suggests, among other actions, the closure of custodial mental hospitals and steps towards integrating mental health care into general health care. Scenario C, for those countries with most resources, proposes improvements in the management of mental disorders in primary health care, easier access to newer drugs, and community care facilities offering 100% coverage.

All of the above recommendations and actions stem from the main body of the report itself.

OUTLINE OF THE REPORT

Chapter 1 introduces the reader to a new understanding of mental health and explains why it is as important as physical health to the overall well-being of individuals, families, societies and communities.

Mental and physical health are two vital strands of life that are closely interwoven and deeply interdependent. Advances in neuroscience and behavioural medicine have shown that, like many physical illnesses, mental and behavioural disorders are the result of a complex interaction between biological, psychological and social factors.

As the molecular revolution proceeds, researchers are becoming able to see the living, feeling, thinking human brain at work and to see and understand why, sometimes, it works less well than it could. Future advances will provide a more complete understanding of how the brain is related to complex mental and behavioural functioning. Innovations in brain imaging and other investigative techniques will permit "real time cinema" of the nervous system in action.

Meanwhile, scientific evidence from the field of behavioural medicine has demonstrated a fundamental connection between mental and physical health – for instance, that depression predicts the occurrence of heart disease. Research shows that there are two main pathways through which mental and physical health mutually influence each other.

Physiological systems, such as neuroendocrine and immune functioning, are one such pathway. Anxious and depressed moods, for example, initiate a cascade of adverse changes in endocrine and immune functioning, and create increased susceptibility to a range of physical illnesses.

Health behaviour is another pathway and concerns activities such as diet, exercise, sexual practices, smoking and adhering to medical therapies. The health behaviour of an individual is highly dependent on that person's mental health. For example, recent evidence has shown that young people with psychiatric disorders such as depression and substance dependence are more likely to engage in smoking and high-risk sexual behaviour.

Individual psychological factors are also related to the development of mental disorders. The relationships between children and their parents or other caregivers during childhood are crucial. Regardless of the specific cause, children deprived of nurture are more likely to develop mental and behavioural disorders either in childhood or later in life. Social factors such as uncontrolled urbanization, poverty and rapid technological change are also important. The relationship between mental health and poverty is particularly important: the poor and the deprived have a higher prevalence of disorders, including substance abuse. The treatment gap for most mental disorders is high, but for the poor population it is indeed massive.

Chapter 2 begins to address the treatment gap as one of the most important issues in mental health today. It does so first of all by describing the magnitude and burden of mental and behavioural disorders. It shows they are common, affecting 20–25% of all people at some time during their life. They are also universal – affecting all countries and societies, and individuals at all ages. The disorders have a large direct and indirect economic impact on societies, including service costs. The negative impact on the quality of life of individuals and families is massive. It is estimated that, in 2000, mental and neurological disorders accounted for 12% of the total disability-adjusted life years (DALYs) lost due to all diseases and injuries. By 2020, it is projected that the burden of these disorders will have increased 15%. Yet only a small minority of all those presently affected receive any treatment.

The chapter introduces a group of common disorders that usually cause severe disability, and describes how they are identified and diagnosed, and their impact on quality of life. The group includes depressive disorders, schizophrenia, substance use disorders, epilepsy, mental retardation, disorders of childhood and adolescence, and Alzheimer's disease. Although epilepsy is clearly a neurological disorder, it is included because it has been seen historically as a mental disorder and is still considered this way in many societies. Like those with mental disorders, people with epilepsy suffer stigma and also severe disability if left untreated.

Factors determining the prevalence, onset and course of all these disorders include poverty, sex, age, conflict and disasters, major physical diseases, and family and social environment. Often, two or more mental disorders occur together in an individual, anxiety and depressive disorders being a common combination.

The chapter discusses the possibility of suicide associated with such disorders. Three aspects of suicide are of public health importance. First, it is one of the main causes of death of young people in most developed countries and in many developing ones as well. Second, there are wide variations in suicide rates across countries, between the sexes and across age groups, an indication of the complex interaction of biological, psychological and sociocultural factors. Third, suicides of younger people and of women are a recent and growing problem in many countries. Suicide prevention is among the issues discussed in the next chapter.

Chapter 3 is concerned with solving mental health problems. It highlights one key issue in the whole report, and one that features strongly in the overall recommendations. This is the positive shift, recommended for all countries and already occurring in some, from institutionalized care, in which the mentally disordered are held in asylums, custodial-type hospitals or prisons, to care in the community backed by the availability of beds in general hospitals for acute cases.

In 19th-century Europe, mental illness was seen on one hand as a legitimate topic for scientific enquiry: psychiatry burgeoned as a medical discipline, and people suffering from mental disorders were considered medical patients. On the other hand, people with these disorders, like those with many other diseases and undesirable social behaviour, were isolated from society in large custodial institutions, the state lunatic asylums, later known as mental hospitals. The trends were later exported to Africa, the Americas and Asia.

During the second half of the 20th century, a shift in the mental health care paradigm took place, largely owing to three independent factors. First, psychopharmacology made significant progress, with the discovery of new classes of drugs, particularly neuroleptics and antidepressants, as well as the development of new forms of psychosocial interventions. Second, the human rights movement became a truly international phenomenon under the sponsorship of the newly created United Nations, and democracy advanced on a global basis. Third, a mental component was firmly incorporated into the concept of health as defined by the newly established WHO. Together these events have prompted the move away from care in large custodial institutions to more open and flexible care in the community.

The failures of asylums are evidenced by repeated cases of ill-treatment to patients, geographical and professional isolation of the institutions and their staff, weak reporting and accounting procedures, bad management and ineffective administration, poorly targeted financial resources, lack of staff training, and inadequate inspection and quality assurance procedures.

In contrast, community care is about providing good care and the empowerment of people with mental and behavioural disorders. In practice, community care implies the development of a wide range of services within local settings. This process, which has not yet begun in many regions and countries, aims to ensure that some of the protective functions of the asylum are fully provided and that the negative aspects of the institutions are not perpetuated.

The following are characteristics of providing care in the community:

- services which are close to home, including general hospital care for acute admissions, and long-term residential facilities in the community;
- interventions related to disabilities as well as symptoms;
- treatment and care specific to the diagnosis and needs of each individual;
- a wide range of services which address the needs of people with mental and behavioural disorders;
- services which are coordinated between mental health professionals and community agencies;
- ambulatory rather than static services, including those which can offer home treatment;
- partnership with carers and meeting their needs;
- legislation to support the above aspects of care.

However, this chapter warns against closing mental hospitals without community alternatives and, conversely, creating community alternatives without closing mental hospitals. Both have to occur at the same time, in a well-coordinated, incremental way. A sound deinstitutionalization process has three essential components:

- prevention of inappropriate mental hospital admissions through the provision of community facilities;
- discharge to the community of long-term institutional patients who have received adequate preparation;
- establishment and maintenance of community support systems for non-institutionalized patients.

In many developing countries, mental health care programmes have a low priority. Provision is limited to a small number of institutions that are usually overcrowded, understaffed and inefficient. Services reflect little understanding of the needs of the ill or the range of approaches available for treatment and care. There is no psychiatric care for the majority of the population. The only services are in large mental hospitals that operate under legislation which is often more penal than therapeutic. They are not easily accessible and become communities of their own, isolated from society at large.

Despite the major differences between mental health care in developing and developed countries, they share a common problem: many people who could benefit do not take advantage of available psychiatric services. Even in countries with well-established services, fewer than half of those individuals needing care make use of such services. This is related both to the stigma attached to individuals with mental and behavioural disorders, and to the inappropriateness of the services provided.

The chapter identifies important principles of care in mental health. These include diagnosis, early intervention, rational use of treatment techniques, continuity of care, and a wide range of services. Additional principles are consumer involvement, partnerships with families, involvement of the local community, and integration into primary health care. The chapter also describes three fundamental ingredients of care – medication, psychotherapy and psychosocial rehabilitation – and says a balanced combination of them is always required. It discusses prevention, treatment, and rehabilitation in the context of the disorders highlighted in the report.

Chapter 4 deals with mental health policy and service provision. To protect and improve the mental health of the population is a complex task involving multiple decisions. It requires priorities to be set among mental health needs, conditions, services, treatments, and prevention and promotion strategies, and choices to be made about their funding. Mental health services and strategies must be well coordinated among themselves and with other services, such as social security, education, and public interventions in employment and housing. Mental health outcomes must be monitored and analysed so that decisions can be continually adjusted to meet emerging challenges.

Governments, as the ultimate stewards of mental health, need to assume the responsibility for ensuring that these complex activities are carried out. One critical role in stewardship is to develop and implement policy. This means identifying the major issues and objectives, defining the respective roles of the public and private sectors in financing and provision, and identifying policy instruments and organizational arrangements required in the public and possibly in the private sectors to meet mental health objectives. It also means prompting action for capacity building and organizational development, and providing guidance for prioritizing expenditure, thus linking analysis of problems to decisions about resource allocation.

The chapter looks in detail at these issues, beginning with options for financing arrangements for the delivery of mental health services, while noting that the characteristics of these should be no different from those for health services in general. People should be protected from catastrophic financial risk, which means minimizing out-of-pocket payments in favour of prepayment methods, whether via general taxation, mandatory social insurance or voluntary private insurance. The healthy should subsidize the sick through prepayment mechanisms, and a good financing system will also mean that the well-off subsidize the poor, at least to some extent.

The chapter goes on to discuss the formulation of mental health policy, which it notes is often developed separately from alcohol and drug policies. It says mental health, alcohol and drug policies must be formulated within the context of a complex body of government health, welfare and general social policies. Social, political and economic realities must be recognized at local, regional and national levels.

Policy formulation must be based upon up-to-date and reliable information concerning the community, mental health indicators, effective treatments, prevention and promotion strategies, and mental health resources. The policy will need to be reviewed periodically.

Policies should highlight vulnerable groups with special mental health needs, such as children, the elderly, and abused women, as well as refugees and displaced persons in countries experiencing civil wars or internal conflicts.

Policies should also include suicide prevention. This means, for example, reducing access to poisons and firearms, and detoxifying domestic gas and car exhausts. Such policies need to ensure not only care for individuals particularly at risk, such as those with depression, schizophrenia or alcohol dependence, but also the control of alcohol and illicit drugs.

The public mental health budget in many countries is mainly spent on maintaining institutional care, with few or no resources being made available for more effective services in the community. In most countries, mental health services need to be assessed, reevaluated and reformed to provide the best available treatment and care. The chapter discusses three ways of improving how services are organized, even with limited resources, so that those who need them can make full use of them. These are: shifting care away from mental hospitals, developing community mental health services, and integrating mental health services into general health care.

Other matters discussed in this chapter include ensuring the availability of psychotropic drugs, creating intersectoral links, choosing mental health interventions, public and private roles in provision of services, developing human resources, defining roles and functions of health workers, and promoting not just mental health but also the human rights of people with mental disorders. In this latter instance, legislation is essential to guarantee that their fundamental human rights are protected.

Intersectoral collaboration between government departments is essential in order for mental health policies to benefit from mainstream government programmes. In addition, mental health input is required to ensure that all government activities and policies contribute to and not detract from mental health. This involves labour and employment, commerce and economics, education, housing, other social welfare services and the criminal justice system.

The chapter says that the most important barriers to overcome in the community are stigma and discrimination, and that a multilevel approach is required, including the role of the mass media and the use of community resources to stimulate change.

Chapter 5 contains the recommendations and three scenarios for action listed at the beginning of this overview. It brings the report to an optimistic end, by emphasizing that solutions for mental disorders do exist and are available. The scientific advances made in the treatment of mental disorders mean that most individuals and families can be helped. In addition to effective treatment and rehabilitation, strategies for the prevention of some disorders are available. Suitable and progressive mental health policy and legislation can go a long way towards delivering services to those in need. There is new understanding, and there is new hope.

CHAPTER ONE

A Public Health
Approach to Mental Health

Mental health is as important as physical health to the overall well-being of individuals, societies and countries. Yet only a small minority of the 450 million people suffering from a mental or behavioural disorder are receiving treatment. Advances in neuroscience and behavioural medicine have shown that, like many physical illnesses, mental and behavioural disorders are the result of a complex interaction between biological, psychological and social factors. While there is still much to be learned, we already have the knowledge and power to reduce the burden of mental and behavioural disorders worldwide.

1

A Public Health Approach to Mental Health

Introduction

*F*or all individuals, mental, physical and social health are vital strands of life that are closely interwoven and deeply interdependent. As understanding of this relationship grows, it becomes ever more apparent that mental health is crucial to the overall well-being of individuals, societies and countries.

Unfortunately, in most parts of the world, mental health and mental disorders are not regarded with anything like the same importance as physical health. Instead, they have been largely ignored or neglected. Partly as a result, the world is suffering from an increasing burden of mental disorders, and a widening "treatment gap". Today, some 450 million people suffer from a mental or behavioural disorder, yet only a small minority of them receive even the most basic treatment. In developing countries, most individuals with severe mental disorders are left to cope as best they can with their private burdens such as depression, dementia, schizophrenia, and substance dependence. Globally, many are victimized for their illness and become the targets of stigma and discrimination.

Further increases in the number of sufferers are likely in view of the ageing of the population, worsening social problems, and civil unrest. Already, mental disorders represent four of the 10 leading causes of disability worldwide. This growing burden amounts to a huge cost in terms of human misery, disability and economic loss.

Mental and behavioural disorders are estimated to account for 12% of the global burden of disease, yet the mental health budgets of the majority of countries constitute less than 1% of their total health expenditures. The relationship between disease burden and disease spending is clearly disproportionate. More than 40% of countries have no mental health policy and over 30% have no mental health programme. Over 90% of countries have no mental health policy that includes children and adolescents. Moreover, health plans frequently do not cover mental and behavioural disorders at the same level as other illnesses, creating significant economic difficulties for patients and their families. And so the suffering continues, and the difficulties grow.

This need not be so. The importance of mental health has been recognized by WHO since its origin, and is reflected by the definition of health in the WHO Constitution as "not merely the absence of disease or infirmity", but rather, "a state of complete physical, mental and social well-being". In recent years this definition has been given sharper focus by many huge advances in the biological and behavioural sciences. These in turn have broadened our understanding of mental functioning, and of the profound relationship between mental, physical and social health. From this new understanding emerges new hope.

Today we know that most illnesses, mental and physical, are influenced by a combination of biological, psychological, and social factors (see Figure 1.1). We know that mental and behavioural disorders have a basis in the brain. We know that they affect people of all ages in all countries, and that they cause suffering to families and communities as well as individuals. And we know that in most cases, they can be diagnosed and treated cost-effectively. From the sum of our understanding, people with mental or behavioural disorders today have new hope of living full and productive lives in their own communities.

This report presents information concerning the current understanding of mental and behavioural disorders, their magnitude and burden, effective treatment strategies, and strategies for enhancing mental health through policy and service development.

The report makes it clear that governments are as responsible for the mental health as for the physical health of their citizens. One of the key messages to governments is that mental asylums, where they still exist, must be closed down and replaced with well-organized community-based care and psychiatric beds in general hospitals. The days of locking up people with mental or behavioural disorders in grim prison-like psychiatric institutions must end. The vast majority of people with mental disorders are not violent. Only a small proportion of mental and behavioural disorders are associated with an increased risk of violence, and comprehensive mental health services can decrease the likelihood of such violence.

As the ultimate stewards of any health system, governments must take the responsibility for ensuring that mental health policies are developed and implemented. This report recommends strategies that countries should pursue, including the integration of mental

Figure 1.1 Interaction of biological, psychological and social factors in the development of mental disorders

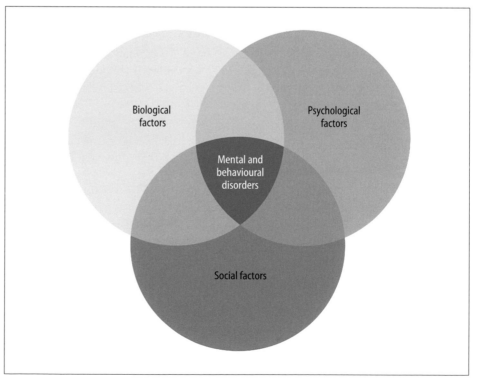

health treatment and services into the general health system, particularly into primary health care. This approach is being successfully applied in a number of countries. In many parts of the world, though, much more remains to be accomplished.

UNDERSTANDING MENTAL HEALTH

Mental health has been defined variously by scholars from different cultures. Concepts of mental health include subjective well-being, perceived self-efficacy, autonomy, competence, intergenerational dependence, and self-actualization of one's intellectual and emotional potential, among others. From a cross-cultural perspective, it is nearly impossible to define mental health comprehensively. It is, however, generally agreed that mental health is broader than a lack of mental disorders.

An understanding of mental health and, more generally, mental functioning is important because it provides the basis on which to form a more complete understanding of the development of mental and behavioural disorders.

In recent years, new information from the fields of neuroscience and behavioural medicine has dramatically advanced our understanding of mental functioning. Increasingly, it is becoming clear that mental functioning has a physiological underpinning, and is fundamentally interconnected with physical and social functioning and health outcomes.

ADVANCES IN NEUROSCIENCE

The World Health Report 2001 appears at an exciting time in the history of neuroscience. This is the branch of science which deals with the anatomy, physiology, biochemistry and molecular biology of the nervous system, especially as related to behaviour and learning. Spectacular advances in molecular biology are providing a more complete view of the building blocks of nerve cells (neurons). These advances will continue to provide a critical platform for the genetic analysis of human disease, and will contribute to new approaches to the discovery of treatments.

The understanding of the structure and function of the brain has evolved over the past 500 years (Figure 1.2). As the molecular revolution proceeds, tools such as neuroimaging and neurophysiology are permitting researchers to see the living, feeling, thinking human brain at work. Used in combination with cognitive neuroscience, imaging technologies make it increasingly possible to identify the specific parts of the brain used for different aspects of thinking and emotion.

The brain is responsible for melding genetic, molecular and biochemical information with information from the world. As such, the brain is an extremely complex organ. Within the brain, there are two types of cells: neurons and neuroglia. Neurons are responsible for sending and receiving nerve impulses or signals. Neuroglia provide neurons with nourishment, protection and structural support. Collectively, there are more than one hundred billion neurons in the brain, comprising thousands of distinct types. Each of these neurons communicates with other neurons via specialized structures called synapses. More than one hundred distinct brain chemicals, called neurotransmitters, communicate across these synapses. In aggregate, there are probably more than 100 trillion synapses in the brain. Circuits, formed by hundreds or thousands of neurons, give rise to complex mental and behavioural processes.

During fetal development, genes drive brain formation. The outcome is a specific and highly organized structure. This early development can also be influenced by environmental factors such as the pregnant woman's nutrition and substance use (alcohol, tobacco, and other psychoactive substances) or exposure to radiation. After birth and throughout life, all types of experience have the power not only to produce immediate communication between and among neurons, but also to initiate molecular processes that remodel synaptic connections (Hyman 2000). This process is described as *synaptic plasticity*, and it literally changes the physical structure of the brain. New synapses can be created, old ones removed, existing ones strengthened or weakened. The result is that information processing within the circuit will be changed to accommodate the new experience.

Prenatally, during childhood and through adulthood, genes and environment are involved in a series of inextricable interactions. Every act of learning – a process that is

Figure 1.2 Understanding the brain

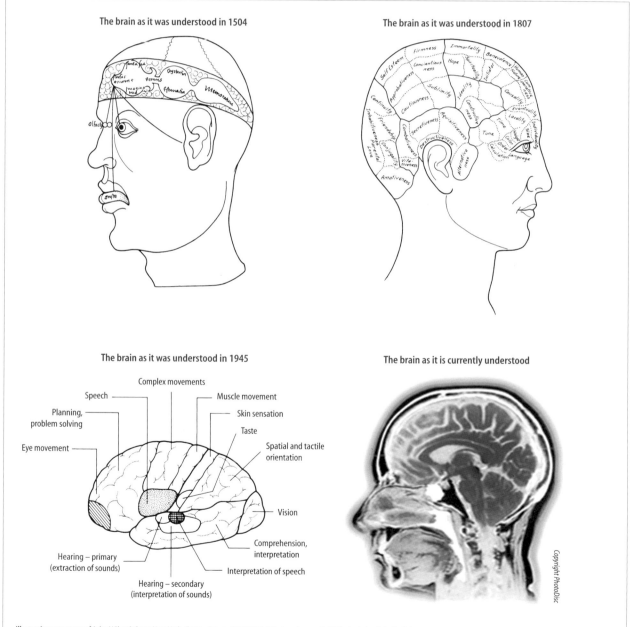

Illustrations courtesy of John Wiley & Sons, New York. From: Czerner TB (2001). *What makes you tick? The brain in plain English.*

dependent both on particular circuits and on the regulation of particular genes – physically changes the brain. Indeed, the remarkable evolutionary success of the human brain is that, within certain limits, it remains plastic across the lifespan. This recent discovery of lifelong synaptic plasticity represents a shift away from earlier theories that held that the structure of the adult brain is static (see Box 1.1).

As notable as discoveries to date have been, neuroscience is yet in its infancy. Future advances will provide a more complete understanding of how the brain is related to complex mental and behavioural functioning. Innovations in brain imaging along with neuropsychological and electrophysiological studies will permit real time cinema of the nervous system at work. Imaging will be combined with a growing ability to record from a large number of neurons at once; in this manner, it will be possible to decode their language. Other advances will be based on progress in genetics. An initial working draft sequence of the human genome is available in the public domain (at http://www.ornl.gov/hgmis/). One of the important uses of genomic information will be to provide a new basis for developing effective treatments for mental and behavioural disorders.

Another important tool that will enhance understanding of the molecular building blocks of development, anatomy, physiology and behaviour is the generation of genetically altered mice. For nearly every human gene there is an analogous mouse gene. This conservation of gene function between humans and mice suggests that mouse models will yield fundamental insights into human physiology and disease (O'Brien et al. 1999). Many laboratories around the world are involved in systematically inserting or deleting identified genes, and others are embarking on projects of generating random mutations throughout the mouse genome. These approaches will help connect genes with their actions in cells, organs and whole organisms.

Integration of the research results of neuroimaging and neurophysiology with those of molecular biology should lead to a greater understanding of the basis of normal and abnormal mental function, and to the development of more effective treatments.

ADVANCES IN BEHAVIOURAL MEDICINE

Advances have occurred not only in our understanding of mental functioning, but also in the knowledge of how these functions influence physical health. Modern science is dis-

---

Box 1.1 The brain: new understanding wins the Nobel Prize

The Nobel Prize in Physiology or Medicine for 2000 was awarded jointly to Professor Arvid Carlsson, Professor Paul Greengard and Professor Eric Kandel for their discoveries concerning how brain cells communicate with each other.[1] Their research is related to signal transduction in the nervous system, which takes place in synapses (points of contact between brain cells). These discoveries are crucial in advancing the understanding of the normal functioning of the brain, and how disturbances in this signal transduction can lead to mental and behavioural disorders. Their findings have already resulted in the development of effective new medications.

Arvid Carlsson's research revealed that dopamine is a transmitter of the brain that helps to control movements and that Parkinson's disease is related to lack of dopamine. As a result of this discovery, there is now an effective treatment (L-DOPA) for Parkinson's disease. Carlsson's work also demonstrated how other medications work, especially drugs used to treat schizophrenia, and has led to the development of a new generation of effective antidepressant medications.

Paul Greengard discovered how dopamine and a number of other neurotransmitters exert their influence in the synapse. His research clarified the mechanism by which several psychoactive medications act.

Eric Kandel showed how changes in synaptic function are central to learning and memory. He discovered that the development of long-term memory requires a change in protein synthesis which can also lead to changes in the shape and function of the synapse. By furthering understanding of the brain mechanisms crucial for memory, this research increases the possibility of developing new types of medications to improve memory functioning.

[1] Butcher J (2000). A Nobel pursuit. *The Lancet*, 356: 1331.

covering that, while it is operationally convenient for purposes of discussion to separate mental health from physical health, this is a fiction created by language. Most "mental" and "physical" illnesses are understood to be influenced by a combination of biological, psychological and social factors. Furthermore, thoughts, feelings and behaviour are now acknowledged to have a major impact on physical health. Conversely, physical health is recognized as considerably influencing mental health and well-being.

Behavioural medicine is a broad interdisciplinary area that is concerned with the integration of behavioural, psychosocial, and biomedical science knowledge relevant to the understanding of health and illness. Over the past 20 years, mounting scientific evidence from the field of behavioural medicine has demonstrated a fundamental connection between mental and physical health (see Box 1.2). Research has shown, for example, that women with advanced breast cancer who participate in supportive group therapy live significantly longer than women who do not participate in group therapy (Spiegel et al. 1989), that depression predicts the incidence of heart disease (Ferketich et al. 2000), and that realistic acceptance of one's own death is associated with decreased survival time in AIDS, even after controlling for a range of other potential predictors of mortality (Reed et al. 1994).

How do mental and physical functioning influence each other? Research has pointed to two main pathways through which mental and physical health mutually influence each other over time. The first key pathway is directly through physiological systems, such as neuroendocrine and immune functioning. The second primary pathway is through health behaviour. The term health behaviour covers a range of activities, such as eating sensibly, getting regular exercise and adequate sleep, avoiding smoking, engaging in safe sexual practices, wearing safety belts in vehicles, and adhering to medical therapies (see Box 1.3).

Although the physiological and behavioural pathways are distinct, they are not independent from one another, in that health behaviour can affect physiology (for example, smoking and sedentary lifestyle decrease immune functioning), while physiological functioning can influence health behaviour (for example, tiredness leads to forgetting medical regimens). What results is a comprehensive model of mental and physical health, in which the various components are related and mutually influential over time.

Box 1.2 Pain and well-being

Persistent pain is a major public health problem, accounting for untold suffering and lost productivity around the world. While specific estimates vary, it is agreed that chronic pain is debilitating and costly, ranking among the top reasons for health care visits and health-related work absences.

A recent WHO study of 5447 individuals across 15 study centres located in Asia, Africa, Europe and the Americas examined the relationship between pain and well-being.[1] Results showed that those with persistent pain were over four times more likely to have an anxiety or depressive disorder than those without pain. This relationship was observed in all study centres, regardless of geographical location. Other studies have suggested that pain intensity, disability, and anxiety/depression interact to develop and maintain chronic pain conditions.

Promisingly, a recent primary care study of 255 people with low-back pain has shown that a skills-based group intervention led by lay people reduces worries, decreasing disability.[2] The intervention was based on a model of chronic disease self-management, and consisted of four two-hour classes, held once a week, with 10–15 participants per class. The lay leaders, who themselves had recurrent or chronic back pain, received two days of formal training by a clinician familiar with the treatment of back pain and the treatment programme. No significant problems arose with the lay leaders, and their capabilities in implementing the intervention were noted as impressive. This study indicates that non-health professionals can successfully deliver structured behavioural interventions, which holds promise for applications to other disease areas.

[1] Gureje O et al. (1998). Persistent pain and well-being: a World Health Organization study in primary care. *Journal of the American Medical Association,* 280(2): 147–151.
[2] Von Korff M et al. (1998). A randomized trial of a lay person-led self-management group intervention for back pain patients in primary care. *Spine,* 23(23): 2608–2615.

Box 1.3 Adhering to medical advice

Patients do not always adhere to, or comply with, the advice of their health care providers. One review of the literature suggests that the average adherence rate for long-term medication use is just over 50%, while the adherence rate to lifestyle changes such as altering one's diet is very low. In general, the more lengthy, complex or disruptive the medical regimen, the less likely patients are to comply. Other important factors in adherence include the provider's communication skills, the patient's beliefs about the usefulness of the recommended regimen, and his or her ability to obtain medications or other recommended treatments at a reasonable cost.

Depression plays an important role in non-adherence to medical treatment. Depressed patients are three times more likely not to comply with medical regimens than non-depressed patients.[1] This means, for example, that depressed diabetic patients are more likely to have a poorer diet, more frequent hyperglycemia, greater disability, and higher health care costs than non-depressed diabetics.[2,3] The treatment of anxiety and depression in diabetic patients results in both improved mental and physical outcomes.[4-6]

The strong relationship between depression and non-adherence suggests that medical patients, particularly those who are noncompliant, should be routinely screened and, if necessary, treated for depression.

[1] DiMatteo MR et al. (2000). Depression is a risk factor for noncompliance with medical treatment. *Archives of Internal Medicine*, 160: 2101–2107.
[2] Ciechanowski PS et al. (2000). Depression and diabetes: impact of depressive symptoms on adherence, function, and costs. *Archives of Internal Medicine*, 160: 3278–3285.
[3] Ziegelstein RC et al. (2000). Patients with depression are less likely to follow recommendations to reduce cardiac risk during recovery from a myocardial infarction. *Archives of Internal Medicine*, 2000, 160: 1818–1823.
[4] Lustman PJ et al. (1995). Effects of alprazolam on glucose regulation in diabetes: results of a double-blind, placebo-controlled trial. *Diabetes Care*, 18(8): 1133–1139.
[5] Lustman PJ et al. (1997). Effects of nortriptyline on depression and glycemic control in diabetes: results of a double-blind, placebo-controlled trial. *Psychosomatic Medicine*, 59(3): 241–250.
[6] Lustman PJ et al. (2000). Fluoxetine for depression in diabetes: a randomized double-blind placebo-controlled trial. *Diabetes Care*, 23(5): 618–623.

Physiological pathway

In an integrated and evidence-based model of health, mental health (including emotions and thought patterns) emerges as a key determinant of overall health. Anxious and depressed moods, for example, initiate a cascade of adverse changes in endocrine and immune functioning, and create increased susceptibility to a range of physical illnesses. It is known, for instance, that stress is related to the development of the common cold (Cohen et al. 1991) and that stress delays wound healing (Kielcot-Glaser et al. 1999).

While many questions remain concerning the specific mechanisms of these relationships, it is clear that poor mental health plays a significant role in diminished immune functioning, the development of certain illnesses, and premature death.

Health behaviour pathway

Understanding the determinants of health behaviour is particularly important because of the role that health behaviour plays in shaping overall health status. Noncommunicable diseases such as cardiovascular disease and cancer take an enormous toll in lives and health worldwide. Many of them are strongly linked to unhealthy behaviour such as alcohol and tobacco use, poor diet and sedentary lifestyle. Health behaviour is also a prime determinant of the spread of communicable diseases such as AIDS, through unsafe sexual practices and needle sharing. Much disease can be prevented by healthy behaviour.

The health behaviour of an individual is highly dependent on that person's mental health. Thus, for example, mental illness or psychological stress affect health behaviour. Recent evidence has shown that young people with psychiatric disorders, for example depression and substance dependence, are more likely to engage in high-risk sexual behaviour, compared to those with no psychiatric disorder. This puts them at risk of a range of sexually transmitted diseases, including AIDS (Ranrakha et al. 2000). But other factors also have an effect on health behaviour. Children and adolescents learn through direct experience, through information and by observing others, and this learning affects health behaviour. For example, it has been established that drug use before the age of 15 years is highly associated with the development of drug and alcohol abuse in adulthood (Jaffe 1995). Environmental influences, such as poverty or societal and cultural norms, also affect health behaviour.

Because of the recent nature of this scientific evidence, the link between mental and physical health has yet to be fully recognized and acted upon by the health care system. Yet the evidence is clear: mental health is fundamentally linked to physical health outcomes.

UNDERSTANDING MENTAL AND BEHAVIOURAL DISORDERS

While the promotion of positive mental health in all members of society is clearly an important goal, much remains to be learned about how to achieve this objective. Conversely, effective interventions exist today for a range of mental health problems. Because of the large number of people affected by mental and behavioural disorders, many of whom never receive treatment, and the burden that results from untreated disorders, this report focuses upon mental and behavioural disorders rather than the broader concept of mental health.

Mental and behavioural disorders are a set of disorders as defined by the *International statistical classification of diseases and related health problems (ICD-10)*. While symptoms vary substantially, these disorders are generally characterized by some combination of abnormal thoughts, emotions, behaviour and relationships with others. Examples include schizophrenia, depression, mental retardation, and disorders due to psychoactive substance use. A more detailed consideration of mental and behavioural disorders appears in Chapters 2 and 3. The continuum from normal mood fluctuations to mental and behavioural disorders is illustrated in Figure 1.3 for the case of depressive symptoms.

The artificial separation of biological from psychological and social factors has been a formidable obstacle to a true understanding of mental and behavioural disorders. In reality, these disorders are similar to many physical illnesses in that they are the result of a complex interaction of all these factors.

For years, scientists have argued over the relative importance of *genetics versus environment* in the development of mental and behavioural disorders. Modern scientific evidence indicates that mental and behavioural disorders are the result of *genetics plus environment* or, in other words, the interaction of biology with psychological and social factors. The brain does not simply reflect the deterministic unfolding of complex genetic programmes, nor is human behaviour the mere result of environmental determinism. Prenatally and throughout life, genes and environment are involved in a set of inextricable interactions. These interactions are crucial to the development and course of mental and behavioural disorders.

Modern science is showing, for example, that exposure to stressors during early development is associated with persistent brain hyper-reactivity and increased likelihood of depression later in life (Heim et al. 2000). Promisingly, behaviour therapy for obsessive–compulsive disorder has been shown to result in changes in brain function that are observable through imaging techniques and equal to those that can be achieved by using drug therapy (Baxter et al. 1992). Nonetheless, the discovery of genes associated with increased risk of disorders will continue to provide critically important tools which, together with improved understanding of neural circuits, will yield important new insights into the development of mental and behavioural disorders. There is still much to be learned about the specific causes of mental and behavioural disorders, but contributions from neuroscience, genetics, psychology and sociology, among others, have played an important role in informing our understanding of these complex relationships. A science-based appreciation of the interactions between the various factors will contribute mightily to eradicating ignorance and putting a stop to the maltreatment of people with these problems.

BIOLOGICAL FACTORS

Age and sex are associated with mental and behavioural disorders, and these associations are discussed in Chapter 2.

Mental and behavioural disorders have been shown to be associated with disruptions of neural communication within specific circuits. In schizophrenia, abnormalities in the maturation of neural circuits may produce detectable changes in pathology at the cellular and gross tissue level that result in inappropriate or maladaptive information processing (Lewis & Lieberman 2000). In depression, however, it is possible that distinct anatomical abnormalities may not occur; rather, risk of illness may be due to variations in the responsiveness of neural circuits (Berke & Hyman 2000). These, in turn, may reflect subtle variations in the

Figure 1.3 The continuum of depressive symptoms in the population

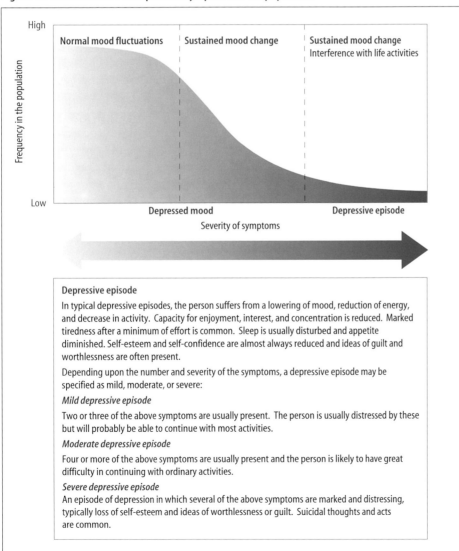

Depressive episode

In typical depressive episodes, the person suffers from a lowering of mood, reduction of energy, and decrease in activity. Capacity for enjoyment, interest, and concentration is reduced. Marked tiredness after a minimum of effort is common. Sleep is usually disturbed and appetite diminished. Self-esteem and self-confidence are almost always reduced and ideas of guilt and worthlessness are often present.

Depending upon the number and severity of the symptoms, a depressive episode may be specified as mild, moderate, or severe:

Mild depressive episode

Two or three of the above symptoms are usually present. The person is usually distressed by these but will probably be able to continue with most activities.

Moderate depressive episode

Four or more of the above symptoms are usually present and the person is likely to have great difficulty in continuing with ordinary activities.

Severe depressive episode

An episode of depression in which several of the above symptoms are marked and distressing, typically loss of self-esteem and ideas of worthlessness or guilt. Suicidal thoughts and acts are common.

structure, location, or expression levels of proteins critical to normal function. Some mental disorders, such as psychoactive substance dependence, may be viewed in part as the result of maladaptive synaptic plasticity. In other words, drug-driven or experience-driven alterations in synaptic connections can produce long-term alterations in thinking, emotion and behaviour.

In parallel with progress in neuroscience has come progress in genetics. Almost all of the common severe mental and behavioural disorders are associated with a significant genetic component of risk. Studies of the mode of transmission of mental disorders within extended multigenerational families, and studies comparing risk of mental disorders in monozygotic (identical) versus dizygotic (fraternal) twins have, however, led to the conclusion that risk of the common forms of mental disorders is genetically complex. Mental and behavioural disorders are predominantly due to the interaction of multiple risk genes with environmental factors. Further, a genetic predisposition to develop a particular mental or behavioural disorder may manifest only in people who also experience specific environmental stressors that elicit the pathology. Examples of environmental factors could range from exposure to psychoactive substances as a fetus, to malnutrition, infections, disrupted family environments, neglect, isolation and trauma.

PSYCHOLOGICAL FACTORS

Individual psychological factors are also related to the development of mental and behavioural disorders. One main finding throughout the 20th century that has shaped current understanding is the crucial importance of relationships with parents or other caregivers during childhood. Affectionate, attentive and stable caring allows infants and young children to develop normally such functions as language, intellect and emotional regulation. Failure may be due to the mental health problems, illness or death of a caregiver. The child may be separated from the caregiver because of poverty, war or population displacement. The child may lack care because of the unavailability of social services in the broader community. Regardless of the specific cause, when children are deprived of nurture from their caregivers they are more likely to develop mental and behavioural disorders, either during childhood or later in life. Evidence for this finding comes from infants living in institutions that did not provide sufficient social stimulation. Although these children received adequate nutrition and bodily care, they were likely to show serious impairments in interactions with others, in emotional expressiveness, and in coping adaptively to stressful life events. In some cases, intellectual deficits also occurred.

Another key finding is that human behaviour is partly shaped through interactions with the natural or social environment. This interaction can result in either desirable or undesirable consequences for the individual. Basically, individuals are more likely to engage in behaviours that are "rewarded" by the environment, and less likely to engage in behaviours that are ignored or punished. Mental and behavioural disorders can thus be viewed as maladaptive behaviour that has been learned – either directly or through observing others over time. Evidence for this theory comes from decades of research on learning and behaviour, and is further substantiated by the success of behaviour therapy, which uses these principles to help people change maladaptive patterns of thinking and behaving.

Finally, psychological science has shown that certain types of mental and behavioural disorders, such as anxiety and depression, can occur as the result of failing to cope adaptively to a stressful life event. Generally, people who try to avoid thinking about or dealing with stressors are more likely to develop anxiety or depression, whereas those who share their problems with others and attempt to find ways of managing stressors function better over time. This finding has prompted the development of interventions that consist of teaching coping skills.

Collectively, these discoveries have contributed to our understanding of mental and behavioural disorders. They have also been the basis for the development of a range of effective interventions, which are discussed in greater detail in Chapter 3.

SOCIAL FACTORS

Although social factors such as urbanization, poverty and technological change have been associated with the development of mental and behavioural disorders, there is no reason to assume that the mental health consequences of social change are the same for all segments of a given society. Changes usually exert differential effects based on economic status, sex, race and ethnicity.

Between 1950 and 2000, the proportion of urban populations in Asia, Africa, and Central and South America increased from 16% to fully one half of the populations of these regions (Harpham & Blue 1995). In 1950, the populations of Mexico City and São Paulo were 3.1 million and 2.8 million, respectively, but by 2000 the estimated population of each was 10 million. The nature of modern urbanization may have deleterious consequences for mental health through the influence of increased stressors and adverse life events, such as overcrowded and polluted environments, poverty and dependence on a cash economy, high levels of violence, and reduced social support (Desjarlais et al. 1995). Approximately half of the urban populations in low and middle income countries live in poverty, and tens of millions of adults and children are homeless. In some areas, economic development is forcing increasing numbers of indigenous peoples to migrate to urban areas in search of a viable livelihood. Usually, migration does not bring improved social well-being; rather, it often results in high rates of unemployment and squalid living conditions, exposing migrants to social stress and increased risk of mental disorders because of the absence of supportive social networks. Conflicts, wars and civil strife are thus associated with higher rates of mental health problems, and these are discussed in Chapter 2.

Rural life is also fraught with problems for many people. Isolation, lack of transport and communications, and limited educational and economic opportunities are common difficulties. Moreover, mental health services tend to concentrate clinical resources and expertise in larger metropolitan areas, leaving limited options for rural inhabitants in need of mental health care. A recent study of suicide in the elderly in some urban and rural areas of Hunan province, China, showed a higher suicide rate in rural areas (88.3 per 100 000) than in urban areas (24.4 per 100 000) (Xu et al. 2000). Elsewhere, rates of depression among rural women have been reported to be more than twice those of general population estimates for women (Hauenstein & Boyd 1994).

The relationship between poverty and mental health is complex and multidimensional (Figure 1.4). In its strictest definition, poverty refers to a lack of money or material possessions. In broader terms, and perhaps more appropriately for discussions related to mental and behavioural disorders, poverty can be understood as the state of having insufficient means, which may include the lack of social or educational resources. Poverty and associated conditions such as unemployment, low education, deprivation and homelessness, are not only widespread in poor countries, but also affect a sizeable minority of rich countries. The poor and the deprived have a higher prevalence of mental and behavioural disorders, including substance use disorders. This higher prevalence may be explainable both by higher

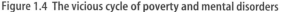

Figure 1.4 The vicious cycle of poverty and mental disorders

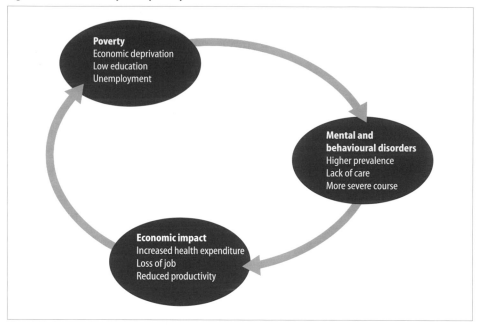

causation of disorders among the poor and by the drift of the mentally ill into poverty. Though there has been controversy about which of these two mechanisms accounts for the higher prevalence among the poor, the available evidence suggests that both are relevant (Patel 2001). For example, the causal mechanism may be more valid for anxiety and depressive disorders, while the drift theory may account more for the higher prevalence of psychotic and substance use disorders among the poor. But the two are not mutually exclusive: individuals may be predisposed to mental disorder because of their social situation and those who develop disorders may face further deprivation as a result of being ill. Such deprivation includes lower levels of educational attainment, unemployment and, in extreme cases, homelessness. Mental disorders may cause severe and sustained disabilities, including an inability to work. If sufficient social support is not available, which is often the case in developing countries without organized social welfare agencies, impoverishment is quick to develop.

There is also evidence that the *course* of mental and behavioural disorders is determined by the socioeconomic status of the individual. This may be the result of an overall lack of mental health services together with the barriers faced by certain socioeconomic groups in accessing care. Poor countries have very few resources for mental health care and these are often unavailable to the poorer segments of society. Even in rich countries, poverty along with associated factors such as lack of insurance coverage, lower educational level, unemployment and minority status in terms of race, ethnicity and language can create insurmountable barriers to care. The treatment gap for most mental disorders is high, but in the poor population it is indeed massive.

Across socioeconomic levels, the multiple roles that women fulfil in society put them at greater risk of experiencing mental and behavioural disorders than others in the community. Women continue to bear the burden of responsibility associated with being wives, mothers, educators and carers of others, while they are increasingly becoming an essential part of the labour force and in one-quarter to one-third of households they are the prime source of income. In addition to the pressures placed on women because of their expanding and often conflicting roles, they face significant sex discrimination and associated poverty, hunger, malnutrition, overwork and domestic and sexual violence. Not surprisingly, therefore, women have been shown to be more likely than men to be prescribed psychotropic drugs (see Figure 1.5). Violence against women constitutes a major social and public health problem, affecting women of all ages, cultural backgrounds, and income levels.

Racism, too raises important issues. Although there is still reluctance in some quarters to discuss racial and ethnic bigotry in the context of mental health concerns, psychological, sociological and anthropological research has shown racism to be related to the perpetuation of mental problems. The available evidence indicates that people long targeted by racism are at heightened risk for developing mental problems or experiencing a worsening of existing ones. And people who practise and perpetuate racism themselves are found to have or to develop certain kinds of mental disorders.

Psychiatrists examining the interplay between racism and mental health in societies where racism is prevalent have observed, for example, that racism may worsen depression. In a recent review of 10 studies of diverse racial groups in North America, amounting in total to over 15 000 respondents, a positive association between experiences of racism and psychological distress was firmly established (Williams & Williams-Morris 2000).

Racism's influence can also be considered at the level of the collective mental health of groups and societies. Racism has fuelled many oppressive social systems around the world and across the ages. In recent history, racism allowed white South Africans to define black South Africans categorically as "the enemy", and thus to commit acts that they would otherwise have found morally reprehensible.

The extraordinary scale and rapidity of technological change in the late 20th century is another factor that has been associated with the development of mental and behavioural disorders. These technological changes, and in particular the communications revolution, offer tremendous opportunities for enhanced diffusion of information and empowerment of users. Telemedicine now makes it possible to provide treatment at a distance.

Figure 1.5 Average female/male ratio of psychotropic drug use, selected countries

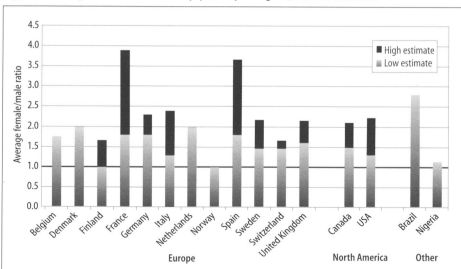

Note: The horizontal bold line at 1.0 indicates where the ratio of female to male use of psychotropic drugs is equal. Above this line women use more such drugs than men. In countries where more than one study was conducted, high and low estimates are provided in darker shade and grey.

Source: *Gender and the use of medications: a systematic review* (2000a). Geneva, World Health Organization (unpublished working document WHO/GHW).

But these advances also have their downside. There is evidence to suggest that media portrayals exert an influence on levels of violence, sexual behaviour and interest in pornography, and that exposure to video game violence increases aggressive behaviour and other aggressive tendencies (Dill & Dill 1998). Advertising spending worldwide is now outpacing the growth of the world's economy by one-third. Aggressive marketing is playing a substantial role in the globalization of alcohol and tobacco use among young people, thus increasing the risk of disorders related to substance use and associated physical conditions (Klein 1999).

AN INTEGRATED PUBLIC HEALTH APPROACH

The essential links between biological, psychological and social factors in the development and progression of mental and behavioural disorders are the grounds for a message of hope for the millions who suffer from these disabling problems. While there is much yet to be learned, the emerging scientific evidence is clear: we have at our disposal the knowledge and power to significantly reduce the burden of mental and behavioural disorders worldwide.

This message is a call to action to reduce the burden of the estimated 450 million people with mental and behavioural disorders. Given the sheer magnitude of the problem, its multifaceted etiology, widespread stigma and discrimination, and the significant treatment gap that exists around the world, a public health approach is the most appropriate method of response.

Stigma can be defined as a mark of shame, disgrace or disapproval which results in an individual being rejected, discriminated against, and excluded from participating in a number of different areas of society.

The United States Surgeon General's Report on Mental Health (DHHS 1999) described the impact of stigma as follows: "Stigma erodes confidence that mental disorders are valid, treatable health conditions. It leads people to avoid socializing, employing or working with, or renting to or living near persons who have a mental disorder." Further, "stigma deters the public from wanting to pay for care and, thus, reduces consumers' access to resources and opportunities for treatment and social services. A consequent inability or failure to obtain treatment reinforces destructive patterns of low self-esteem, isolation, and hopelessness. Stigma tragically deprives people of their dignity and interferes with their full participation in society."

From a public health perspective, there is much to be accomplished in reducing the burden of mental disorders:

- formulating policies designed to improve the mental health of populations;
- assuring universal access to appropriate and cost-effective services, including mental health promotion and prevention services;
- ensuring adequate care and protection of human rights for institutionalized patients with most severe mental disorders;
- assessment and monitoring of the mental health of communities, including vulnerable populations such as children, women and the elderly;
- promoting healthy lifestyles and reducing risk factors for mental and behavioural disorders, such as unstable family environments, abuse and civil unrest;
- supporting stable family life, social cohesion and human development;
- enhancing research into the causes of mental and behavioural disorders, the development of effective treatments, and the monitoring and evaluation of mental health systems.

The remainder of this report is devoted to these crucial issues. Through the presentation of scientific information on mental and behavioural disorders, WHO hopes that stigma and discrimination will be reduced, that mental health will be recognized as an urgent public health issue, and that steps will be taken by governments across the world to improve mental health.

Chapter 2 provides the latest epidemiological information on the magnitude, burden, and economic consequences of mental and behavioural disorders worldwide.

Chapter 3 presents information on effective treatments for people with mental and behavioural disorders. It outlines general principles of care and specific strategies for treating disorders.

Chapter 4 offers strategies for policy-makers to overcome common barriers and improve mental health in their communities.

Chapter 5 highlights the priority activities to be undertaken, depending on the level of resources available.

CHAPTER TWO

Burden of Mental and Behavioural Disorders

Mental and behavioural disorders are common, affecting more than 25% of all people at some time during their lives. They are also universal, affecting people of all countries and societies, individuals at all ages, women and men, the rich and the poor, from urban and rural environments. They have an economic impact on societies and on the quality of life of individuals and families. Mental and behavioural disorders are present at any point in time in about 10% of the adult population. Around 20% of all patients seen by primary health care professionals have one or more mental disorders. One in four families is likely to have at least one member with a behavioural or mental disorder. These families not only provide physical and emotional support, but also bear the negative impact of stigma and discrimination. It was estimated that, in 1990, mental and neurological disorders accounted for 10% of the total DALYs lost due to all diseases and injuries. This was 12% in 2000. By 2020, it is projected that the burden of these disorders will have increased to 15%. Common disorders, which usually cause severe disability, include depressive disorders, substance use disorders, schizophrenia, epilepsy, Alzheimer's disease, mental retardation, and disorders of childhood and adolescence. Factors associated with the prevalence, onset and course of mental and behavioural disorders include poverty, sex, age, conflicts and disasters, major physical diseases, and the family and social environment.

2

Burden of Mental
and Behavioural Disorders

Identifying disorders

*M*ental and behavioural disorders are understood as clinically significant conditions characterized by alterations in thinking, mood (emotions) or behaviour associated with personal distress and/or impaired functioning. Mental and behavioural disorders are not just variations within the range of "normal", but are clearly abnormal or pathological phenomena. One incidence of abnormal behaviour or a short period of abnormal mood does not, of itself, signify the presence of a mental or behavioural disorder. In order to be categorized as disorders, such abnormalities must be sustained or recurring and they must result in some personal distress or impaired functioning in one or more areas of life. Mental and behavioural disorders are also characterized by specific symptoms and signs, and usually follow a more or less predictable natural course, unless interventions are made. Not all human distress is mental disorder. Individuals may be distressed because of personal or social circumstances; unless all the essential criteria for a particular disorder are satisfied, such distress is not a mental disorder. There is a difference, for example, between depressed mood and diagnosable depression (see Figure 1.3).

Diverse ways of thinking and behaving across cultures may influence the way mental disorders manifest but are not, of themselves, indicative of a disorder. Thus, culturally determined normal variations must not be labelled mental disorders. Nor can social, religious, or political beliefs be taken as evidence of mental disorder.

The ICD-10 classification of mental and behavioural disorders: clinical descriptions and diagnostic guidelines (WHO 1992b) gives a complete list of all mental and behavioural disorders (see Box 2.1). Additional diagnostic criteria for research are also available for a more precise definition of these disorders (WHO 1993a).

Any classification of mental disorders classifies syndromes and conditions, but not individuals. Individuals may suffer from one or more disorders during one or more periods of their lives, but a diagnostic label should not be used to describe an individual. A person should never be equated with a disorder – physical or mental.

Diagnosing disorders

Mental and behavioural disorders are identified and diagnosed using clinical methods that are similar to those used for physical disorders. These methods include a careful and detailed collection of historical information from the individual and others, including the family; a systematic clinical examination for mental status; and specialized tests and investigations, as needed. Advances have been made during recent decades in standardizing clinical assessment and improving the reliability of diagnosis. Structured interview schedules, uniform definitions of symptoms and signs, and standard diagnostic criteria have now made it possible to achieve a high degree of reliability and validity in the diagnosis of mental disorders. Structured interview schedules and diagnostic symptom/sign checklists allow mental health professionals to collect information using standard questions and pre-coded responses. The symptoms and signs have been defined in detail to allow for uniform application. Finally, diagnostic criteria for disorders have been standardized internationally. Mental disorders can now be diagnosed as reliably and accurately as most of the common physical disorders. Concordance between two experts in the diagnosis of mental disorders averages 0.7 to 0.9 (Wittchen et al. 1991; Wing et al.1974; WHO 1992; APA 1994; Andrews et al. 1995). These figures are in the same range as those for physical disorders such as diabetes mellitus, hypertension or coronary artery disease.

Since a reliable diagnosis is a prerequisite to appropriate intervention at the individual level as well as to accurate epidemiology and monitoring at the community level, advances in diagnostic methods have greatly facilitated the application of clinical and public health principles to the field of mental health.

Box 2.1 Mental and behavioural disorders classified in ICD-10

A complete list of all mental and behavioural disorders is given in *The ICD-10 classification of mental and behavioural disorders: clinical descriptions and diagnostic guidelines*.[1] Additional diagnostic criteria for research are also available for a more precise definition of these disorders.[2] These materials, which are applicable cross culturally, were developed from Chapter V(F) of the *Tenth Revision of the International Classification of Diseases* (ICD-10)[3] on the basis of an international review of scientific literature, worldwide consultations and consensus. Chapter V of ICD-10 is exclusively devoted to mental and behavioural disorders. Besides giving the names of diseases and disorders, like the rest of the chapters, Chapter V has been further developed to give clinical descriptions and diagnostic guidelines as well as diagnostic criteria for research. The broad categories of mental and behavioural disorders covered in ICD-10 are as follows.

- **Organic, including symptomatic, mental disorders** – e.g., dementia in Alzheimer's disease, delirium.
- **Mental and behavioural disorders due to psychoactive substance use** – e.g., harmful use of alcohol, opioid dependence syndrome.
- **Schizophrenia, schizotypal and delusional disorders** – e.g., paranoid schizophrenia, delusional disorders, acute and transient psychotic disorders.
- **Mood [affective] disorders** – e.g., bipolar affective disorder, depressive episode.
- **Neurotic, stress-related and somatoform disorders** – e.g., generalized anxiety disorders, obsessive–compulsive disorders.

- **Behavioural syndromes associated with physiological disturbances and physical factors** – e.g., eating disorders, non-organic sleep disorders.
- **Disorders of adult personality and behaviour** – e.g., paranoid personality disorder, transsexualism.
- **Mental retardation** – e.g., mild mental retardation.
- **Disorders of psychological development** – e.g., specific reading disorders, childhood autism.
- **Behavioural and emotional disorders with onset usually occurring in childhood and adolescence** – e.g., hyperkinetic disorders, conduct disorders, tic disorders.
- **Unspecified mental disorder.**

This report focuses on a selection of disorders that usually cause severe disability when not treated adequately and which place a heavy burden on communities. These include: depressive disorders, substance use disorders, schizophrenia, epilepsy, Alzheimer's disease, mental retardation, and disorders of childhood and adolescence. The inclusion of epilepsy is explained later in this chapter.

Some of the mental, behavioural and neurological disorders are included under "neuropsychiatric disorders" in the statistical annex of this report. This group includes unipolar major depression, bipolar affective disorder, psychoses, epilepsy, alcohol dependence, Alzheimer's and other dementias, Parkinson disease, multiple sclerosis, drug dependence, post-traumatic stress disorder, obsessive–compulsive disorders, panic disorder, migraine and sleep disorders.

[1] *The ICD-10 classification of mental and behavioural disorders: clinical descriptions and diagnostic guidelines* (1992b). Geneva, World Health Organization.
[2] *The ICD-10 classification of mental and behavioural disorders: diagnostic criteria for research* (1993a). Geneva, World Health Organization.
[3] *International statistical classification of diseases and related health problems, Tenth revision 1992 (ICD-10). Vol.1: Tabular list. Vol.2: Instruction manual. Vol.3: Alphabetical index* (1992a). Geneva, World Health Organization.

PREVALENCE OF DISORDERS

Mental disorders are not the exclusive preserve of any special group; they are truly universal. Mental and behavioural disorders are found in people of all regions, all countries and all societies. They are present in women and men at all stages of the life course. They are present among the rich and poor, and among people living in urban and rural areas. The notion that mental disorders are problems of industrialized and relatively richer parts of the world is simply wrong. The belief that rural communities, relatively unaffected by the fast pace of modern life, have no mental disorders is also incorrect.

Recent analyses done by WHO show that neuropsychiatric conditions which included a selection of these disorders had an aggregate point prevalence of about 10% for adults (GBD 2000). About 450 million people were estimated to be suffering from neuropsychiatric conditions. These conditions included unipolar depressive disorders, bipolar affective disorder, schizophrenia, epilepsy, alcohol and selected drug use disorders, Alzheimer's and other dementias, post traumatic stress disorder, obsessive and compulsive disorder, panic disorder, and primary insomnia.

The prevalence rates differ depending on whether they refer to people who have a condition at a point in time (point prevalence) or at any time during a period of time (period prevalence), or at any time in their lifetime (lifetime prevalence). Though point prevalence figures are often quoted, including in this report, one-year period prevalence figures are more useful for giving an indication of the number of people who may require services in a year. Prevalence figures also vary based on the concept and definitions of the disorders included in the study. When all the disorders included in ICD-10 (see Box 2.1) are considered, higher prevalence rates have been reported. Surveys conducted in developed as well as developing countries have shown that, during their entire lifetime, more than 25% of individuals develop one or more mental or behavioural disorders (Regier et al. 1988; Wells et al. 1989; Almeida-Filho et al. 1997).

Most studies have found the overall prevalence of mental disorders to be about the same among men and women. Whatever differences exist are accounted for by the differential distribution of disorders. The severe mental disorders are about equally common, with the exception of depression, which is more common among women, and substance use disorders, which are more common among men.

The relationship between poverty and mental disorders is discussed later in this chapter.

DISORDERS SEEN IN PRIMARY HEALTH CARE SETTINGS

Mental and behavioural disorders are common among patients attending primary health care settings. An assessment of the extent and pattern of such disorders in these settings is useful because of the potential for identifying individuals with disorders and providing the needed care at that level.

Epidemiological studies in primary care settings have been based on identification of mental disorders by the use of screening instruments, or clinical diagnosis by primary care professionals or by psychiatric diagnostic interview. The cross-cultural study conducted by WHO at 14 sites (Üstün & Sartorius 1995; Goldberg & Lecrubier 1995) used three different methods of diagnosis: a short screening instrument, a detailed structured interview, and a clinical diagnosis by the primary care physician. Though the prevalence of mental disorders across the sites varied considerably, the results clearly demonstrate that a substantial proportion (about 24%) of all patients in these settings had a mental disorder (see Table 2.1). The most common diagnoses in primary care settings are depression, anxiety and substance abuse disorders. These disorders are present either alone or in addition to one or more physical disorders. There are no consistent differences in prevalence between developed and developing countries.

IMPACT OF DISORDERS

Mental and behavioural disorders have a large impact on individuals, families and communities. Individuals suffer the distressing symptoms of disorders. They also suffer because they are unable to participate in work and leisure activities, often as a result of discrimination. They worry about not being able to shoulder their responsibilities towards family and friends, and are fearful of being a burden for others.

It is estimated that one in four families has at least one member currently suffering from a mental or behavioural disorder. These families are required not only to provide physical and emotional support, but also to bear the negative impact of stigma and discrimination present in all parts of the world. While the burden of caring for a family member with a mental or behavioural disorder has not been adequately studied, the available evidence suggests that it is indeed substantial (Pai & Kapur 1982; Fadden et al. 1987; Winefield & Harvey 1994). The burden on families ranges from economic difficulties to emotional reactions to the illness, the stress of coping with disturbed behaviour, the disruption of household routine and the restriction of social activities (WHO 1997a). Expenses for the treatment of mental illness often are borne by the family either because insurance is unavailable or because mental disorders are not covered by insurance.

Table 2.1 Prevalence of major psychiatric disorders in primary health care

Cities	Current depression (%)	Generalized anxiety (%)	Alcohol dependence (%)	All mental disorders (according to CIDI[a]) (%)
Ankara, Turkey	11.6	0.9	1.0	16.4
Athens, Greece	6.4	14.9	1.0	19.2
Bangalore, India	9.1	8.5	1.4	22.4
Berlin, Germany	6.1	9.0	5.3	18.3
Groningen, Netherlands	15.9	6.4	3.4	23.9
Ibadan, Nigeria	4.2	2.9	0.4	9.5
Mainz, Germany	11.2	7.9	7.2	23.6
Manchester, UK	16.9	7.1	2.2	24.8
Nagasaki, Japan	2.6	5.0	3.7	9.4
Paris, France	13.7	11.9	4.3	26.3
Rio de Janeiro, Brazil	15.8	22.6	4.1	35.5
Santiago, Chile	29.5	18.7	2.5	52.5
Seattle, USA	6.3	2.1	1.5	11.9
Shanghai, China	4.0	1.9	1.1	7.3
Verona, Italy	4.7	3.7	0.5	9.8
Total	**10.4**	**7.9**	**2.7**	**24.0**

[a]CIDI: Composite International Diagnostic Interview.

Source: Goldberg DP, Lecrubier Y (1995). Form and frequency of mental disorders across centres. In: Üstün TB, Sartorius N, eds. *Mental illness in general health care: an international study.* Chichester, John Wiley & Sons on behalf of WHO: 323–334.

In addition to the direct burden, lost opportunities have to be taken into account. Families in which one member is suffering from a mental disorder make a number of adjustments and compromises that prevent other members of the family from achieving their full potential in work, social relationships and leisure (Gallagher & Mechanic 1996). These are the human aspects of the burden of mental disorders, which are difficult to assess and quantify; they are nevertheless important. Families often have to set aside a major part of their time to look after the mentally ill relative, and suffer economic and social deprivation because he or she is not fully productive. There is also the constant fear that recurrence of illness may cause sudden and unexpected disruption of the lives of family members.

The impact of mental disorders on communities is large and manifold. There is the cost of providing care, the loss of productivity, and some legal problems (including violence) associated with some mental disorders, though violence is caused much more often by "normal" people than by individuals with mental disorders.

One specific variety of burdens is the health burden. This has traditionally been measured – in national and international health statistics – only in terms of incidence/prevalence and mortality. While these indices are well suited to acute diseases that either cause death or result in full recovery, their use for chronic and disabling diseases poses serious limitations. This is particularly true for mental and behavioural disorders, which more often cause disability than premature death. One way to account for the chronicity of disorders and the disability caused by them is the Global Burden of Disease (GBD) methodology. The methodology of GBD 2000 is described briefly in Box 2.2. In the original estimates developed for 1990, mental and neurological disorders accounted for 10.5% of the total DALYs lost due to all diseases and injuries. This figure demonstrated for the first time the high burden due to these disorders. The estimate for 2000 is 12.3% for DALYs (see Figure 2.1). Three neuropsychiatric conditions rank in the top twenty leading causes of DALYs for all ages, and six in the age group 15-44 (see Figure 2.2). In the calculation of DALYs, recent estimates from

---

Box 2.2 Global Burden of Disease 2000

In 1993 the Harvard School of Public Health in collaboration with the World Bank and WHO assessed the Global Burden of Disease (GBD).[1] Aside from generating the most comprehensive and consistent set of estimates of mortality and morbidity by age, sex and region ever produced, GBD also introduced a new metric – disability-adjusted life year (DALY) – to quantify the burden of disease.[2,3] The DALY is a health gap measure, which combines information on the impact of premature death and of disability and other nonfatal health outcomes. One DALY can be thought of as one lost year of 'healthy' life, and the burden of disease as a measurement of the gap between current health status and an ideal situation where everyone lives into old age free of disease and disability. For a review of the development of DALYs and recent advances in the measurement of burden of disease see Murray & Lopez (2000).[4]

The World Health Organization has undertaken a new assessment of the Global Burden of Disease for the year 2000, GBD 2000, with the following specific objectives:

• to quantify the burden of premature mortality and disability by age, sex, and region for 135 major causes or groups of causes;

• to analyse the contribution to this burden of selected risk factors using a comparable framework;

• to develop various projection scenarios of the burden of disease over the next 30 years.

DALYs for a disease are the sum of the years of life lost due to premature mortality (YLL) in the population and the years lost due to disability (YLD) for incident cases of the health condition. The DALY is a health gap measure that extends the concept of potential years of life lost due to premature death (PYLL) to include equivalent years of 'healthy' life lost in states of less than full health, broadly termed disability.

GBD 2000 results for neuropsychiatric disorders given in this report are based on an extensive analysis of mortality data for all regions of the world, together with systematic reviews of epidemiological studies and population-based mental health surveys. Final results of GBD 2000 will be published in 2002.

[1] World Bank (1993). *World development report 1993: investing in health*. New York, Oxford University Press for the World Bank.

[2] Murray CJL, Lopez AD, eds (1996a). *The global burden of disease: a comprehensive assessment of mortality and disability from diseases, injuries and risk factors in 1990 and projected to 2020*. Cambridge, MA, Harvard School of Public Health on behalf of the World Health Organization and the World Bank (Global Burden of Disease and Injury Series, Vol. I).

[3] Murray CJL, Lopez AD (1996b). *Global health statistics*. Cambridge, MA, Harvard School of Public Health on behalf of the World Health Organization and the World Bank (Global Burden of Disease and Injury Series, Vol. II).

[4] Murray CJL, Lopez AD (2000). Progress and directions in refining the global burden of disease approach: a response to Williams. *Health Economics*, 9: 69–82.

Figure 2.1 Burden of neuropsychiatric conditions as a proportion of the total burden of disease, globally and in WHO Regions, estimates for 2000

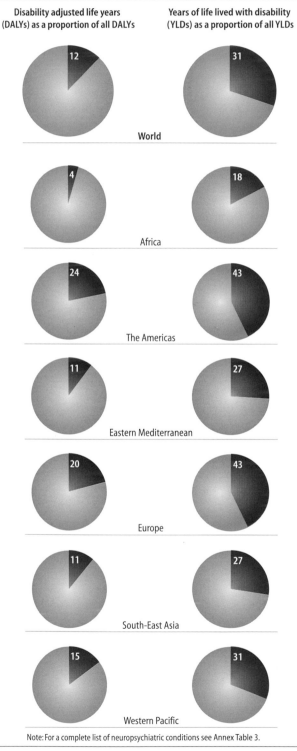

Disability adjusted life years (DALYs) as a proportion of all DALYs

Years of life lived with disability (YLDs) as a proportion of all YLDs

World
Africa
The Americas
Eastern Mediterranean
Europe
South-East Asia
Western Pacific

Note: For a complete list of neuropsychiatric conditions see Annex Table 3.

Australia based on detailed methods and different data sources have confirmed mental disorders as the leading cause of disability burden (Vos & Mathers 2000). From an analysis of trends, it is evident that this burden will increase rapidly in the future. Projections indicate that it will increase to 15% in the year 2020 (Murray & Lopez 1996a). The proportion of DALYs and YLDs for neuropsychiatric conditions globally and regionally are given in Figure 2.1.

Taking the disability component of burden alone, GBD 2000 estimates show that mental and neurological conditions account for 30.8% of all years lived with disability (YLDs). Indeed, depression causes the largest amount of disability, accounting for almost 12% of all disability. Six neuropsychiatric conditions figured in the top twenty causes of disability (YLDs) in the world, these being unipolar depressive disorders, alcohol use disorders, schizophrenia, bipolar affective disorder, Alzheimer's and other dementias, and migraine. (see Figure 2.3).

The disability caused by mental and neurological disorders is high in all regions of the world. As a proportion of the total, however, it is comparatively less in the developing countries, mainly because of the large burden of communicable, maternal, perinatal and nutritional conditions in those regions. Even so, neuropsychiatric disorders cause 17.6% of all YLDs in Africa.

There are varying degrees of uncertainty in GBD 2000 estimates of DALYs and YLDs for mental and neurological disorders, reflecting uncertainty in the prevalence of the various conditions in different regions of the world, and uncertainty in the variation of their severity distributions. In particular, there is considerable uncertainty in the estimates of prevalence of mental disorders in many regions, reflecting the limitations of self-report instruments for classifying mental health symptoms in a comparable way across populations, limitations in the generalizability of surveys in subpopulations to broader population groups, and limitations in the information available to classify the severity of disabling symptoms of mental health conditions.

ECONOMIC COSTS TO SOCIETY

The economic impact of mental disorders is wide ranging, long lasting and huge. These disorders impose a range of costs on individuals, families and communities as a whole. Part of this economic burden is obvious and measurable, while part is almost impossible to measure. Among the measurable components of the economic burden are health and social service needs, lost employment and reduced productivity, impact on families and caregivers, levels of crime and public safety, and the negative impact of premature mortality.

Some studies, mainly from industrialized countries, have estimated the aggregate economic costs of mental disorders. One such study (Rice et al. 1990) concluded that the aggregate yearly cost for the United States accounted for about 2.5% of gross national product. A few studies from Europe have estimated expenditure on mental disorders as a proportion of all health service costs: in the Netherlands, this was 23.2% (Meerding et al. 1998) and in the United Kingdom, for inpatient expenditure only, it was 22% (Patel & Knapp

Figure 2.2 Leading causes of disability-adjusted life years (DALYs), in all ages and in 15–44-year-olds, by sex, estimates for 2000[a]

	Both sexes, all ages	% total		Males, all ages	% total		Females, all ages	% total
1	Lower respiratory infections	6.4	1	Perinatal conditions	6.4	1	HIV/AIDS	6.5
2	Perinatal conditions	6.2	2	Lower respiratory infections	6.4	2	Lower respiratory infections	6.4
3	HIV/AIDS	6.1	3	HIV/AIDS	5.8	3	Perinatal conditions	6.0
4	Unipolar depressive disorders	4.4	4	Diarrhoeal diseases	4.2	4	Unipolar depressive disorders	5.5
5	Diarrhoeal diseases	4.2	5	Ischaemic heart disease	4.2	5	Diarrhoeal diseases	4.2
6	Ischaemic heart disease	3.8	6	Road traffic accidents	4.0	6	Ischaemic heart disease	3.3
7	Cerebrovascular disease	3.1	7	Unipolar depressive disorders	3.4	7	Cerebrovascular disease	3.2
8	Road traffic accidents	2.8	8	Cerebrovascular disease	3.0	8	Malaria	3.0
9	Malaria	2.7	9	Tuberculosis	2.9	9	Congenital abnormalities	2.2
10	Tuberculosis	2.4	10	Malaria	2.5	10	Chronic obstructive pulmonary disease	2.1
11	Chronic obstructive pulmonary disease	2.3	11	Chronic obstructive pulmonary disease	2.4	11	Iron-deficiency anaemia	2.1
12	Congenital abnormalities	2.2	12	Congenital abnormalities	2.2	12	Tuberculosis	2.0
13	Measles	1.9	13	Alcohol use disorders	2.1	13	Measles	2.0
14	Iron-deficiency anaemia	1.8	14	Measles	1.8	14	Hearing loss, adult onset	1.7
15	Hearing loss, adult onset	1.7	15	Hearing loss, adult onset	1.8	15	Road traffic accidents	1.5
16	Falls	1.3	16	Violence	1.6	16	Osteoarthritis	1.4
17	Self-inflicted injuries	1.3	17	Iron-deficiency anaemia	1.5	17	Protein–energy malnutrition	1.2
18	Alcohol use disorders	1.3	18	Falls	1.5	18	Self-inflicted injuries	1.1
19	Protein–energy malnutrition	1.1	19	Self-inflicted injuries	1.5	19	Diabetes mellitus	1.1
20	Osteoarthritis	1.1	20	Cirrhosis of the liver	1.4	20	Falls	1.1

	Both sexes, 15–44-year-olds	% total		Males, 15–44-year-olds	% total		Females, 15–44-year-olds	% total
1	HIV/AIDS	13.0	1	HIV/AIDS	12.1	1	HIV/AIDS	13.9
2	Unipolar depressive disorders	8.6	2	Road traffic accidents	7.7	2	Unipolar depressive disorders	10.6
3	Road traffic accidents	4.9	3	Unipolar depressive disorders	6.7	3	Tuberculosis	3.2
4	Tuberculosis	3.9	4	Alcohol use disorders	5.1	4	Iron-deficiency anaemia	3.2
5	Alcohol use disorders	3.0	5	Tuberculosis	4.5	5	Schizophrenia	2.8
6	Self-inflicted injuries	2.7	6	Violence	3.7	6	Obstructed labour	2.7
7	Iron-deficiency anaemia	2.6	7	Self-inflicted injuries	3.0	7	Bipolar affective disorder	2.5
8	Schizophrenia	2.6	8	Schizophrenia	2.5	8	Abortion	2.5
9	Bipolar affective disorder	2.5	9	Bipolar affective disorder	2.4	9	Self-inflicted injuries	2.4
10	Violence	2.3	10	Iron-deficiency anaemia	2.1	10	Maternal sepsis	2.1
11	Hearing loss, adult onset	2.0	11	Hearing loss, adult onset	2.0	11	Road traffic accidents	2.0
12	Chronic obstructive pulmonary disease	1.5	12	Ischaemic heart disease	1.9	12	Hearing loss, adult onset	2.0
13	Ischaemic heart disease	1.5	13	War	1.7	13	Chlamydia	1.9
14	Cerebrovascular disease	1.4	14	Falls	1.7	14	Panic disorder	1.6
15	Falls	1.3	15	Cirrhosis of the liver	1.6	15	Chronic obstructive pulmonary disease	1.5
16	Obstructed labour	1.3	16	Drug use disorders	1.6	16	Maternal haemorrhage	1.5
17	Abortion	1.2	17	Cerebrovascular disease	1.5	17	Osteoarthritis	1.4
18	Osteoarthritis	1.2	18	Chronic obstructive pulmonary disease	1.5	18	Cerebrovascular disease	1.3
19	War	1.2	19	Asthma	1.4	19	Migraine	1.2
20	Panic disorder	1.2	20	Drownings	1.1	20	Ischaemic heart disease	1.1

[a]Neuropsychiatric conditions and self-inflicted injuries (see Annex Table 3) are highlighted.

Figure 2.3 Leading causes of years of life lived with disability (YLDs), in all ages and in 15–44-year-olds, by sex, estimates for 2000[a]

	Both sexes, all ages	% total		Males, all ages	% total		Females, all ages	% total
1	Unipolar depressive disorders	11.9	1	Unipolar depressive disorders	9.7	1	Unipolar depressive disorders	14.0
2	Hearing loss, adult onset	4.6	2	Alcohol use disorders	5.5	2	Iron-deficiency anaemia	4.9
3	Iron-deficiency anaemia	4.5	3	Hearing loss, adult onset	5.1	3	Hearing loss, adult onset	4.2
4	Chronic obstructive pulmonary disease	3.3	4	Iron-deficiency anaemia	4.1	4	Osteoarthritis	3.5
5	Alcohol use disorders	3.1	5	Chronic obstructive pulmonary disease	3.8	5	Chronic obstructive pulmonary disease	2.9
6	Osteoarthritis	3.0	6	Falls	3.3	6	Schizophrenia	2.7
7	Schizophrenia	2.8	7	Schizophrenia	3.0	7	Bipolar affective disorder	2.4
8	Falls	2.8	8	Road traffic accidents	2.7	8	Falls	2.3
9	Bipolar affective disorder	2.5	9	Bipolar affective disorder	2.6	9	Alzheimer's and other dementias	2.2
10	Asthma	2.1	10	Osteoarthritis	2.5	10	Obstructed labour	2.1
11	Congenital abnormalities	2.1	11	Asthma	2.3	11	Cataracts	2.0
12	Perinatal conditions	2.0	12	Perinatal conditions	2.2	12	Migraine	2.0
13	Alzheimer's and other dementias	2.0	13	Congenital abnormalities	2.2	13	Congenital abnormalities	1.9
14	Cataracts	1.9	14	Cataracts	1.9	14	Asthma	1.8
15	Road traffic accidents	1.8	15	Protein–energy malnutrition	1.8	15	Perinatal conditions	1.8
16	Protein–energy malnutrition	1.7	16	Alzheimer's and other dementias	1.8	16	Chlamydia	1.8
17	Cerebrovascular disease	1.7	17	Cerebrovascular disease	1.7	17	Cerebrovascular disease	1.8
18	HIV/AIDS	1.5	18	HIV/AIDS	1.6	18	Protein–energy malnutrition	1.6
19	Migraine	1.4	19	Lymphatic filariasis	1.6	19	Abortion	1.6
20	Diabetes mellitus	1.4	20	Drug use disorders	1.6	20	Panic disorder	1.6

	Both sexes, 15–44-year-olds	% total		Males, 15–44-year-olds	% total		Females, 15–44-year-olds	% total
1	Unipolar depressive disorders	16.4	1	Unipolar depressive disorders	13.9	1	Unipolar depressive disorders	18.6
2	Alcohol use disorders	5.5	2	Alcohol use disorders	10.1	2	Iron-deficiency anaemia	5.4
3	Schizophrenia	4.9	3	Schizophrenia	5.0	3	Schizophrenia	4.8
4	Iron-deficiency anaemia	4.9	4	Bipolar affective disorder	5.0	4	Bipolar affective disorder	4.4
5	Bipolar affective disorder	4.7	5	Iron-deficiency anaemia	4.2	5	Obstructed labour	4.0
6	Hearing loss, adult onset	3.8	6	Hearing loss, adult onset	4.1	6	Hearing loss, adult onset	3.6
7	HIV/AIDS	2.8	7	Road traffic accidents	3.8	7	Chlamydia	3.3
8	Chronic obstructive pulmonary disease	2.4	8	HIV/AIDS	3.2	8	Abortion	3.1
9	Osteoarthritis	2.3	9	Drug use disorders	3.0	9	Panic disorder	2.8
10	Road traffic accidents	2.3	10	Chronic obstructive pulmonary disease	2.6	10	HIV/AIDS	2.5
11	Panic disorder	2.2	11	Asthma	2.5	11	Osteoarthritis	2.5
12	Obstructed labour	2.1	12	Falls	2.4	12	Maternal sepsis	2.3
13	Chlamydia	2.0	13	Osteoarthritis	2.1	13	Chronic obstructive pulmonary disease	2.2
14	Falls	1.9	14	Lymphatic filariasis	2.1	14	Migraine	2.1
15	Asthma	1.9	15	Panic disorder	1.6	15	Alcohol use disorders	1.5
16	Drug use disorders	1.8	16	Tuberculosis	1.6	16	Rheumatoid arthritis	1.4
17	Abortion	1.6	17	Gout	1.3	17	Obsessive–compulsive disorder	1.4
18	Migraine	1.6	18	Obsessive–compulsive disorder	1.3	18	Falls	1.4
19	Obsessive–compulsive disorder	1.4	19	Violence	1.2	19	Post-traumatic stress disorder	1.4
20	Maternal sepsis	1.2	20	Gonorrhoea	1.1	20	Asthma	1.3

[a]Neuropsychiatric conditions (see Annex Table 3) are highlighted.

1998). Though scientific estimates are not available for other regions of the world, it is likely that the costs of mental disorders as a proportion of the overall economy are high there too. Although estimates of direct costs may be low in countries where there is low availability and coverage of mental health care, these estimates are spurious. Indirect costs arising from productivity loss account for a larger proportion of overall costs than direct costs. Furthermore, low treatment costs (because of lack of treatment) may actually increase the indirect costs by increasing the duration of untreated disorders and associated disability (Chisholm et al. 2000).

All these estimates of economic evaluations are most certainly underestimates, since lost opportunity costs to individuals and families are not taken into account.

IMPACT ON THE QUALITY OF LIFE

Mental and behavioural disorders cause massive disruption in the lives of those who are affected and their families. Though the whole range of unhappiness and suffering is not measurable, one of the methods to assess its impact is by using quality of life (QOL) instruments (Lehman et al. 1998). QOL measures use the subjective ratings of the individual in a variety of areas to assess the impact of symptoms and disorders on life (Orley et al. 1998). A number of studies have reported on the quality of life of individuals with mental disorders, concluding that the negative impact is not only substantial but sustained (UK700 Group 1999). It has been shown that quality of life continues to be poor even after recovery from mental disorders as a result of social factors that include continued stigma and discrimination. Results from QOL studies also suggest that individuals with severe mental disorders living in long-term mental hospitals have a poorer quality of life than those living in the community. A recent study clearly demonstrated that unmet basic social and functioning needs were the largest predictors of poor quality of life among individuals with severe mental disorders (UK700 Group 1999).

The impact on quality of life is not limited to severe mental disorders. Anxiety and panic disorders also have a major effect, in particular with regard to psychological functioning (Mendlowicz & Stein 2000; Orley & Kuyken 1994).

SOME COMMON DISORDERS

Mental and behavioural disorders present a varied and heterogeneous picture. Some disorders are mild while others are severe. Some last just a few weeks while others may last a lifetime. Some are not even discernible except by detailed scrutiny while others are impossible to hide even from a casual observer. This report focuses on a few common disorders that place a heavy burden on communities and that are generally regarded with a high level of concern. These include depressive disorders, substance use disorders, schizophrenia, epilepsy, Alzheimer's disease, mental retardation, and disorders of childhood and adolescence. The inclusion of epilepsy needs some explanation. Epilepsy is a neurological disorder and is classified under Chapter VI of ICD-10 with other diseases of the nervous system. However, epilepsy was historically seen as a mental disorder and is still considered this way in many societies. Like those with mental disorders, people with epilepsy suffer stigma and severe disability if left untreated. The management of epilepsy is often the responsibility of mental health professionals because of the high prevalence of this disorder and the relative scarcity of specialist neurological services, especially in developing countries. In addition, many countries have laws that prevent individuals with mental disorders and epilepsy from undertaking certain civil responsibilities.

The following section briefly describes the basic epidemiology, burden, course/outcome and special characteristics of some disorders, as examples, to provide background to the discussion of available interventions (in Chapter 3) and mental health policy and programmes (in Chapter 4).

DEPRESSIVE DISORDERS

Depression is characterized by sadness, loss of interest in activities, and decreased energy. Other symptoms include loss of confidence and self-esteem, inappropriate guilt, thoughts of death and suicide, diminished concentration, and disturbance of sleep and appetite. A variety of somatic symptoms may also be present. Though depressive feelings are common, especially after experiencing setbacks in life, depressive disorder is diagnosed only when the symptoms reach a threshold and last at least two weeks. Depression can vary in severity from mild to very severe (see Figure 1.3). It is most often episodic but can be recurrent or chronic. Depression is more common in women than in men. GBD 2000 estimates the point prevalence of unipolar depressive episodes to be 1.9% for men and 3.2% for women, and that 5.8% of men and 9.5% of women will experience a depressive episode in a 12-month period. These prevalence figures vary across populations and may be higher in some populations.

GBD 2000 analysis also shows that unipolar depressive disorders place an enormous burden on society and are ranked as the fourth leading cause of burden among all diseases, accounting for 4.4% of the total DALYs and the leading cause of YLDs, accounting for 11.9% of total YLDs. In the age group 15–44 years it caused the second highest burden, amounting to 8.6% of DALYs lost. While these estimates clearly demonstrate the current very high level of burden resulting from depression, the outlook for the future is even grimmer. By the year 2020, if current trends for demographic and epidemiological transition continue, the burden of depression will increase to 5.7% of the total burden of disease, becoming the second leading cause of DALYs lost. Worldwide it will be second only to ischaemic heart disease for DALYs lost for both sexes. In the developed regions, depression will then be the highest ranking cause of burden of disease.

Depression can affect individuals at any stage of the life span, although the incidence is highest in the middle ages. There is, however, an increasing recognition of depression during adolescence and young adulthood (Lewinsohn et al. 1993). Depression is essentially an episodic recurring disorder, each episode lasting usually from a few months to a few years, with a normal period in between. In about 20% of cases, however, depression follows a chronic course with no remission (Thornicroft & Sartorius 1993), especially when adequate treatment is not available. The recurrence rate for those who recover from the first episode is around 35% within 2 years and about 60% at 12 years. The recurrence rate is higher in those who are more than 45 years of age. One of the particularly tragic outcomes of a depressive disorder is suicide. Around 15–20% of depressive patients end their lives by committing suicide (Goodwin & Jamison 1990). Suicide remains one of the common and avoidable outcomes of depression.

Bipolar affective disorder refers to patients with depressive illness along with episodes of mania characterized by elated mood, increased activity, over-confidence and impaired concentration. According to GBD 2000, the point prevalence of bipolar disorder is around 0.4%.

To summarize, depression is a common mental disorder, causing a very high level of disease burden, and is expected to show a rising trend during the coming 20 years.

SUBSTANCE USE DISORDERS

Mental and behavioural disorders resulting from psychoactive substance use include disorders caused by the use of alcohol, opioids such as opium or heroin, cannabinoids such as marijuana, sedatives and hypnotics, cocaine, other stimulants, hallucinogens, tobacco and volatile solvents. The conditions include intoxication, harmful use, dependence and psychotic disorders. Harmful use is diagnosed when damage has been caused to physical or mental health. Dependence syndrome involves a strong desire to take the substance, difficulty in controlling use, a physiological withdrawal state, tolerance, neglect of alternative pleasures and interests, and persistence of use despite harm to oneself and others.

Though the use of substances (along with their associated disorders) varies from region to region, tobacco and alcohol are the substances that are used most widely in the world as a whole and that have the most serious public health consequences.

Use of tobacco is extremely common. Most of the use is in the form of cigarettes. The World Bank estimates that, in high income countries, smoking-related health care accounts for 6–15.1% of all annual health care costs (World Bank 1999).

Today, about one in three adults, or 1.2 billion people, smoke. By 2025, the number is expected to rise to more than 1.6 billion. Tobacco was estimated to account for over 3 million annual deaths in 1990, rising to 4 million annual deaths in 1998. It is estimated that tobacco-attributable deaths will rise to 8.4 million in 2020 and reach 10 million annual deaths in about 2030. This increase will not, however, be shared equally: deaths in developed regions are expected to rise 50% from 1.6 to 2.4 million, while those in Asia will soar almost fourfold from 1.1 million in 1990 to an estimated 4.2 million in 2020 (Murray & Lopez 1997).

In addition to the social and behavioural factors associated with the onset of tobacco use, a clear dependence on nicotine is found in the majority of chronic smokers. This dependence prevents these individuals from giving up tobacco use and staying away from it. Box 2.3 describes the link between mental disorders and tobacco use.

Alcohol is also a commonly used substance in most regions of the world. Point prevalence of alcohol use disorders (harmful use and dependence) in adults has been estimated to be around 1.7% globally according to GBD 2000 analysis. The rates are 2.8% for men and 0.5% for women. The prevalence of alcohol use disorders varies widely across different

---

Box 2.3 Tobacco use and mental disorders

The link between tobacco use and mental disorders is a complex one. Research findings strongly suggest that mental health professionals need to pay much greater attention to tobacco use by patients during and after their treatment, in order to prevent related problems.

People with mental disorders are about twice as likely to smoke as others; those with schizophrenia and alcohol dependence are particularly likely to be heavy smokers, with rates as high as 86%.[1-3] A recent study in the USA showed that individuals with current mental disorders had a smoking rate of 41% compared with 22.5% in the general population, and estimated that 44% of all cigarettes smoked in the US are consumed by people with mental disorders.[4]

Regular smoking starts earlier in male adolescents with attention deficit disorder,[5] and individuals with depression are also more likely to be smokers.[6] Though the traditional thinking has been that depressed individuals tend to smoke more because of their symptoms, new evidence reveals that it may be the other way round. A study of teenagers showed that those who became depressed had a higher prevalence of smoking beforehand – suggesting that smoking actually resulted in depression in this age group.[7]

Alcohol and drug use disorder patients also show systematic changes in their smoking behaviour during treatment. A recent study found that though heavy smokers decreased their smoking while hospitalized for detoxification, light smokers actually increased their smoking substantially.[8]

The reasons for the high rate of smoking by persons with mental and behavioural disorders are not clearly known, but neurochemical mechanisms have been suggested to account for it.[9] Nicotine is a highly psychoactive chemical that has a variety of effects in the brain: it has reinforcing properties and activates the reward systems of the brain; it also leads to increased dopamine release in parts of the brain that are intimately related to mental disorders. Nicotine may also be consumed in an attempt to decrease the distress and other undesirable effects of mental symptoms. Social environment, including isolation and boredom, may also play a role; these aspects are particularly evident in an institutional setting. Whatever the reasons, the fact that people with mental disorders further jeopardize their health by excessive smoking is not in doubt.

[1]Hughes JR et al. (1986). Prevalence of smoking among psychiatric outpatients. *American Journal of Psychiatry*, 143: 993–997.
[2]Goff DC et al. (1992). Cigarette smoking in schizophrenia: relationship to psychopathology and medication side-effects. *American Journal of Psychiatry*, 149: 1189–1194.
[3]True WR et al. (1999). Common genetic vulnerability for nicotine and alcohol dependence in men. *Archives of General Psychiatry*, 56: 655–661.
[4]Lasser K et al. (2000). Smoking and mental illness: a population-based prevalence study. *Journal of the American Medical Association*, 284: 2606–2610.
[5]Castellanos FX et al. (1994). Quantitative morphology of the caudate nucleus in attention deficit hyperactivity disorder. *American Journal of Psychiatry*, 151(12): 1791–1796.
[6]Pomerleau OF et al. (1995). Cigarette smoking in adult patients diagnosed with attention deficit hyperactivity disorder. *Journal of Substance Abuse*, 7(3): 373–368.
[7]Goodman E, Capitman J (2000). Depressive symptoms and cigarette smoking among teens. *Pediatrics* 106(4): 748–755.
[8]Harris J et al. (2000). Changes in cigarette smoking among alcohol and drug misusers during inpatient detoxification. *Addiction Biology*, 5: 443–450.
[9]Batra A (2000). Tobacco use and smoking cessation in the psychiatric patient. *Fortschritte de Neurologie-Psychiatrie*, 68: 80–92.

regions of the world, ranging from very low levels in some Middle Eastern countries to over 5% in North America and parts of Eastern Europe.

Alcohol use is rising rapidly in some of the developing regions of the world (Jernigan et al. 2000; Riley & Marshall 1999; WHO 1999) and this is likely to escalate alcohol-related problems (WHO 2000b). Alcohol use is also a major reason for concern among the indigenous people around the world, who show a higher prevalence of use and associated problems.

Alcohol ranks high as a cause of disease burden. The global burden of disease project (Murray & Lopez 1996a) estimated alcohol to be responsible for 1.5% of all deaths and 3.5% of the total DALYs. This burden includes physical disorders (such as cirrhosis), and injuries (for example, motor vehicle crash injuries) attributable to alcohol.

Alcohol imposes a high economic cost on society. One estimate puts the yearly economic cost of alcohol abuse in the United States to be US$ 148 billion, including US$ 19 billion for health care expenditure (Harwood et al. 1998). In Canada, the economic costs of alcohol amount to approximately US$ 18.4 billion, representing 2.7% of the gross domestic product. Studies in other countries have estimated the cost of alcohol-related problems to be around 1% of the gross domestic product (Collins & Lapsely 1996; Rice et al. 1991). A recent study demonstrated that alcohol-related hospital charges in 1998 in New Mexico, USA, were US$ 51 million in comparison to US$ 35 million collected as alcohol taxes (New Mexico Department of Health 2001), clearly showing that communities spend more money on taking care of alcohol problems than they earn from alcohol.

Besides tobacco and alcohol, a large number of other substances – generally grouped under the broad category of drugs – are also abused. These include illicit drugs such as heroin, cocaine and cannabis. The period prevalence of drug abuse and dependence ranges from 0.4% to 4%, but the type of drugs used varies greatly from region to region. GBD 2000 analysis suggests that the point prevalence of heroin and cocaine use disorders is 0.25%. Injecting drugs involves considerable risk of infections, including hepatitis B, hepatitis C and HIV. It has been estimated that there are about 5 million people in the world who inject illicit drugs. The prevalence of HIV infection among injecting drug users is 20–80% in many cities. The increasing role of injecting drug use in HIV transmission has attracted serious concern all over the world, especially in Central and Eastern European countries (UNAIDS 2000).

The burden attributable to illicit drugs (heroin and cocaine) was estimated at 0.4% of the total disease burden according to GBD 2000. The economic cost of harmful drug use and dependence in the United States has been estimated to be US$ 98 billion (Harwood et al. 1998). These disease burden and cost estimates do not take into account a variety of negative social effects that are caused by drug use. Tobacco and alcohol use typically starts during youth and acts as a facilitator to the use of other drugs. Thus tobacco and alcohol contribute indirectly to a large amount of the burden of other drugs and the consequent diseases.

Questions are often raised as to whether substance use disorders are genuine disorders or should rather be seen as deviant behaviour by people who deliberately indulge in an activity that causes them harm. While deciding to experiment with a psychoactive substance is usually a personal decision, developing dependence after repeated use is not a conscious and informed decision by the individual or the result of a moral weakness, but the outcome of a complex combination of genetic, physiological and environmental factors. It is very difficult to distinguish exactly when a person becomes dependent on a substance (regardless of its legal status), and there is evidence that dependence is not a clearly demarcated category but that it happens along a continuum, from early problems without significant dependence to severe dependence with physical, mental and socioeconomic consequences.

There is also increasing evidence of neurochemical changes in the brain that are associated with and indeed cause many of the essential characteristics of substance dependence. Even the clinical evidence suggests that substance dependence should be seen as both a chronic medical illness and a social problem (Leshner 1997; McLellan et al. 2000). Common roots of dependence for a variety of substances and the high prevalence of multiple dependence also suggest that substance dependence should be viewed as a complex mental disorder with a possible basis in brain functioning.

SCHIZOPHRENIA

Schizophrenia is a severe disorder that typically begins in late adolescence or early adulthood. It is characterized by fundamental distortions in thinking and perception, and by inappropriate emotions. The disturbance involves the most basic functions that give the normal person a feeling of individuality, uniqueness and self-direction. Behaviour may be seriously disturbed during some phases of the disorder, leading to adverse social consequences. Strong belief in ideas that are false and without any basis in reality (delusions) is another feature of this disorder.

Schizophrenia follows a variable course, with complete symptomatic and social recovery in about one-third of cases. Schizophrenia can, however, follow a chronic or recurrent course, with residual symptoms and incomplete social recovery. Individuals with chronic schizophrenia constituted a large proportion of all residents of mental institutions in the past, and still do where these institutions continue to exist. With modern advances in drug therapy and psychosocial care, almost half the individuals initially developing schizophrenia can expect a full and lasting recovery. Of the remainder, only about one-fifth continue to face serious limitations in their day-to-day activities.

Schizophrenia is found approximately equally in men and women, though the onset tends to be later in women, who also tend to have a better course and outcome of this disorder.

GBD 2000 reports a point prevalence of 0.4% for schizophrenia. Schizophrenia causes a high degree of disability. In a recent 14-country study on disability associated with physical and mental conditions, active psychosis was ranked the third most disabling condition, higher than paraplegia and blindness, by the general population (Üstün et al. 1999).

In the global burden of disease study, schizophrenia accounted for 1.1% of the total DALYs and 2.8% of YLDs. The economic cost of schizophrenia to society is also high. It has been estimated that, in 1991, the cost of schizophrenia to the United States was US$ 19 billion in direct expenditure and US$ 46 billion in lost productivity.

Even after the more obvious symptoms of this disorder have disappeared, some residual symptoms may remain. These include lack of interest and initiative in daily activities and work, social incompetence, and inability to take interest in pleasurable activities. These can cause continued disability and poor quality of life. These symptoms can place a considerable burden on families (Pai & Kapur 1982). It has been repeatedly demonstrated that schizophrenia follows a less severe course in developing countries (Kulhara & Wig 1978; Thara & Eaton 1996). For example, in one of the multi-site international studies, the proportion of patients showing full remission at 2 years was 63% in developing countries compared to 37% in developed countries (Jablensky et al. 1992). Though attempts have been made to explain this better outcome on the basis of stronger family support and fewer demands on the patients, the exact reasons for these differences are not clear.

A substantial number of individuals with schizophrenia attempt suicide at some time during the course of their illness. A recent study showed that 30% of patients diagnosed with this disorder had attempted suicide at least once during their lifetime (Radomsky et al. 1999). About 10% of persons with schizophrenia die by suicide (Caldwell & Gottesman 1990). Globally, schizophrenic illness reduces an affected individual's lifespan by an average of 10 years.

EPILEPSY

Epilepsy is the most common brain disorder in the general population. It is characterized by recurrence of seizures, caused by outbursts of excessive electrical activity in part or the whole of the brain. The majority of individuals with epilepsy do not have any obvious or demonstrable abnormality in the brain, besides the electrical changes. However, a proportion of individuals with this disorder may have accompanying brain damage, which may cause other physical dysfunctions such as spasticity or mental retardation.

The causes of epilepsy include genetic predisposition, brain damage caused by birth complications, infections and parasitic diseases, brain injuries, intoxication and tumours. Cysticercosis (tapeworm), schistosomiasis, toxoplasmosis, malaria, and tubercular and viral encephalitis are some of the common infectious causes of epilepsy in developing countries (Senanayake & Román 1993). Epileptic seizures vary greatly in frequency, from several a day to once every few months. The manifestation of epilepsy depends on the brain areas involved. Usually the individual undergoes sudden loss of consciousness and may experience spasmodic movements of the body. Injuries can result from a fall during the seizure.

GBD 2000 estimates that about 37 million individuals globally suffer from primary epilepsy. When epilepsy caused by other diseases or injury is also included, the total number of persons affected increases to about 50 million. It is estimated that more than 80% individuals with epilepsy live in developing countries.

Epilepsy places a significant burden on communities, especially in developing countries where it may remain largely untreated. GBD 2000 estimates the aggregate burden due to epilepsy to be 0.5% of the total disease burden. In addition to physical and mental disability, epilepsy often results in serious psychosocial consequences for the individual and the family. The stigma attached to epilepsy prevents individuals with epilepsy from participating in normal activities, including education, marriage, work and sports.

Epilepsy typically arises during childhood and can (though does not always) follow a chronic course. The rate of spontaneous recovery is substantial, with many of those initially identified as suffering from epilepsy being free from seizure after three years.

ALZHEIMER'S DISEASE

Alzheimer's disease is a primary degenerative disease of the brain. Dementia in Alzheimer's disease is classified as a mental and behavioural disorder in ICD-10. It is characterized by progressive decline of cognitive functions such as memory, thinking, comprehension, calculation, language, learning capacity and judgement. Dementia is diagnosed when these declines are sufficient to impair personal activities of daily living. Alzheimer's disease shows insidious onset with slow deterioration. This disease needs to be clearly differentiated from age-related normal decline of cognitive functions. The normal decline is much less, much more gradual and leads to milder disabilities. The onset of Alzheimer's disease is usually after 65 years of age, though earlier onset is not uncommon. As age advances, the incidence increases rapidly (it roughly doubles every 5 years). This has obvious implications for the total number of individuals living with this disorder as life expectancy increases in the population.

The incidence and prevalence of Alzheimer's disease have been studied extensively. The population samples are usually composed of people over 65 years of age, although some studies have included younger populations, especially in countries where the expected life span is shorter (for example, India). The wide range of prevalence figures (1–5%) is partly explained by the different age samples and diagnostic criteria. In GBD 2000, Alzheimer's and other dementias have an overall point prevalence of 0.6%. The prevalence among those above 60 years is about 5% for men and 6% for women. There is no evidence of any sex difference in incidence, but more women are encountered with Alzheimer's disease because of greater female longevity.

The exact cause of Alzheimer's disease remains unknown, although a number of factors have been suggested. These include disturbances in the metabolism and regulation of amyloid precursor protein, plaque-related proteins, tau proteins, zinc and aluminium (Drouet et al. 2000; Cuajungco & Lees 1997).

GBD 2000 estimates the DALYs due to dementias as 0.84% and YLDs as 2.0%. With the ageing of populations, especially in the industrialized regions, this percentage is likely to show a rapid increase in the next 20 years.

The cost of Alzheimer's disease to society is already massive (Rice et al. 1993) and will continue to increase (Brookmeyer & Gray 2000). The direct and total costs of this disorder in the United States have been estimated to be US$ 536 million and US$ 1.75 billion, respectively, for the year 2000.

MENTAL RETARDATION

Mental retardation is a condition of arrested or incomplete development of the mind characterized by impairment of skills and overall intelligence in areas such as cognition, language, and motor and social abilities. Also referred to as intellectual disability or handicap, mental retardation can occur with or without any other physical or mental disorders. Although reduced level of intellectual functioning is the characteristic feature of this disorder, the diagnosis is made only if it is associated with a diminished ability to adapt to the daily demands of the normal social environment. Mental retardation is further categorized as mild (IQ levels 50-69), moderate (IQ levels 35–49), severe (IQ levels 20–34), and profound (IQ levels below 20).

The prevalence figures vary considerably because of the varying criteria and methods used in the surveys, as well as differences in the age range of the samples. The overall prevalence of mental retardation is believed to be between 1% and 3%, with the rate for moderate, severe and profound retardation being 0.3%. It is more common in developing countries because of the higher incidence of injuries and anoxia around birth, and early childhood brain infections. A common cause of mental retardation is endemic iodine deficiency, which leads to cretinism (Sankar et al. 1998). Iodine deficiency constitutes the world's greatest single cause of preventable brain damage and mental retardation (Delange 2000).

Mental retardation places a severe burden on the individual and the family. For more severe retardation, this involves assistance in carrying out daily life activities and self care. No estimates are available for the overall disease burden of mental retardation, but all evidence points towards a substantial burden caused by this condition. In most cases, this burden continues throughout life.

DISORDERS OF CHILDHOOD AND ADOLESCENCE

Contrary to popular belief, mental and behavioural disorders are common during childhood and adolescence. Inadequate attention is paid to this area of mental health. In a recent report, the Surgeon General of the United States (DHHS 2001) has said that the United States is facing a public crisis in mental health of infants, children and adolescents. According to the report, one in ten young people suffers from mental illness severe enough to cause some level of impairment, yet fewer than one in five receives the needed treatment. The situation in large parts of the developing world is likely to be even more unsatisfactory.

ICD-10 identifies two broad categories specific to childhood and adolescence: disorders of psychological development, and behavioural and emotional disorders. The former are characterized by impairment or delay in the development of specific functions such speech and language (dyslexias) or overall pervasive development (for example, autism). The course of these disorders is steady, without remission or relapses, though most tend to improve with time. The broad group of dyslexias consists of reading and spelling disorders. The prevalence of these disorders is still uncertain, but it may be about 4% for the school-age population (Spagna et al. 2000). The second category, behavioural and emotional disorders, includes hyperkinetic disorders (in ICD-10), attention deficit/hyperactivity disorder (in DSM-IV, APA 1994), conduct disorders and emotional disorders of childhood. In addition, many of the disorders more commonly found among adults can begin during childhood. An example is depression, which is increasingly being identified among children.

The overall prevalence of mental and behavioural disorders among children has been investigated in several studies from developed and developing countries. The results of selected studies are summarized in Table 2.2. Though the prevalence figures vary considerably between studies, it seems that 10–20% of all children have one or more mental or behavioural problems. A caveat must be made to these high estimates of morbidity among children and adolescents. Childhood and adolescence being developmental phases, it is difficult to draw clear boundaries between phenomena that are part of normal development and others that are abnormal. Many studies have used behavioural checklists completed by parents and teachers to detect cases. This information, though useful in identifying children who may need special attention, may not always correspond to a definite diagnosis.

Mental and behavioural disorders of childhood and adolescence are very costly to society in both human and financial terms. The aggregate disease burden of these disorders has not been estimated, and it would be complex to calculate because many of these disorders can be precursors to much more disabling disorders during later life.

Table 2.2 Prevalence of child and adolescent disorders, selected studies

Country	Age (years)	Prevalence (%)
Ethiopia[1]	1–15	17.7
Germany[2]	12–15	20.7
India[3]	1–16	12.8
Japan[4]	12–15	15.0
Spain[5]	8, 11, 15	21.7
Switzerland[6]	1–15	22.5
USA[7]	1–15	21.0

[1] Tadesse B et al. (1999). Childhood behavioural disorders in Ambo district, Western Ethiopia: I. Prevalence estimates. *Acta Psychiatrica Scandinavica*, 100(Suppl): 92–97.

[2] Weyerer S et al. (1988). Prevalence and treatment of psychiatric disorders in 3–14-year-old children: results of a representative field study in the small rural town region of Traunstein, Upper Bavaria. *Acta Psychiatrica Scandinavica*, 77: 290–296.

[3] Indian Council of Medical Research (2001). *Epidemiological study of child and adolescent psychiatric disorders in urban and rural areas*. New Delhi, ICMR (unpublished data).

[4] Morita H et al. (1993). Psychiatric disorders in Japanese secondary school children. *Journal of Child Psychology and Psychiatry*, 34: 317–332.

[5] Gomez-Beneyto M et al. (1994). Prevalence of mental disorders among children in Valencia, Spain. *Acta Psychiatrica Scandinavica*, 89: 352–357.

[6] Steinhausen HC et al. (1998). Prevalence of child and adolescent psychiatric disorders: the Zurich Epidemiological Study. *Acta Psychiatrica Scandinavica*, 98: 262–271.

[7] Shaffer D et al. (1996). The NIMH Diagnostic Interview Schedule for Children version 2.3 (DISC-2.3): description acceptability, prevalence rates, and performance in the MECA study. *Journal of the American Academy of Child and Adolescent Psychiatry*, 35: 865–877.

COMORBIDITY

It is common for two or more mental disorders to occur together in an individual. This is not unlike the situation with physical disorders, which also tend to occur together much more frequently than can be explained by chance. It is especially common with advancing age, when a number of physical and mental disorders occur together. Physical health problems not only coexist with mental disorders such as depression, but can also predict the onset and persistence of depression (Geerlings et al. 2000).

One of the methodologically sound studies of a nationally representative sample was done in the United States (Kessler et al. 1994) and showed that 79% of all ill people were comorbid. In other words, only in 21% of patients did a mental disorder occur singly. More than half of all lifetime disorders occurred in 14% of the population. Similar findings have been obtained in studies from other countries, although not much information is available from developing countries.

Anxiety and depressive disorders commonly occur together. Such comorbidity is found among about half of all the individuals with these disorders (Zimmerman et al. 2000). Another common situation is the presence of mental disorders associated with substance use and dependence. Among those attending alcohol and drug services, between 30% and 90% have a "dual disorder" (Gossop et al. 1998). The rate of alcohol use disorders is also high among those attending mental health services (65% reported by Rachliesel et al. 1999). Alcohol use disorders are also common (12–50%) among persons with schizophrenia.

The presence of substantial comorbidity has serious implications for the identification, treatment and rehabilitation of affected individuals. The disability of individual sufferers and the burden on families also increase correspondingly.

SUICIDE

Suicide is the result of an act deliberately initiated and performed by a person in the full knowledge or expectation of its fatal outcome. Suicide is now a major public health problem. Taken as an average for 53 countries for which complete data is available, the age-standardized suicide rate for 1996 was 15.1 per 100 000. The rate for males was 24.0 per 100 000 and for females 6.8 per 100 000. The rate of suicide is almost universally higher among men compared to women by an aggregate ratio of 3.5 to 1.

Over the past 30 years, for the 39 countries for which complete data is available for the period 1970-96, the suicide rates seem to have remained quite stable, but the current aggregate rates hide important differences regarding the sexes, age groups, geography and longer time trends.

Geographically, changes in suicide rates vary considerably. Trends in the mega-countries of the world – those with a population of more than 100 million – are likely to provide reliable information on suicide mortality. Information is available for seven of eleven such countries for the last 15 years. The trends range from an almost 62% increase in Mexico to a 17% decrease in China, with the United States and the Russian Federation going in opposite directions by the same 5.3%, as shown in Figure 2.4. Two remarks are needed: first, probably only the size of their populations puts these countries in the same category, as they differ virtually in every other aspect. Second, the magnitude of the change does not reflect the actual magnitude of suicide rates in those countries. In the most recent year for which data are available, suicide rates range from 3.4 per 100 000 in Mexico to 14.0 per 100 000 in China and 34.0 per 100 000 in the Russian Federation.

It is very difficult, if not impossible, to find a common explanation for this diverse variation. Socioeconomic change (in any direction) is often suggested as a factor contributing to
an increase in suicide rates. However, although this has been documented on several occa-
sions, increases in suicide rates have also been observed in periods of socioeconomic stability, while stable suicide rates have been seen during periods of major socioeconomic changes.
Nevertheless, these aggregate figures may hide important differences across some population segments. For instance, a flat evolution of suicide rates may hide an increase in men's
rates statistically compensated for by a decrease in women's rates (as occurred, for example,
in Australia, Chile, Cuba, Japan and Spain); the same would apply to extreme age groups,
such as adolescents and the elderly (for example, in New Zealand). It has been shown that
an increase in unemployment rates is usually, but not always, accompanied by a decrease in
suicide rates of the general population (for example, in Finland), but by an increase in
suicide rates of elderly and retired people (for example, in Switzerland).

Alcohol consumption (for example, in the Baltic States and the Russian Federation) and
easy access to some toxic substances (for example, in China, India and Sri Lanka) and to
firearms (for example, in El Salvador and the United States) seem to be positively correlated with suicide rates across all countries – industrialized or developing – so far studied.
Once again, aggregate figures can hide major discrepancies between, for example, rural
and urban areas (for example, in China and the Islamic Republic of Iran).

Suicide is a leading cause of death for young adults. It is among the top three causes of
death in the population aged 15–34 years. As shown in two examples in Figure 2.5, suicide
is predominant in the 15–34-year-old age group, where it ranks as the first or second cause
of death for both the sexes. This represents a massive loss to societies of young persons in
their productive years of life. Data on suicide attempts are only available from a few countries; they indicate that the number of suicide attempts may be up to 20 times higher than
the number of completed suicides.

Self-inflicted injuries including suicide accounted for about 814 000 deaths in 2000. They
were responsible for 1.3% of all DALYs according to GBD 2000.

**Figure 2.4 Changes in age-standardized suicide rates over specific time periods in countries
with a population over 100 million**

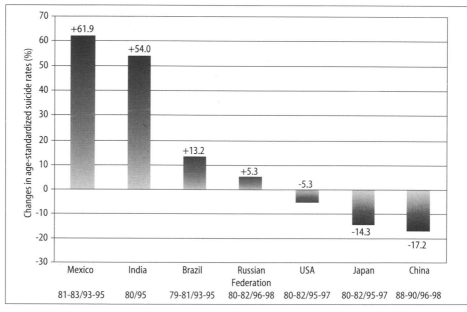

Figure 2.5 Suicide as a leading cause of death, selected countries of the European Region and China, 15–34-year-olds, 1998

European Region (selected countries)[a]

Both sexes	Males	Females
1. Transport accidents	1. Transport accidents	1. All cancers
2. Suicide	2. Suicide	2. Transport accidents
3. All cancers	3. All cancers	3. Suicide

China (selected areas)[b]

Both sexes (rural and urban areas)	Males (rural areas)	Females (rural areas)
1. Suicide	1. Motor vehicle accidents	1. Suicide
2. Motor vehicle accidents	2. All cancers	2. All cancers
3. All cancers	3. Suicide	3. All cardiovascular diseases

[a] Albania, Austria, Bulgaria, Croatia, Czech Republic, Estonia, Finland, France, Germany, Greece, Hungary, Israel, Italy, Kazakhstan, Latvia, Lithuania, Luxembourg, Macedonia, Malta, Netherlands, Norway, Portugal, Republic of Moldova, Romania, Slovakia, Slovenia, Spain, United Kingdom.

[b] Cause-of-death statistics and vital rates, civil registration systems and alternative sources of information. *World Health Statistics Annual 1993*, Geneva, World Health Organization, 1994 (Section A/B: China 11–17).

The most common mental disorder leading to suicide is depression, although the rates are also high for schizophrenia. In addition, suicide is often related to substance use – either in the person who commits it or within the family. The major proportion of suicides in some countries of Central and Eastern Europe have recently been attributed to alcohol use (Rossow 2000).

It is well known that availability of means to commit suicide has a major impact on actual suicides in any region. This has been best studied for firearm availability, the finding being that there is a high mortality by suicide among people purchasing firearms in the recent past (Wintemute et al. 1999). Of all the persons who died from firearm injuries in the United States in 1997, a total of 54% died by suicide (Rosenberg et al. 1999).

The precise explanation for variations in suicide rates must always be considered in the local context. There is a pressing need for epidemiological surveillance and appropriate local research to contribute to a better understanding of this major public health problem and improve the possibilities of prevention.

DETERMINANTS OF MENTAL AND BEHAVIOURAL DISORDERS

A variety of factors determine the prevalence, onset and course of mental and behavioural disorders. These include social and economic factors, demographic factors such as sex and age, serious threats such as conflicts and disasters, the presence of major physical diseases, and the family environment, which are briefly described here to illustrate their impact on mental health.

POVERTY

Poverty and associated conditions of unemployment, low educational level, deprivation and homelessness are not only widespread in poor countries, but also affect a sizeable minority of rich countries. Data from cross-national surveys in Brazil, Chile, India and Zimbabwe show that common mental disorders are about twice as frequent among the poor as among the rich (Patel et al. 1999). In the United States, children from the poorest families were found to be at increased risk of disorders in the ratio of 2:1 for behavioural disorders and 3:1 for comorbid conditions (Costello et al. 1996). A review of 15 studies found the median ratio for overall prevalence of mental disorders between the lowest and the highest socioeconomic categories was 2.1:1 for one year and 1.4:1 for lifetime prevalence (Kohn et al. 1998). Similar results have been reported from recent studies carried out in North America, Latin America and Europe (WHO International Consortium of Psychiatric Epidemiology 2000). Figure 2.6 shows that depression is more common among the poor than the rich.

There is also evidence that the course of disorders is determined by the socioeconomic status of the individual (Kessler et al. 1994; Saraceno & Barbui 1997). This may be a result of service-related variables, including barriers to accessing care. Poor countries have few resources for mental health care and these resources are often unavailable to the poorer segments of society. Even in rich countries, poverty and associated factors such as lack of insurance coverage, lower levels of education, unemployment, and racial, ethnic and language minority status create insurmountable barriers to care. The treatment gap for most mental disorders is large, but for the poor population it is massive. In addition, poor people often raise mental health concerns when seeking treatment for physical problems, as shown in Box 2.4.

Figure 2.6 Prevalence of depression in low versus high income groups, selected countries

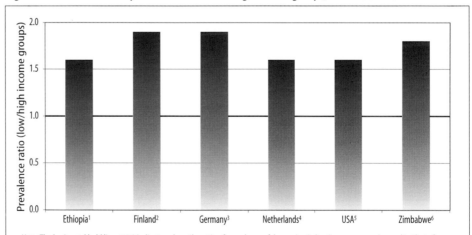

Note: The horizontal bold line at 1.0 indicates where the ratio of prevalence of depression in low income groups is equal to that of high income groups. Above this line people with a low income have a higher prevalence of depression.

[1] Awas M et al. (1999). Major mental disorders in Butajira, southern Ethiopia. *Acta Psychiatrica Scandinavica,* 100 (Suppl 397): 56–64.

[2] Lindeman S et al. (2000). The 12-month prevalence and risk factors for major depressive episode in Finland: representative sample of 5993 adults. *Acta Psychiatrica Scandinavica,* 102: 178–184.

[3] Wittchen HU et al. (1998). Prevalence of mental disorders and psychosocial impairments in adolescents and young adults. *Psychological Medicine,* 28: 109–126.

[4] Bijl RV et al. (1998). Prevalence of psychiatric disorders in the general population: results of the Netherlands Mental Health Survey and Incidence Study (NEMESIS). *Social Psychiatry and Psychiatric Epidemiology,* 33: 587–595.

[5] Kessler RC et al. (1994). Lifetime and 12-month prevalence of DSM-III-R psychiatric disorders in the United States. Results from the National Comorbidity Survey. *Archives of General Psychiatry,* 51: 8–19.

[6] Abas MA, Broadhead JC (1997). Depression and anxiety among women in an urban setting in Zimbabwe. *Psychological Medicine,* 27: 59–71.

The relationship between mental and behavioural disorders, including those related to alcohol use, and the economic development of communities and countries has not been explored in a systematic way. It appears, however, that the vicious cycle of poverty and mental disorders at the family level (see Figure 1.4) may well be operative at the community and country levels.

SEX

There has been an increasing focus on sex differences in studying the prevalence, causation and course of mental and behavioural disorders. A higher proportion of women among the inmates of asylums and other treatment facilities was noted in earlier centuries, but it is not clear whether mental disorders were indeed more prevalent among women or whether women were brought in more frequently for treatment.

Recent community studies using sound methodology have revealed some interesting differences. The overall prevalence of mental and behavioural disorders does not seem to be different between men and women. Anxiety and depressive disorders are, however, more common among women, while substance use disorders and antisocial personality disorders are more common among men (Gold 1998). Almost all studies show a higher prevalence of depressive and anxiety disorders among women, the usual ratio being between 1.5:1 and 2:1. These findings have been seen not only in developed but also in a number of developing countries (Patel et al. 1999; Pearson 1995). It is interesting to note that sex differences in rates of depression are strongly age-related; the greatest differences occur in adult life, with no reported differences in childhood and few in the elderly.

Many reasons for the higher prevalence of depressive and anxiety disorders among women have been proposed. Genetic and biological factors certainly play some role, as indicated in particular by the close temporal relationship between higher prevalence and reproductive age range with associated hormonal changes. Mood swings related to hormonal changes as part of the menstrual cycle and following childbirth are well documented. Indeed, depression within a few months of childbirth can be the beginning of a recurrent depressive disorder. Psychological and social factors are, however, also significant for the

---

Box 2.4 Poor people's views on sickness of body and mind

When questioned about their health,[1] poor people mention a broad range of injuries and illnesses: broken limbs, burns, poisoning from chemicals and pollution, diabetes, pneumonia, bronchitis, tuberculosis, HIV/AIDS, asthma, diarrhoea, typhoid, malaria, parasitic diseases from contaminated water, skin infections, and other debilitating diseases. Mental health problems are often raised jointly with physical concerns, and hardships associated with drug and alcohol abuse are also frequently discussed. Stress,

anxiety, depression, lack of self-esteem and suicide are among the effects of poverty and ill-health commonly identified by discussion groups. A recurring theme is the stress of not being able to provide for one's family. People associate many forms of sickness with stress, anguish and being ill at ease, but often pick out three for special mention: HIV/AIDS, alcoholism and drugs.

HIV/AIDS has a marked impact: in Zambia a youth group made a causal link between poverty and prostitution, AIDS and, finally, death.

Group discussions in Argentina, Ghana, Jamaica, Thailand, Viet Nam, and several other countries also mention HIV/AIDS and related diseases as problems that affect their livelihoods and strain the extended family.

People regard drug use and alcoholism as causes of violence, insecurity and theft, and see money spent on alcohol or other drugs, male drunkenness, and domestic violence as syndromes of poverty. Many discussion groups from all regions report problems of physical abuse of women when husbands

bands come home drunk, and several groups find that beer-drinking leads to promiscuity and disease. Alcoholism is especially prevalent among men. In both urban and rural Africa, poor people mention it more frequently than drugs.

Drug abuse is mentioned frequently in urban areas, especially in Latin America, Thailand and Viet Nam. It is also raised in parts of Bulgaria, Kyrgyzstan, the Russian Federation and Uzbekistan. People addicted to drugs are miserable, and so are their families.

[1]Narayan D et al. (2000). *Voices of the poor, crying out for change.* New York, Oxford University Press for the World Bank.

gender difference in depressive and anxiety disorders. There may be more actual as well as perceived stressors among women. The traditional role of women in societies exposes women to greater stresses as well as making them less able to change their stressful environment.

Another reason for the sex differences in common mental disorders is the high rate of domestic and sexual violence to which women are exposed. Domestic violence is found in all regions of the world and women bear the major brunt of it (WHO 2000b). A review of studies (WHO 1997a) found the lifetime prevalence of domestic violence to be between 16% and 50%. Sexual violence is also common; it has been estimated that one in five women suffer rape or attempted rape in their lifetime. These traumatic events have their psychological consequences, depressive and anxiety disorders being the most common. A recent study in Nicaragua found that women with emotional distress were six times more likely to report spousal abuse compared with women without such distress (Ellsberg et al. 1999). Also, women who had experienced severe abuse during the past year were 10 times more likely to experience emotional distress than women who had never experienced abuse.

The WHO Multi-country Study on Women's Health and Domestic Violence and the World Studies of Abuse in Family Environments (WorldSAFE) by the International Network of Clinical Epidemiologists (INCLEN 2001) are studying the prevalence and health consequences for women of intimate partner violence in population-based samples in different settings. In both studies, women are asked if they have contemplated or attempted suicide. Preliminary results indicate a highly significant relationship between such violence and contemplation of suicide (see Table 2.3). Moreover, the same significant patterns were found for sexual violence alone and in combination with physical violence.

In contrast to depressive and anxiety disorders, severe mental disorders such as schizophrenia and bipolar affective disorder do not show any clear differences of incidence or prevalence (Kessler et al. 1994). Schizophrenia, however, seems to have an earlier onset and a more disabling course among men (Sartorius et al. 1986). Almost all the studies show that substance use disorders and antisocial personality disorders are much more common among men than among women.

Comorbidity is more common among women than men. Most often, it takes the form of a co-occurrence of depressive, anxiety and somatoform disorders, the latter being the presence of physical symptoms that are not accounted for by physical diseases. There is evidence that women report a higher number of physical and psychological symptoms than men.

There is also evidence that the prescription of psychotropic medicines is higher among women (see Figure 1.5); these drugs include anti-anxiety, antidepressant, sedative, hyp-

Table 2.3 Relationship between domestic violence and contemplation of suicide

Experience of physical violence by intimate partner	% of women who have ever thought of committing suicide (P<0.001)							
	Brazil[1] (n=940)	Chile[2] (n=422)	Egypt[2] (n=631)	India[2] (n=6327)	Indonesia[3] (n=765)	Philippines[2] (n=1001)	Peru[1] (n=1088)	Thailand[1] (n=2073)
Never	21	11	7	15	1	8	17	18
Ever	48	36	61	64	11	28	40	41

[1] WHO Multi-country Study on Women's Health and Domestic Violence (preliminary results, 2001). Geneva, World Health Organization (unpublished document).

[2] International Network of Clinical Epidemiologists (INCLEN) (2001). *World Studies of Abuse in Family Environments (WorldSAFE)*. Manila, International Network of Clinical Epidemiologists. This survey questioned women about "severe physical violence".

[3] Hakimi M et al. (2001). *Silence for the sake of harmony: domestic violence and women's health in Central Java.* Yogyakarta, Indonesia, Program for Appropriate Technology in Health.

notic and antipsychotic drugs. This higher use of drugs may be partly explained by the higher prevalence of common mental disorders and a higher rate of help-seeking behaviour. A significant factor is likely to be the prescribing behaviour of physicians, who may take the easier path of prescription when faced with a complex psychosocial situation that actually requires psychological intervention.

The higher prevalence of substance use disorders and antisocial personality disorder among men is a consistent finding across the world. In many regions of the world, however, substance use disorders are increasing rapidly among women.

Women also bear the brunt of care for the mentally ill within the family. This is becoming increasingly crucial, as more and more individuals with chronic mental disorders are being looked after in the community.

To summarize, mental disorders have clear sex determinants that need to be better understood and researched in the context of assessing the overall burden.

AGE

Age is an important determinant of mental disorders. Mental disorders during childhood and adolescence have been briefly described above. A high prevalence of disorders is also seen in old age. Besides Alzheimer's disease, discussed above, elderly people also suffer from a number of other mental and behavioural disorders. Overall, the prevalence of some disorders tends to rise with age. Predominant among these is depression. Depressive disorder is common among elderly people: studies show that 8–20% being cared for in the community and 37% being cared for at the primary level are suffering from depression. A recent study on a community sample of people over 65 years of age found depression among 11.2% of this population (Newman et al. 1998). Another recent study, however, found the point prevalence of depressive disorders to be 4.4% for women and 2.7% for men, although the corresponding figures for lifetime prevalence were 20.4% and 9.6%. Depression is more common among older people with physically disabling disorders (Katona & Livingston 2000). The presence of depression further increases the disability among this population. Depressive disorders among elderly people go undetected even more often than among younger adults because they are often mistakenly considered a part of the ageing process.

CONFLICTS AND DISASTERS

Conflicts, including wars and civil strife, and disasters affect a large number of people and result in mental problems. It is estimated that globally about 50 million people are refugees or are internally displaced. In addition, millions are affected by natural disasters including earthquakes, floods, typhoons, hurricanes and similar large-scale calamities (IFRC 2000). Such situations take a heavy toll on the mental health of the people involved, most of whom live in developing countries, where capacity to take care of these problems is extremely limited. Between a third and half of all the affected persons suffer from mental distress. The most frequent diagnosis made is post-traumatic stress disorder (PTSD), often along with depressive or anxiety disorders. In addition, most individuals report psychological symptoms that do not amount to disorders. PTSD arises after a stressful event of an exceptionally threatening or catastrophic nature and is characterized by intrusive memories, avoidance of circumstances associated with the stressor, sleep disturbances, irritability and anger, lack of concentration and excessive vigilance. The point prevalence of PTSD in the general population, according to GBD 2000, is 0.37%. The specific diagnosis of PTSD has been questioned as being culture-specific and also as being made too often. Indeed,

PTSD has been called a diagnostic category that has been invented based on sociopolitical needs (Summerfield 2001). Even if the suitability of this specific diagnosis is uncertain, the overall significance of mental morbidity among individuals exposed to severe trauma is generally accepted.

Studies on victims of natural disasters have also shown a high rate of mental disorders. A recent study from China found a high rate of psychological symptoms and a poor quality of life among earthquake survivors. The study also showed that post-disaster support was effective in the improvement of well-being (Wang et al. 2000).

MAJOR PHYSICAL DISEASES

The presence of major physical diseases affects the mental health of individuals as well as of entire families. Most of the seriously disabling or life-threatening diseases, including cancers in both men and women, have this impact. The case of HIV/AIDS is described here as an illustration of this effect.

HIV is spreading very rapidly in many parts of the world. At the end of 2000, a total of 36.1 million people were living with HIV/AIDS and 21.8 million had already died (UNAIDS 2000). Of the 5.3 million new infections in 2000, 1 in 10 occurred in children and almost half among women. In 16 countries of sub-Saharan Africa more than 10% of the population of reproductive age is now infected with HIV. The HIV/AIDS epidemics has lowered economic growth and is reducing life expectancy by up to 50% in the hardest hit countries. In many countries HIV/AIDS is now considered a threat to national security. With neither cure nor vaccine, prevention of transmission remains the principal response, with care and support for those infected with HIV offering a critical entry point.

The mental health consequences of this epidemic are substantial. A proportion of individuals suffer psychological consequences (disorders as well as problems) as a result of their infection. The effects of intense stigma and discrimination against people with HIV/AIDS also play a major role in psychological stress. Disorders range from anxiety or depressive disorders to adjustment disorder (Maj et al. 1994a). Cognitive deficits are also detected if looked for specifically (Maj et al. 1994b; Starace et al. 1998). In addition, family members also suffer the consequences of stigma and, later, of the premature deaths of their infected family members. The psychological effects on members of families broken and on children orphaned by AIDS have not been studied in any detail, but are likely to be substantial.

These complex situations, where a physical condition leads to psychosocial consequences at individual, family and community levels, require comprehensive assessment in order to determine their full impact on mental health. There is a need for further research in this area.

FAMILY AND ENVIRONMENTAL FACTORS

Mental disorders are firmly rooted in the social environment of the individual. A variety of social factors influence the onset, course and outcome of these disorders.

People go through a series of significant events in life – minor as well as major. These may be desirable (such as a promotion at work) or undesirable (for example, bereavement or business failure). It has been observed that there is an accumulation of life events immediately before onset of mental disorders (Brown et al. 1972; Leff et al. 1987). Though undesirable events predominate before onset or relapse in depressive disorders, a higher occurrence of all events (undesirable and desirable) precedes other mental disorders. Studies suggest that all significant events in life act as stressors and, coming in quick succession, predispose the individual to mental disorders. This effect is not limited to mental disorders and has also been demonstrated to be associated with a number of physical diseases, for example myocardial infarction.

Of course, life events are only one of several interacting factors (such as genetic predisposition, personality, and coping skills) in the causation of disorders.

The relevance of life events research lies mainly in identifying individuals who are at a higher risk because of experiencing major life events in quick succession (for example, loss of job, loss of spouse, and change of residence). Initially this effect was observed for depression and schizophrenia, but subsequently an association has been found between life events and a variety of other mental and behavioural disorders and conditions. Notable among these is suicide.

The social and emotional environment within the family also plays a role in mental disorders. Although attempts to link serious mental disorders such as schizophrenia and depression to the family environment have been made for a long time (Kuipers & Bebbington 1990), some definitive advances have been made in the recent past. The social and emotional environment within the family has clearly been correlated with relapses in schizophrenia but not necessarily with the onset of the disorder. The initial observation was that patients with schizophrenia who went back to stay with parents after a period of hospitalization relapsed more frequently. This led to some research on the cause of this phenomenon. Most studies have used the concept of "expressed emotions" of family members towards the individual with schizophrenia. Expressed emotions in these studies have included critical comments, hostility, emotional over-involvement and warmth.

A large number of studies from all regions of the world have demonstrated that expressed emotionality can predict the course of schizophrenia, including relapses (Butzlaff & Hooley 1998). There is also evidence that changing the emotional environmental within families can have an additive effect on prevention of relapses by antipsychotic drugs. These findings are useful for improving the care of selected patients within their family environment and also recall the importance of social factors in the course and treatment of serious mental disorders such as schizophrenia.

CHAPTER THREE

Solving Mental Health Problems

Over the past half century, the model for mental health care has changed from the institutionalization of individuals suffering from mental disorders to a community care approach backed by the availability of beds in general hospitals for acute cases. This change is based both on respect for the human rights of individuals with mental disorders, and on the use of updated interventions and techniques. A correct objective diagnosis is fundamental for planning individual care and choice of appropriate treatment. The earlier a proper course of treatment starts, the better the prognosis. Appropriate treatment of mental and behavioural disorders implies the rational use of pharmacological, psychological and psychosocial interventions in a clinically meaningful and integrated way. The management of specific conditions consists of interventions in the areas of prevention, treatment and rehabilitation.

3

SOLVING MENTAL
HEALTH PROBLEMS

THE SHIFTING PARADIGM

*T*he care of people with mental and behavioural disorders has always reflected prevailing social values related to the social perception of mental illness. Through the ages, people with mental and behavioural disorders have been treated in different ways (see Box 3.1). They have been given a high status in societies which believe them to intermediate with gods and the dead. In medieval Europe and elsewhere they were beaten and burnt at the stake. They have been locked up in large institutions. They have been explored as scientific objects. And they have been cared for and integrated into the communities to which they belong.

In Europe, the 19th century witnessed diverging trends. On one hand, mental illness was seen as a legitimate topic for scientific enquiry; psychiatry burgeoned as a medical discipline, and people with mental disorders were considered medical patients. On the other hand, people with mental disorders, like those with many other diseases and undesirable social behaviour, were isolated from society in large custodial institutions, the state mental hospitals, formerly known as lunatic asylums. These trends were later exported to Africa, the Americas and Asia.

During the second half of the 20th century, a shift in the mental health care paradigm took place, largely owing to three independent factors.

- Psychopharmacology made significant progress, with the discovery of new classes of drugs, particularly neuroleptics and antidepressants, as well as the development of new forms of psychosocial interventions.
- The human rights movement became a truly international phenomenon under the sponsorship of the newly created United Nations, and democracy advanced on a global basis, albeit at different speeds in different places (Merkl 1993).
- Social and mental components were firmly incorporated in the definition of health (see Chapter 1) of the newly established WHO in 1948.

These technical and sociopolitical events contributed to a change in emphasis: from care in large custodial institutions, which over time had become repressive and regressive, to more open and flexible care in the community.

The failures of asylums are evidenced by repeated cases of ill-treatment to patients, geographical and professional isolation of the institutions and their staff, weak reporting and accounting procedures, bad management, ineffective administration, poorly targeted financial resources, lack of staff training, and inadequate inspection and quality assurance

Box 3.1 Mental care: then or now?

The following three statements give vivid insights into how attitudes and policies towards the treatment of the mentally ill have changed, or been called into question, over the last 150 years.

"It is now sixteen years since the use of all mechanical restraint [of mental patients] – strait-waistcoat, muff, leg-lock, handcuff, coercion-chair or other – was abolished. Wherever the attempt has been resolutely made it has succeeded. [...] no fallacy can be greater than that of imagining what is called a moderate use of restraint to be consistent with a general plan of treatment in all other respects complete, and un-objectionable, and humane. [Its] abolition must be absolute, or it cannot be efficient."

1856. John Conolly (1794–1866), English physician, director of Asylum for the Insane at Hanwell. In: *The treatment of the insane without mechanical restraints.* London, Smith, Elder & Co.

"When the National Committee was organized, its chief concern was to humanize the care of the insane: to eradicate the abuses, brutalities and neglect from which the mentally sick have traditionally suffered; to focus public attention on the need for reform; to hospitalize "asylums", extend treatment facilities, and raise standards of care; in short, to secure for the mentally ill the same high standards of medical attention as that generally accorded to the physically ill."

1908. Clifford Beers (1976–1943), US founder of the international movement of mental hygiene, himself admitted several times to mental hospitals. In: *A mind that found itself: an autobiography.* New York, Longmans Green.

"We stand against the right given to some men, narrow-minded or not, of concluding their investigations in the realm of the mind by a life imprisonment sentence. And what imprisonment! We know – in fact, we don't – that asylums, far from being a place of *asylum*, are frightening gaols, where inmates are a cheap and convenient workforce, where abuse is the rule, all tolerated by you. The mental hospital, under the cover of science and justice, is comparable to a barracks, a penitentiary, a penal colony."

1935. Antonin Artaud (1896–1948), French poet, actor and playwright, who spent many years in mental hospitals. In: *Open letter to medical directors of madhouses.* Paris, *La Révolution Surréaliste*, No. 3.

procedures. Also, the living conditions in psychiatric hospitals throughout the world are poor, leading to human rights violations and chronicity. In terms of absolute standards, it could be argued that conditions in hospitals in developed countries are better than living standards in many developing countries. However, in terms of relative standards – comparing hospital standards with general community standards in a particular country – it is fair to say that the conditions in all psychiatric hospitals are poor. Some examples have been documented of human rights abuse in psychiatric hospitals (Box 3.2).

In contrast, community care is about the empowerment of people with mental and behavioural disorders. In practice, community care implies the development of a wide range of services within local settings. This process, which has not yet begun in many regions and countries, aims to ensure that some of the protective functions of the asylum are fully provided in the community, and the negative aspects of the institutions are not perpetuated. Care in the community, as an approach, means:

- services which are close to home, including general hospital care for acute admissions, and long-term residential facilities in the community;
- interventions related to disabilities as well as symptoms;
- treatment and care specific to the diagnosis and needs of each individual;
- a wide range of services which address the needs of people with mental and behavioural disorders;
- services which are coordinated between mental health professionals and community agencies;
- ambulatory rather than static services, including those which can offer home treatment;
- partnership with carers and meeting their needs;
- legislation to support the above aspects of care.

The accumulating evidence of the inadequacies of the psychiatric hospital, coupled with the appearance of "institutionalism" – the development of disabilities as a consequence of social isolation and institutional care in remote asylums – led to the de-institutionalization movement. While de-institutionalization is an important part of mental health care reform, it is not synonymous with de-hospitalization. De-institutionalization is a complex process leading to the implementation of a solid network of community alternatives. Closing mental hospitals without community alternatives is as dangerous as creating community alternatives without closing mental hospitals. Both have to occur at the same time, in a well-coordinated incremental way. A sound de-institutionalization process has three essential components:

- prevention of inappropriate mental hospital admissions through the provision of community facilities;
- discharge to the community of long-term institutional patients who have received adequate preparation;
- establishment and maintenance of community support systems for non-institutionalized patients.

De-institutionalization has not been an unqualified success, and community care still faces some operational problems. Among the reasons for the lack of better results are that governments have not allocated resources saved by closing hospitals to community care; professionals have not been adequately prepared to accept their changing roles; and the stigma attached to mental disorders remains strong, resulting in negative public attitudes towards people with mental disorders. In some countries, many people with severe mental disorders are shifted to prisons or become homeless.

Reflecting the paradigm shift from hospital to community, far-reaching policy changes have been introduced in a number of countries. For example, Law 180, enacted in Italy in 1978, closing down all mental hospitals, formalized and accelerated a pre-existing trend in the care of the mentally ill. The major provisions of the Italian law state that no new patients are to be admitted to the large state hospitals nor should there be any readmissions. No new psychiatric hospitals are to be built. Psychiatric wards in general hospitals are not to exceed 15 beds and must be affiliated to community mental health centres. Community-based facilities, staffed by existing mental health personnel, are responsible for a specified catchment area. Law 180 has had an impact far beyond Italian jurisdiction.

Box 3.2 Human rights abuse in psychiatric hospitals

Human Rights Commissions found "appalling and unacceptable" conditions when they visited several psychiatric hospitals in Central America[1] and India[2] during the last five years. Similar conditions exist in many other psychiatric hospitals in other regions, in both industrialized and developing countries. They include filthy living conditions, leaking roofs, overflowing toilets, eroded floors, and broken doors and windows. Most of the patients visited were kept in pyjamas or naked.

Some were penned into small areas of residential wards where they were left to sit, pace, or lie on the concrete floor all day. Children were left lying on mats on the floor, some covered with urine and faeces. Physical restraint was commonly misused: many patients were observed tied to beds.

At least one-third of the individuals were people with epilepsy or mental retardation, for whom psychiatric institutionalization is unnecessary and confers no benefit. They could well return to live in the community if they could be provided with appropriate medication and a full range of community-based services and support systems.

Many hospitals retained the jail-like structure of their construction in colonial times. Patients were referred to as *inmates* and were for most of the day in the care of *warders*, whose supervisors were called *overseers*, while the wards were referred to as *enclosures*. Seclusion rooms were used in the majority of the hospitals.

In over 80% of the hospitals visited, routine blood and urine tests were unavailable. At least one-third of the individuals did not have a psychiatric diagnosis to justify their presence there. In most hospitals, case file recording was extremely inadequate. Trained psychiatric nurses were present in less than 25% of the hospitals, and less than half the hospitals had clinical psychologists and psychiatric social workers.

[1] Levav I, Gonzalez VR (2000). Rights of persons with mental illness in Central America. *Acta Psychiatrica Scandinavica*, 101: 83–86.
[2] National Human Rights Commission (1999). *Quality assurance in mental health*. New Delhi, National Human Rights Commission of India.

The dominant model in the organization of comprehensive psychiatric care in many European countries has been the creation of geographically defined areas, known as *sectors*. This concept was developed in France in the mid-20th century and, from the 1960s on, the organizing principle of sectorization has been widely applied in almost all countries in Western Europe, with sector size ranging from populations of 25 000 to 30 000. The concept of the health district in the primary health care strategy has many points in common with this sector approach.

In many developing countries, care programmes for the individuals with mental and behavioural problems have a low priority. Provision of care is limited to a small number of institutions – usually overcrowded, understaffed and inefficient – and services reflect little understanding of the needs of the ill individuals or the range of approaches available for treatment and care.

In most developing countries, there is no psychiatric care for the majority of the population; the only services available are in mental hospitals. These mental hospitals are usually centralized and not easily accessible, so people often seek help there only as a last resort. The hospitals are large in size, built for economy of function rather than treatment. In a way, the asylum becomes a community of its own with very little contact with society at large. The hospitals operate under legislation which is more penal than therapeutic. In many countries, laws that are more than 40 years old place barriers to admission and discharge. Furthermore, most developing countries do not have adequate training programmes at national level to train psychiatrists, psychiatric nurses, clinical psychologists, psychiatric social workers and occupational therapists. Since there are few specialized professionals, the community turns to the available traditional healers (Saeed et al. 2000).

A result of these factors is a negative institutional image of the people with mental disorders, which adds to the stigma of suffering from a mental or behavioural disorder. Even now, these institutions are not in step with the developments concerning the human rights of people with mental disorders.

Box 3.3 The Declaration of Caracas[1]

The legislators, associations, health authorities, mental health professionals and jurists assembled at the Regional Conference on the Restructuring of Psychiatric Care in Latin America within the Local Health Systems Model, ...

DECLARE

1. That the restructuring of psychiatric care on the basis of Primary Health Care and within the framework of the Local Health Systems Model will permit the promotion of alternative service models that are community-based and integrated into social and health care networks.
2. That the restructuring of psychiatric care in the Region implies a critical review of the dominant and centralizing role played by the mental hospital in mental health service delivery.
3. That the resources, care and treatment that are made available must:
(a) safeguard personal dignity and human and civil rights;
(b) be based on criteria that are rational and technically appropriate; and
(c) strive to ensure that patients remain in their communities.
4. That national legislation must be redrafted if necessary so that:
(a) the human and civil rights of mental patients are safeguarded; and
(b) the organization of [community mental health] services guarantees the enforcement of these rights.

5. That training in mental health and psychiatry should use a service model that is based on the community health center and encourages psychiatric admission in general hospitals, in accordance with the principles that underlie the restructuring movement.
6. That the organizations, associations, and other participants in this Conference hereby undertake to advocate and develop programs at the country level that will promote the restructuring desired, and at the same time that they commit themselves to monitoring and defending the human rights of mental patients in accordance with national legislation and international agreements.

To this end, they call upon the Ministries of Health and Justice, the Parliaments, Social Security and other care-providing institutions, professional organizations, consumer associations, universities and other training facilities, and the media to support the restructuring of psychiatric care, thus assuring its successful development for the benefit of the population in the Region.

[1] Extract from the text adopted on 14 November 1990 by the Regional Conference on the Restructuring of Psychiatric Care in Latin America, convened in Caracas, Venezuela, by the Pan American Health Organization/WHO Regional Office for the Americas. *International Digest of Health Legislation*, 1991, 42(2): 336–338.

Some developing countries, particularly in the Eastern Mediterranean Region, have attempted to formulate national plans for mental health services, develop human resources and integrate mental health with general health care, in accordance with the recommendations of a 1974 WHO expert committee (WHO 1975; Mohit 1999).

In 1991, the United Nations General Assembly adopted the principles for the protection of persons with mental illness and the improvement of mental health care, emphasizing care in the community and the rights of individuals with mental disorders (United Nations 1991). It is now recognized that violation of human rights can be perpetrated both by neglecting the patient through discrimination, carelessness and lack of access to services, as well as by intrusive, restrictive and regressive interventions.

In 1990, WHO/PAHO launched an initiative for the restructuring of psychiatric care in the Region of the Americas, which resulted in the Declaration of Caracas (Box 3.3). The declaration called for the development of psychiatric care closely linked with primary health care and within the framework of the local health system. The above developments helped stimulate the organization of mental health care in developing countries.

Where organized mental health services have been initiated in developing countries in recent times, such services are usually part of primary health care. At one level, this can be seen as necessity in the face of the lack of trained professionals and resources to provide specialized services. At another level, it is a reflection of the opportunity to organize mental health services in a manner that avoids isolation, stigma and discrimination. The approach of utilizing all the available community resources has the attraction of empowering individuals, families and communities to make mental health an agenda of people rather than of professionals. Currently, however, in developing countries mental health care is not receiving the attention that is needed. Even in countries where pilot programmes have shown the value of integrating mental health care into primary health care (for example, in Brazil, China, Colombia, India, the Islamic Republic of Iran, Pakistan, Philippines, Senegal, South Africa and Sudan), that approach has not been expanded to cover the whole country.

Table 3.1 Utilization of professional services for mental problems, Australia, 1997

Consultations for mental problems	No disorder %	Any disorder %	> 3 disorders %
General practitioner only[a]	2.2	13.2	18.1
Mental health professional only[b]	0.5	2.4	3.9
Other health professional only[c]	1.0	4.0	5.7
Combination of health professionals	1.0	15.0	36.4
Any health professional[d]	4.6	34.6	64.0

[a] Refers to persons who had at least one consultation with a general practitioner in the previous 12 months but did not consult any other type of health professional.

[b] Refers to persons who had at least one consultation with a mental health professional (psychiatrist/psychologist/mental health team) in the previous 12 months but did not consult any other type of health professional.

[c] Refers to persons who had at least one consultation with another health professional (nurse/non-psychiatric medical specialist/ pharmacist/ambulance officer/welfare worker or counsellor) in the previous 12 months but did not consult any other type of health professional.

[d] Refers to persons who had at least one consultation with any health professional in the previous 12 months.

Source: Andrews G et al. (2001). Prevalence, comorbidity, disability and service utilisation: overview of the Australian National Mental Health Survey. *British Journal of Psychiatry*, 178: 145–153.

Despite the major differences between mental health care in developing and developed countries, they share a common problem: the poor utilization of available psychiatric services. Even in countries with well-established services, fewer than half of those individuals needing care make use of available services. This is related both to the stigma attached to individuals with mental and behavioural disorders and to the inadequacy of the services provided (see Table 3.1).

This stigma issue was highlighted in the US Surgeon General's Report of 1999 (DHHS 1999). The report noted that: "Despite the efficacy of treatment options and the many possible ways of obtaining a treatment of choice, nearly half of all Americans who have a severe mental illness do not seek treatment. Most often, reluctance to seek care is an unfortunate outcome of very real barriers. Foremost among these is the stigma that many in our society attach to mental illness and to people who have a mental illness."

In summary, the past half century witnessed an evolution of care towards a community care paradigm. This is based on two main pillars: first, respect of the human rights of individuals with mental disorders; and second, the use of updated interventions and techniques. In the best cases, this has been translated into a responsible process of de-institutionalization, supported by health workers, consumers, family members and other progressive community groups.

PRINCIPLES OF CARE

The idea of community-based mental health care is a global approach rather than an organizational solution. Community-based care means that the large majority of patients requiring mental health care should have the possibility of being treated at community level. Mental health care should not only be local and accessible, but should also be able to address the multiple needs of individuals. It should ultimately aim at empowerment and use efficient treatment techniques which enable people with mental disorders to enhance their self-help skills, incorporating the informal family social environment as well as formal support mechanisms. Community-based care (unlike hospital-based care) is able to identify resources and create healthy alliances that would otherwise remain hidden and inactivated.

Use of those hidden resources can prevent situations in which discharged patients are abandoned by health services to the care of their unequipped families (with the well-known negative psychosocial consequences and burden for both). It allows for quite effective management of the social and family burden, traditionally alleviated by institutional care. This kind of service is spreading in some European countries, in some states of the United States, in Australia, Canada and China. Some countries in Latin America, Africa, the Eastern Mediterranean, South-East Asia and the Western Pacific have introduced innovative services (WHO 1997b).

Good care, however and wherever it is applied, flows from basic guiding principles, some of which are particularly relevant to mental health care. These are: diagnosis; early intervention; rational use of treatment techniques; continuity of care; wide range of services; consumer involvement; partnership with families; involvement of the local community; and integration into primary health care.

DIAGNOSIS AND INTERVENTION

A correct objective diagnosis is fundamental for the planning of individual care, and for the choice of an appropriate treatment. Mental and behavioural disorders can be diagnosed with a high level of reliability. Since different treatments are indicated for different diseases, diagnosis is an important starting point of any intervention.

A diagnosis can be made in nosological terms (that is, according to an international classification and nomenclature of diseases and disorders), in terms of the type and level of disability experienced by an individual, or preferably in terms of both.

Early intervention is fundamental in preventing progress towards a full-blown disease, in controlling symptoms and improving outcomes. The earlier the institution of a proper course of treatment, the better the prognosis. The importance of early intervention is highlighted by the following examples.

- In schizophrenia, the duration of untreated psychosis is proving to be important. Delays in treatment are likely to result in poorer outcomes (McGorry 2000; Thara et al. 1994).

- Screening and brief interventions for those at high risk of developing alcohol-related problems are effective in reducing alcohol consumption and related harm (Wilk et al. 1997).

The appropriate treatment of mental disorders implies the rational use of pharmacological, psychological and psychosocial interventions in a clinically meaningful, balanced, and well-integrated way. In view of the extreme importance of the ingredients of care, they are dealt with at length later in this chapter.

CONTINUITY OF CARE

Some mental and behavioural disorders follow a chronic course, albeit with periods of remission and relapses which may mimic acute disorders. Nevertheless, as far as management is concerned, they are similar to chronic physical illnesses. The chronic care paradigm is therefore more appropriate to them than the one generally used for acute, communicable disease. This has particular implications concerning access to services, staff availability, and costs to patients and families.

The needs of patients and their families are complex and changing, and continuity of care is important. This calls for changes in the way care is currently organized. Some of the measures to ensure continuity of care include:

- special clinics for groups of patients with the same diagnosis or problems;
- imparting caring skills to carers;
- the same treatment team providing care to patients and their families;
- group education of patients and their families;
- decentralization of services;
- integration of care into primary health care.

WIDE RANGE OF SERVICES

The needs of people with mental illness and their families are multiple and varied and differ at different stages of illness. A wide variety of services are required to provide comprehensive care for some of the people with mental illness. Those recovering from illness need help to regain their skills and resume their roles in society. Those who recover only partially need assistance to compete in an open society. Some patients, especially in developing countries, who have had sub-optimum care can nevertheless benefit from rehabilitation programmes. These services may dispense medication or provide special rehabilitation programmes, housing, judicial assistance or other forms of socioeconomic support. Specialized personnel, such as nurses, clinical psychologists, social workers, occupational therapists and volunteers, have demonstrated their value as intrinsic elements of flexible care teams. Multidisciplinary teams are especially relevant in the management of mental disorders, owing to the complex needs of patients and their families at different points during the illness.

PARTNERSHIPS WITH PATIENTS AND FAMILIES

The emergence of consumer movements in a number of countries has changed the way stakeholders' views are seen. These consumer groups are generally composed of people with mental disorders and their families. In many countries, consumer movements have grown in parallel with traditional mental health advocacy, such as that of family movements. The consumer movement is based on a belief in individual patient choice regarding treatment and other decisions (see Box 3.4).

Probably the best example of a consumer movement is Alcoholics Anonymous, which has become popular around the world and has achieved recovery rates comparable to those obtained by formal psychiatric care. The availability of computer-assisted treatment and online support from ex-patients have opened up new ways of getting care. Patients with mental disorders can be very successful in helping themselves, and peer support has been important in a number of conditions for recovery and reintegration into society.

The consumer movement has substantially influenced mental health policy in a number of countries. In particular, it has increased the employment of people with disorders in the traditional mental health system as well as in other social service agencies. For example, in the Ministry of Health of the Province of British Columbia, Canada, the position of Director of Alternative Care was recently assigned to a person with a mental disorder, who is thus in a strong position to influence mental health policy and services.

Consumer advocacy has targeted involuntary treatment, self-managed care, the role of consumers in research, service delivery and access to care. Programmes run by the consumers include drop-in centres, case management programmes, outreach programmes and crisis services.

The positive role of families in mental health care programmes has been recognized relatively recently. The earlier view of the family as a causative factor is not valid. The role of

---

Box 3.4 The role of consumers in mental health care

People using mental health services have traditionally been viewed within the system as passive recipients, unable to articulate their own needs and wishes, and subjected to forms of care or treatment decided on and designed by others. However, over the past 30 years, as consumers they have begun to articulate their own visions of what services they need and want.

Among the strongest themes that have emerged are: the right to self-determination; the need for information about medication and other treatment; the need for services to facilitate active community participation; an end to stigma and discrimination; improved laws and public attitudes, removing barriers to community integration; the need for alternative, consumer-run services; better legal rights and legal protection of existing rights; and an end to keeping people in large institutions, often for life.

Opinions vary among consumers and their organizations about how best to achieve their goals. Some groups want active cooperation and collaboration with mental health professionals, while others want complete separation from them. There are also major differences as to how closely to cooperate, if at all, with organizations representing family members of patients.

It is clear that consumer organizations around the world want their voices to be heard and considered as decisions are made about their lives. People diagnosed with mental illness are entitled to be heard in the discussions on mental health policy and practice that involve professionals, family members, legislators, and opinion leaders. Behind the labels and diagnoses are real people, who, no matter what others may think, have ideas, thoughts, opinions, and ambitions. Those who have been diagnosed with mental illness are no different from other people, and want the same basic things out of life: adequate incomes; decent places to live; educational opportunities; job training leading to real, meaningful jobs; participation in the lives of their communities; friends and social relationships; and loving personal relationships.

Contributed by Judi Chamberlin (MadPride@aol.com), National Empowerment Center, Lawrence, MA, USA (http://www.power2u.org).

families now extends beyond day-to-day care to organized advocacy on behalf of the mentally ill. Such advocacy has been pivotal in changing mental health legislation in some countries, and improving services and developing support networks in others.

Substantial evidence demonstrates the benefits of involving families in the treatment and management of schizophrenia, mental retardation, depression, alcohol dependence and childhood behaviour disorders. The role of the family in the treatment of other conditions remains to be more firmly established by further controlled trials. There are indications that the outcome for patients living with their families is better than for those in institutions. However, many international studies have established a strong relationship between high "expressed emotion" attitudes in relatives and an increased relapse rate for patients living with them. By changing the emotional atmosphere in the home, the relapse rate can be reduced (Leff & Gamble 1995; Dixon et al. 2000).

Work with families to reduce relapses was always seen as an adjunct to maintenance medication and not as a substitute for it. Indeed, family therapy, when added to antipsychotic medication, has been shown to be more efficacious than medication alone in preventing relapse in schizophrenia. A meta-analysis by the Cochrane Collaboration (Pharaoh et al. 2000) showed relapse rates being reduced on average by half over both one year and two years. The question remains, however, whether ordinary clinical teams can reproduce the striking results of the pioneering research groups which have conducted their work mostly in developed countries. In developing countries, the family is usually involved in the treatment of the individual psychiatric patient, both by traditional healers and biomedical services.

Family networking locally and nationally has brought carers into partnership with professionals (Box 3.5). In addition to providing mutual support, many networks have become

---

Box 3.5 Partnerships with families

Mental health care workers, the families of individuals with mental illness, and family support organizations have a great deal to learn from each other. Through regular contact, health staff are able to learn from families what knowledge, attitudes and skills are needed to enable them to work together effectively. They also learn about problems such as limited resources, huge caseloads, and inadequate training, which prevent clinicians and clinical services from delivering effective services. In such cases, advocacy by a family organization may be seen to have a greater value than the "vested interest" of the professional worker.

When mental illness occurs, professional workers benefit from developing an early partnership with the family. Through such a joint engagement, information on a wide range of issues related to the illness can be discussed, family reactions explored, and a treatment plan formulated. Families, in turn, benefit from learning a process of problem-solving in order to manage the illness most effectively.

Two family support associations which have been very successful in meeting the needs of their respective constituencies, and in connecting with professionals, are briefly described below.

Alzheimer's Disease International (ADI) is an umbrella organization of 57 national Alzheimer's associations worldwide. Its purpose is to support the development and increased effectiveness of new and existing national Alzheimer's associations through such activities as World Alzheimer's Day, an annual conference, and the Alzheimer's University (a series of workshops addressing basic organizational issues). It also provides information through its web site (http://www.alz.co.uk), fact sheets, booklets and newsletters.

National Alzheimer's associations are dedicated to supporting people with dementia and their families. They provide information as well as practical and emotional help such as help lines, support groups and respite care. They also provide training for carers and professionals and advocacy to governments.

The *World Fellowship for Schizophrenia and Allied Disorders (WSF)* stresses that the mutual sharing of knowledge – the professional knowledge of mental health workers, and the knowledge gained by families and consumers through their lived experiences – is vital for the development of trust. Without trust, an effective therapeutic alliance is often not possible and clinicians, families and consumers can find themselves at odds with each other.

This continuing partnership aims at developing assertiveness in family carers so that they are able to resolve the many complicated challenges with which they are confronted, rather than having to rely always on professional support. This process is known as "moving from passive minding to active caring". It is reinforced by referral to family support organizations, which professionals should strongly recommend to family members as an important part of the long-term treatment and care plan. More information about this association can be obtained by email from info@worldschizophrenia.org.

advocates, educating the general public, increasing support by policy-makers, and fighting stigma and discrimination.

INVOLVEMENT OF THE LOCAL COMMUNITY

Societal beliefs, attitudes and responses decide many aspects of mental health care. People with mental illness are members of society, and the social environment is an important determinant of outcome. If the social environment is favourable, it contributes to recovery and reintegration; if negative, it can reinforce stigma and discrimination. Efforts to enhance the involvement of local communities include disseminating accurate information about mental disorders and using community resources for specific initiatives, such as volunteers in suicide prevention and collaboration with traditional healers. Shifting care from institutions to the community itself can alter community attitudes and responses, and help people with mental illness lead a better life.

Studies in many African and Asian countries show that about 40% of the clients of traditional healers suffer from mental illnesses (Saeed et al. 2000). This is not much different from the picture revealed by many studies conducted in general health care settings. Working with traditional healers is thus an important mental health initiative. Professionals give healers accurate information about mental and behavioural disorders, encourage them to function as referral agents, and discourage practices such as starvation and punishment. For their part, professionals come to understand the healers' skills in dealing with psychosocial disorders.

Nongovernmental organizations have been important in mental health movements throughout history. It was a consumer, Clifford Beers, who in 1906 created the first successful nongovernmental organization dealing with mental health, the forerunner of the World Federation for Mental Health. The contributions of these organizations are unquestionable.

There are a number of avenues for bringing about changes in the community. The most important of these is the use of mass media for educational campaigns directed to the general public. "Defeat depression", "Changing minds – every family in the land", and the World Health Day 2001 slogan "Stop exclusion – Dare to care" are examples. Massive public awareness programmes in countries such as Australia, Canada, India, the Islamic Republic of Iran, Malaysia, the United Kingdom and the United States have changed the attitudes of the population to mental disorders. The World Psychiatric Association (WPA) has launched a programme in a number of countries to fight stigma and discrimination against persons suffering from schizophrenia (see Box 4.9). The programme uses the mass media, schools and family members as change agents.

Although in many developing countries the community does not necessarily discriminate against people with mental illness, beliefs in witchcraft, supernatural forces, fate, ill will of gods and so forth can interfere with seeking help and adherence to treatment. One of the best examples of how communities can become carers of the mentally ill is to be found in the Belgian town of Geel, the site of what is undoubtedly the oldest community mental health programme in the western world. Since the 13th century, and originating perhaps as early as the 8th century, severely mentally ill people have been welcomed by the Church of St Dympha or by foster families in the town, with whom they have lived, often for several decades. Today, such families in Geel care for some 550 patients, about half of whom have jobs in sheltered workshops.

INTEGRATION INTO PRIMARY HEALTH CARE

Another important principle which plays a crucial role in the organization of mental health care is integration into primary health care. The fundamental role of primary care for the entire health system in any country was clearly stated in the Alma-Ata Declaration. This basic level of care acts as a filter between the general population and specialized health care.

Mental disorders are common and most patients are only seen in primary care; but their disorders are often not detected (Üstün & Sartorius 1995). Also, psychological morbidity is a common feature of physical disease, and emotional distress is often seen (but not always recognized) by the primary health care professionals. Training primary care and general health care staff in the detection and treatment of common mental and behavioural disorders is an important public health measure. This training can be facilitated by liaison with local community-based mental health staff, who are almost always keen to share their expertise.

The quality and quantity of specialist mental health services needed depend upon the services that are provided at the primary health care level. In other words, the provision of services needs to be balanced between community care and hospital care.

Patients discharged from psychiatric wards (in either general or specialized hospitals) can be effectively followed up by primary health care doctors. It is clear that primary health care plays a major role in countries where community-based mental health services do not exist. In many developing countries, well-trained primary health care workers provide adequate treatment for the mentally ill. It is interesting to note that the poverty of a country does not necessarily mean that mentally ill people will receive poor care. Experiences in some African, Asian and Latin American countries show that adequate training of primary health care workers in the early recognition and management of mental disorders can reduce institutionalization and improve clients' mental health.

INGREDIENTS OF CARE

The management of mental and behavioural disorders – perhaps more particularly than that of other medical conditions – calls for the balanced combination of three fundamental ingredients: medication (or pharmacotherapy); psychotherapy; and psychosocial rehabilitation.

The rational management of mental and behavioural disorders needs a skilful titration of each of these ingredients. The amounts needed will vary as a function not only of the main diagnosis, but also of any physical and mental comorbidity, the age of the patient and the current stage of the disease. In other words, treatment should be tailored to individual needs; but these change as the disease evolves and as the patient's living conditions change (see Figure 3.1).

A balanced combination of interventions implies adherence to the following guiding principles:

- each intervention has a specific indication according to the diagnosis, that is, should be used in specific clinical conditions;
- each intervention should be used in a given amount, that is, the level of the intervention should be proportional to the severity of the condition;
- each intervention should have a determined duration, that is, it should last for the time required by the nature and severity of the condition, and should be discontinued as soon as possible;

Figure 3.1 Needs of people with mental disorders

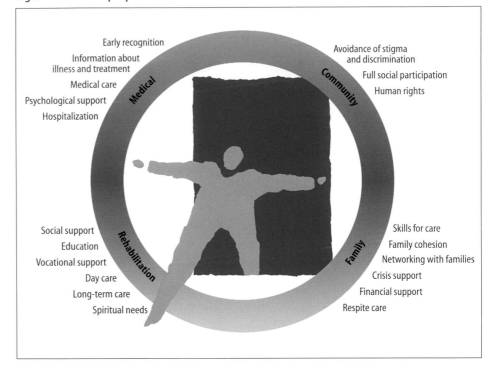

- each intervention should be periodically monitored for adherence and expected results, as well as for adverse effects, and the recipient of the intervention should always be an active partner in this monitoring.

Effective management of mental and behavioural disorders includes paying careful attention to treatment adherence. Mental disorders are, at times, chronic conditions and thus often require treatment regimes that span the period of adulthood. Compliance with longer-term treatment is harder to achieve than compliance with short-term treatment. A further complication is that the existence of a mental or behavioural disorder has been shown to be associated with poor compliance to treatment regimes.

There has been considerable research on factors that improve compliance with treatment. These include:
- a trusting physician–patient relationship;
- time and energy spent on educating the patient regarding the goals of therapy and the consequences of good or poor adherence;
- a negotiated treatment plan;
- recruitment of family and friends to support the therapeutic plan and its implementation;
- simplification of the treatment regimen;
- reduction of the adverse consequences of the treatment regimen.

Over the years, a consensus has arisen among clinicians about the effectiveness of some interventions for the management of mental disorders; these interventions are described below. The information available on cost-effectiveness is disappointingly limited. The main limitations are: first, the chronic nature of some mental disorders, which calls for very long term follow-up for the information to be meaningful; second, the different clinical and methodological criteria employed in the few studies conducted on the cost-effectiveness of these interventions; and third, the fact that most studies available have compared advanced approaches to the management of a given disorder, few of which are feasible in developing countries. The interventions described below were therefore selected on the basis of evidence of their effectiveness – despite the fact that many people do not have access to them – rather than on the criterion of cost-effectiveness. Up-to-date information on the cost-effectiveness of interventions is, however, included where available.

PHARMACOTHERAPY

The discovery and improvement of medicines useful for the management of mental disorders, which occurred in the second half of the 20th century, have been widely acknowledged as a revolution in the history of psychiatry.

There are basically three classes of psychotropic drugs that target specific symptoms of mental disorders: antipsychotics for psychotic symptoms; antidepressants for depression; anti-epileptics for epilepsy, and anxiolytics or tranquillizers for anxiety. Different types are used for drug-related and alcohol-related problems. It is important to remember that these medicinal drugs address the symptoms of diseases, not the diseases themselves or their causes. The drugs are therefore not meant to cure the diseases, but rather to reduce or control their symptoms or to prevent relapse.

In view of the effectiveness of most of these drugs, which was evident before the widespread use of controlled clinical trials, most recent economic studies have focused not on the cost-effectiveness of active pharmacotherapy over placebo or no care at all, but on the relative cost-effectiveness of newer classes of medication over their older counterparts. This is particularly true for the newer antidepressants and antipsychotics with regard, respectively, to tricyclic antidepressants and conventional neuroleptics.

A synthesis of the available evidence indicates that, while these newer psychotropic drugs have fewer adverse side-effects, they are not significantly more efficacious, and they are usually more expensive. The considerably higher acquisition costs of the newer drugs are, however, offset by a reduced need for other care and treatment. Drugs in the newer class of antidepressants, for example, may represent a more attractive and affordable prescribing option in lower-income countries as their patents expire or where they are already available at a cost similar to that of older drugs.

The WHO Essential Drugs List currently includes those drugs necessary, at a minimum level, for the satisfactory management of mental and neurological disorders of public health importance. Nevertheless, patients in poor or developing countries should not be deprived, on economic grounds only, of the benefits of advances in psychopharmacology. It is necessary to work towards making available to all the best drugs for the treatment of the condition. This requires a flexible approach to the essential drugs list.

PSYCHOTHERAPY

Psychotherapy refers to planned and structured interventions aimed at influencing behaviour, mood and emotional patterns of reaction to different stimuli through verbal and non-verbal psychological means. Psychotherapy does not comprise the use of any biochemical or biological means.

Several techniques and approaches – derived from different theoretical foundations – have shown their effectiveness in relation to various mental and behavioural disorders. Among these are behaviour therapy, cognitive therapy, interpersonal therapy, relaxation techniques and supportive therapy (counselling) techniques (WHO 1993b).

Behaviour therapy consists of the application of scientifically based psychological principles to the solution of clinical problems (Cottraux 1993). It is based on the principles of learning.

Cognitive behavioural interventions are aimed at changing thought patterns and behaviour through the practice of new ways of thinking and acting, whereas interpersonal therapy stems from a different conceptual model that centres around four common problem areas: role disputes, role transitions, unresolved grief, and social deficits.

Relaxation aims at a reduction of the arousal state – hence, of anxiety – to acceptable levels through a variety of techniques of muscular relaxation, derived from such methods as yoga, transcendental meditation, autogenic training and biofeedback. It can be an important adjunct to other forms of treatment, is easily accepted by patients, and can be self-learned (WHO 1988).

Supportive therapy, probably the simplest form of psychotherapy, is based on the doctor–patient relationship. Other important components of this technique include reassurance, clarification, abreaction, advice, suggestion and teaching. Some see this modality of treatment as the very foundation of good clinical care and suggest its inclusion as an intrinsic component of training programmes for all those involved with clinical duties.

Various types of psychotherapies – particularly cognitive behavioural interventions and interpersonal therapy – are effective in the treatment of phobias, drug and alcohol dependence, and psychotic symptoms such as delusions and hallucinations. They also help depressed patients to learn how to improve coping strategies and lessen symptom distress.

Encouraging evidence has recently emerged in relation to the cost-effectiveness of psychotherapeutic approaches to the management of psychosis and a range of mood and stress-related disorders, in combination with or as an alternative to pharmacotherapy. A consistent research finding is that psychological interventions lead to improved satisfaction and treatment concordance, which can contribute significantly to reduced rates of relapse, less hospitalization and decreased unemployment. The additional costs of psychological treatments are countered by decreased levels of other health service support or contact (Schulberg et al. 1998; Rosenbaum & Hylan 1999).

PSYCHOSOCIAL REHABILITATION

Psychosocial rehabilitation is a process that offers the opportunity for individuals who are impaired, disabled or handicapped by a mental disorder to reach their optimal level of independent functioning in the community. It involves both improving individual competencies and introducing environmental changes (WHO 1995). Psychosocial rehabilitation is a comprehensive process not just a technique.

The strategies of psychosocial rehabilitation vary according to consumers' needs, the setting where the rehabilitation is provided (hospital or community), and the cultural and socioeconomic conditions of the country in which it is undertaken. Housing, vocational rehabilitation, employment, and social support networks are all aspects of psychosocial rehabilitation. The main objectives are consumers' empowerment, the reduction of discrimination and stigma, the improvement of individual social competence, and the creation of a long-term system of social support. Psychosocial rehabilitation is one of the components of comprehensive community-based mental health care. For example, in

Shanghai, China, psychosocial rehabilitation models have been developed using primary care, family support, back-up psychiatric support, community supervisors and factory rehabilitation intervention.

Psychosocial rehabilitation enables many individuals to acquire or regain the practical skills needed to live and socialize in the community, and teaches them how to cope with their disabilities. It includes assistance in developing the social skills, interests and leisure activities that provide a sense of participation and personal worth. It also teaches living skills, such as diet, personal hygiene, cooking, shopping, budgeting, housekeeping and using various means of transport.

VOCATIONAL REHABILITATION AND EMPLOYMENT

Labour cooperatives have been organized by psychiatric patients, health and social workers and, sometimes, other disabled non-psychiatric patients in such countries as Argentina, Brazil, China, Côte d'Ivoire, Germany, Italy, the Netherlands and Spain. These vocational opportunities do not seek to create an artificially protected environment, but provide psychiatric patients with professional training in order to allow them to be engaged in economically efficient activities. Some of these examples are described in Box 3.6.

Activating the hidden resources of the community creates a new model with profound public health implications. This model, known as the "social enterprise", has reached a sophisticated level of development in some Mediterranean countries (de Leonardis et al. 1994). Cooperation between the public and private sectors in a social enterprise is promising from a public health point of view. It also offsets a lack of resources and creates an alternative solution to conventional psychosocial rehabilitation. People with disorders can be more actively involved in a healthy process of cooperative work and consequently in the generation of resources.

Box 3.6 Work opportunities in the community

Many thousands of good examples can be found around the world of people with mental disorders not merely integrated into their own communities but actually playing a productive and economically important role. In Europe alone, some 10 000 such individuals are working in businesses and enterprises that were established to provide them with employment. Several examples of opportunities in the community are given here.[1]

Starting with a handful of people with mental illness, some of whom had been chained up for years, a chicken farm was established in Bouaké, Côte d'Ivoire. Initially regarded with suspicion by the local community, it has grown to become an important enterprise on which the local community now depends. The early resistance to it was gradually transformed into wholehearted support, particularly when the farm was short of workers and started to hire people from the local community, becoming the most important employer in the area.

In Spain, a major nongovernmental organization has created 12 service centres employing more than 800 people with mental disorders. One such centre, in Cabra, Andalusia, is a commercially run furniture factory employing 212 persons, the vast majority of whom have had long stays in psychiatric hospitals. The factory is very modern and has several different assembly lines, where the needs and capabilities of individual workers are taken into account. Only a few years ago these workers were locked up in hospitals, like many others with mental disorders continue to be elsewhere. Today, their products are being sold throughout Europe and the United States.

An employment cooperative for people with mental disorders that was founded in Italy in 1981 with just nine people now has more than 500 members who have returned to a productive life and are integrated into mainstream society. One of hundreds like it in Italy, the cooperative provides cleaning services; social services for elderly people and handicapped adults and children; work training programmes; upkeep of parks and gardens; and general maintenance activities.

In Beijing, China, one of the country's largest cotton factories has several hundred apartments for its employees as well as a 140-bed hospital and two schools. Recently, a young employee was diagnosed with schizophrenia and hospitalized for one year. Upon discharge, she returned to her apartment and her former job with full pay. However, after a month, she found she could not keep up with the pace of her co-workers and was transferred to an office job. This solution is the result of her employer fulfilling a legal obligation to take the woman back following her illness.

[1] Harnois G, Gabriel P (2000). *Mental health and work: impact, issues and good practices*. Geneva, World Health Organization and International Labour Office (WHO/MSD/MPS/00.2).

Housing

Housing, in addition to being a basic right, is in many places the crucial limiting factor in the process of de-institutionalization and psychiatric reform. Everybody needs decent housing. The need for psychiatric beds for people with mental disorders is beyond question.

Specific mental disorders make the use of beds unavoidable in two circumstances: first, in the acute phase; and second, during convalescence or the chronic irreversible stage that some patients present. Experience from many countries in the Americas, Asia and Europe has demonstrated that, in the first case, a bed located in a general hospital is the most adequate resource. In the second case, community residential facilities have successfully replaced the old asylums. There will always be a need, in some situations, for short hospitalizations in general hospitals. A smaller group of patients will need other residential settings. These are non-contradictory components of total care, and are fully in accordance with the strategy of primary health care.

In addition to the examples mentioned above, interesting experiments in the field of psychosocial rehabilitation are taking place in Botswana, Brazil, China, Greece, India, the Islamic Republic of Iran, Malaysia, Mali, Mexico, Pakistan, Senegal, South Africa, Spain, Sri Lanka and Tunisia (Mohit 1999; Mubbashar 1999; WHO 1997b). In these countries, the approach is mostly oriented towards vocational activities and community social support. It is a matter of fact that psychosocial rehabilitation very often does not deal with housing simply because no housing is available. Thus patients with severe disorders who need a shelter have no alternative to institutionalization. Current housing strategies are too expensive for many developing countries, so innovative solutions must be found.

Examples of effectiveness

Interventions for the management of mental and behavioural disorders can be classified in three major categories: prevention, treatment and rehabilitation. These correspond approximately to the concepts of primary, secondary and tertiary prevention (Leavell & Clark 1965).

- *Prevention* (primary prevention or specific protection) comprises measures applicable to a particular disease or group of diseases in order to intercept their causes before they involve the individual; in other words, to avoid the occurrence of the condition.
- *Treatment* (secondary prevention) refers to measures to arrest a disease process already initiated, in order to prevent further complications and sequelae, limit disability, and prevent death.
- *Rehabilitation* (tertiary prevention) involves measures aimed at disabled individuals, restoring their previous situation or maximizing the use of their remaining capacities. It comprises both interventions at the level of the individual and modifications of the environment.

The following examples present a range of effective interventions of public health importance. For some of these disorders, the most effective intervention is preventive action, whereas for others treatment or rehabilitation is the most efficient approach.

Depression

Currently, there is no evidence that interventions proposed for primary prevention of depression are effective except in a few isolated studies. There is, however, evidence of the effectiveness of certain interventions, such as setting up supportive network systems for vulnerable groups, specific event-centred interventions, and interventions that target vulnerable families and individuals, as well as adequate screening and treatment facilities for mental disorders as part of primary care for physical disability (Paykel 1994). A number of screening, education and treatment programmes for mothers have been shown to reduce depression in mothers and prevent adverse health outcomes for their children. These programmes can be delivered in the primary health care setting by, for example, health visitors or community health workers. However, they have not been widely disseminated in primary care, even in industrialized countries (Cooper & Murray 1998).

The goals of therapy are reduction of symptoms, prevention of relapses and, ultimately, complete remission. The first-line treatment for most people with depression today consists of antidepressant medication, psychotherapy, or a combination of the two.

Antidepressant drugs are effective across the full range of severity of major depressive episodes. With mild depressive episodes, the overall response rate is about 70%. With severe depressive episodes, the overall response rate is lower, and medication is more effective than the placebo. Studies have shown that the older antidepressants (tricyclics), known as ADTs, are as effective as the newer drugs and less expensive: the cost of ADTs is about US$ 2–3 per month in many developing countries. New antidepressant drugs are effective treatments for severe depressive episodes, with fewer unwanted effects and greater patient acceptance, but their availability remains limited in many developing countries. These drugs may have advantages in older age groups.

The acute phase requires 6 to 8 weeks of medication during which patients are seen every one or two weeks – and more frequently in the initial stages – for the monitoring of symptoms and side-effects, dosage adjustments, and support.

The successful acute phase of antidepressant drug treatment or psychotherapy should almost always be followed by at least 6 months of continued treatment. Patients are seen once or twice a month. The primary goal of this continuation phase is to prevent relapse; it can cut the relapse rate from 40–60% to 10–20%. The ultimate goal is complete remission and subsequent recovery. There is some evidence, albeit weak, that relapse is less common following successful treatment with cognitive behavioural therapy than with antidepressants (see Table 3.2).

The phase known as maintenance pharmacotherapy is intended to prevent future recurrences of mood disorders, and is typically recommended for individuals with a history of three or more depressive episodes, chronic depression, or persistent depressive symptoms. This phase may extend for years, and typically requires monthly or quarterly visits.

Some people prefer psychotherapy or counselling to medication for the treatment of depression. Twenty years of research have found several forms of time-limited psychotherapy as effective as drugs in mild-to-moderate depressions. These depression-specific therapies include cognitive behavioural therapy and interpersonal psychotherapy, and emphasize active collaboration and patient education. A number of studies from Afghanistan, India, Pakistan, the Netherlands, Sri Lanka, Sweden, the United Kingdom and the United States show the feasibility of training general practitioners to provide this care and its cost-effectiveness (Sriram et al. 1990; Mubbashar 1999; Mohit et al. 1999; Tansella & Thornicroft 1999; Ward et al. 2000; Bower et al. 2000).

Table 3.2 Effectiveness of interventions for depression

Intervention	% remission after 3–8 months
Placebo	27
Tricyclics	48-52
Psychotherapy (cognitive or interpersonal)	48-60

Sources:

Mynors-Wallis L et al. (1996). Problem-solving treatment: evidence for effectiveness and feasibility in primary care. *International Journal of Psychiatric Medicine*, 26: 249–262.

Schulberg HC et al. (1996). Treating major depression in primary care practice: eight-month clinical outcomes. *Archives of General Psychiatry*, 58: 112–118.

Even in industrialized countries, only a minority of people suffering from depression seek or receive treatment. Part of the explanation lies in the symptoms themselves. Feelings of worthlessness, excessive guilt and lack of motivation deter individuals from seeking help. In addition, such individuals are unlikely to appreciate the potential benefits of treatment. Financial difficulties and the fear of stigmatization are also deterrents. Beyond the individuals themselves, health care providers may fail to recognize symptoms and to follow best practice recommendations, because they may not have the time or the resources to provide evidence-based treatment in primary care settings.

ALCOHOL DEPENDENCE

The prevention of alcohol dependence needs to be seen within the context of the broader goal of preventing and reducing alcohol-related problems at the population level (alcohol-related accidents, injuries, suicide, violence, etc). This comprehensive approach is discussed in Chapter 4. Cultural and religious values are associated with low levels of alcohol use.

The goals of therapy are the reduction of alcohol-related morbidity and mortality, and the reduction of other social and economic problems related to chronic and excessive alcohol consumption.

Early recognition of problem drinking, early intervention for problem drinking, psychological interventions, treatment of the harmful effects of alcohol (including withdrawal and other medical consequences), teaching new coping skills in situations associated with a risk of drinking and relapse, family education and rehabilitation are the main strategies proven to be effective for the treatment of alcohol-related problems and dependence.

Epidemiological research has shown that most problems arise among those who are not significantly dependent, such as individuals who get intoxicated and drive or engage in risky behaviours , or those who are drinking at risk levels but continue to have jobs or go to school, and maintain relationships and relatively stable lifestyles. Among patients attending primary health care clinics and drinking at hazardous levels, only 25% are alcohol dependent.

Brief interventions comprise a variety of activities directed at persons who engage in hazardous drinking, but who are not alcohol dependent. These interventions are of low intensity and short duration, typically consisting of 5–60 minutes of counselling and education, usually with no more than three to five sessions. They are intended to prevent the onset of alcohol-related problems. The content of such brief interventions varies, but most are instructional and motivational, designed to address the specific behaviour of drinking, with feedback from screening, education, skill-building, encouragement and practical advice, rather than intensive psychological analysis or extended treatment techniques (Gomel et al. 1995).

For early drinking problems, the effectiveness of brief interventions by primary care professionals has been demonstrated in numerous studies (WHO 1996; Wilk et al. 1997). Such interventions have reduced up to 30% of alcohol consumption and heavy drinking, over periods of 6–12 months or longer. Studies have also demonstrated that these interventions are cost-effective (Gomel et al. 1995).

For patients with more severe alcohol dependence, both outpatient and inpatient treatment options are available and have been shown to be effective, although outpatient treatment is substantially less costly. Several psychological treatments have proved to be equally effective: these include cognitive behavioural treatment, motivational interviewing, and "Twelve Steps" approaches associated with professional treatment. Community reinforce-

ment approaches, such as that of Alcoholics Anonymous, during and following professional treatment are consistently associated with better outcomes than treatment alone.
Therapy for spouses and family members, or simply their involvement, have benefits for
both initiation and maintenance of alcohol treatment.

Detoxification (treatment of alcohol withdrawal) within the community is preferable,
except for those with severe dependence, a history of delirium tremens or withdrawal seizures, an unsupportive home environment, or previous failed attempts at detoxification
(Edwards et al. 1997). Inpatient care remains a choice for patients with serious comorbid
medical or psychiatric conditions. Psychosocial ancillary and family interventions are also
important elements in the recovery process, particularly when other problems occur along
with alcohol dependence.

No evidence indicates that coercive treatment is effective. It is unlikely that such treatment (whether it follows civil commitment, a decision of the criminal justice system, or any
other intervention) will be beneficial (Heather 1995).

Medication cannot replace psychological treatment for people with alcohol dependence, but a few drugs have shown to be effective as a complementary treatment to reduce
relapse rates (NIDA 2000).

DRUG DEPENDENCE

The prevention of drug dependence needs to be seen within the context of the broader
goal of preventing and reducing drug-related problems at the population level. This broad
approach is discussed in Chapter 4.

The goals of therapy are to reduce morbidity and mortality caused by or associated with
the use of psychoactive substances, until patients can achieve a drug-free life. Strategies
include early diagnosis, identification and management of risk of infectious diseases as
well as other medical and social problems, stabilization and maintenance with pharmacotherapy (for opioid dependence), counselling, access to services, and opportunities to achieve
social integration.

Persons with drug dependence often have complex needs. They are at risk of HIV and
other bloodborne pathogens, comorbid physical and mental disorders, problems with
multiple psychoactive substances, involvement in criminal activities, and problems with
personal relationships, employment and housing. Their needs demand links between health
professionals, social services, the voluntary sector and the criminal justice system.

Shared care and integration of services are examples of good practice in caring for substance dependents. General practitioners can identify and treat acute episodes of intoxication and withdrawal, and provide brief counselling as well as immunization, HIV testing,
cervical screening, family planning advice and referral.

Counselling and other behavioural therapies are critical components of effective treatment of dependence, as they can deal with motivation, coping skills, problem-solving abilities, and difficulties in interpersonal relationship. Particularly for opioid dependents,
substitution pharmacotherapies are effective adjuncts to counselling. As the majority of
drug dependents smoke, tobacco cessation counselling and nicotine replacement therapies must be provided. Self-help groups can also complement and extend the effectiveness
of treatment by health professionals.

Medical detoxification is only the first stage of treatment for dependence, and by itself
does not change long-term drug use. Long-term care needs to be provided, and comorbid
psychiatric disorders treated as well, in order to decrease rates of relapse. Most patients
require a minimum of three months of treatment to obtain significant improvement.

Injection of illicit drugs poses a particular threat to public health. Sharing of injection equipment is associated with transmission of bloodborne pathogens (especially HIV and hepatitis B and C) and has been responsible for the spread of HIV in many countries, wherever injecting drug use is widespread.

People who inject drugs and who do not enter treatment are up to six times more likely to become infected with HIV than those who enter and remain in treatment. Treatment services should therefore provide assessment for HIV/AIDS, hepatitis B and C, tuberculosis and other infectious diseases and, whenever possible, treatment for these conditions and counselling to help patients stop unsafe injecting practices.

Drug dependence treatment is cost-effective in reducing drug use (40–60%), and the associated health and social consequences, such as HIV infection and criminal activity. The effectiveness of drug dependence treatment is comparable to the success rates for the treatment of other chronic diseases such as diabetes, hypertension and asthma (NIDA 2000). Treatment has been shown to be less expensive than other alternatives, such as not treating dependents or simply incarcerating them. For example, in the United States, the average cost for one full year of methadone maintenance treatment is approximately US$ 4700 per patient, whereas one full year of imprisonment costs approximately US$18 400 per person.

SCHIZOPHRENIA

Currently, primary prevention of schizophrenia is not possible. Recently, however, research efforts have focused on developing ways of detecting people at risk of schizophrenia in the very early stages or even before the onset of the illness. Early detection would increase the chances of early interventions, possibly diminishing the risk for a chronic course or serious residua. The effectiveness of programmes for early detection or early intervention must be evaluated through long-term follow-up (McGorry 2000).

The treatment of schizophrenia has three main components. First, there are medications to relieve symptoms and prevent relapse. Second, education and psychosocial interventions help patients and families cope with the illness and its complications, and help prevent relapse. Third, rehabilitation helps patients reintegrate into the community and regain educational or occupational functioning. The real challenge in the care of people suffering from schizophrenia is the need to organize services that lead seamlessly from early identification to regular treatment and rehabilitation.

The goals of care are to identify the illness as early as possible, treat the symptoms, provide skills to patients and their families, maintain the improvement over a period of time, prevent relapses and reintegrate the ill persons in the community so that they can lead a normal life. There is conclusive evidence to show that treatment decreases the duration of illness and chronicity, along with the control of relapses.

Two groups of drugs are currently used to treat schizophrenia: standard antipsychotics (previously referred to as neuroleptics), and novel antipsychotics (also referred to as second generation or "atypical" antipsychotics). The first standard antipsychotic medicines were introduced 50 years ago and have proved useful in reducing, and sometimes eliminating, such symptoms of schizophrenia as thought disorder, hallucinations and delusions. They can also decrease associated symptoms such as agitation, impulsiveness and aggressiveness. This can be achieved in a matter of days or weeks in about 70% of patients. If taken consistently, these

Table 3.3 Effectiveness of interventions for schizophrenia

Intervention	% relapses after 1 year
Placebo	55
Chlorpromazine	20-25
Chlorpromazine + Family intervention	2-23

Sources:
Dixon LB, Lehman AF (1995). Family interventions for schizophrenia. *Schizophrenia Bulletin*, 21(4):631–643.

Dixon LB et al. (1995). Conventional antipsychotic medications for schizophrenia. *Schizophrenia Bulletin*, 21(4):567–577.

medicines can also reduce the risk of relapses by half. Currently available drugs appear to be less effective in reducing such symptoms as apathy, social withdrawal and poverty of ideas. First generation drugs are inexpensive and do not cost more than US$ 5 per month of treatment in developing countries. Some of them can be given in long-acting injections at 1–4 week intervals.

Antipsychotic drugs can help sufferers to benefit from psychosocial forms of treatment. The latest antipsychotic drugs are less likely to induce some side effects while improving certain symptoms. There is no clear evidence that the newer antipsychotic medications differ appreciably from the older drugs in their effectiveness, although there are differences in their most common side-effects.

The average duration of treatment is 3–6 months. Maintenance treatment continues for at least one year after the first episode of illness, for 2–5 years after the second episode, and for longer periods in patients with multiple episodes. In developing countries, response to treatment is more positive, medicine dosages are lower, and duration of treatment is shorter. In the total care of the patients, the support of the families is important. Some studies have shown that a combination of regular medication, family education and support can reduce relapses from 50% to less than 10% (see Table 3.3) (Leff & Gamble 1995; Dixon et al. 2000; Pharaoh et al. 2000).

Psychosocial rehabilitation for people with schizophrenia encompasses a variety of measures that range from improving social competence and social support networking to family support. Central to this are consumer empowerment and the reduction of stigma and discrimination, through the enlightenment of public opinion and by introducing pertinent legislation. Respect for human rights is a guiding principle of this strategy.

Currently, few patients with schizophrenia need long-term hospitalization; when they do, the average duration of stay is only 2–4 weeks, compared with a period of years before the introduction of modern therapies. Rehabilitation in day care centres, sheltered workshops and halfway homes improves recovery for patients with long-standing illnesses or residual disabilities of slowness, lack of motivation and social withdrawal.

EPILEPSY

Effective actions for the prevention of epilepsy are adequate prenatal and postnatal care, safe delivery, control of fever in children, control of parasitic and infectious diseases, and prevention of brain injury (for example, control of blood pressure and the use of safety belts and helmets).

The goals of therapy are to control fits by preventing them for at least two years, and to reintegrate people with epilepsy into educational and community life. Early diagnosis and the steady provision of maintenance drugs are fundamental for a positive outcome.

Epilepsy is almost always treated using anti-epileptic drugs (AEDs). Recent studies in both developed and developing countries have shown that up to 70% of newly diagnosed cases of children and adults with epilepsy can be successfully treated with AEDs, so that the people concerned will be seizure free, provided they take their medicines regularly (see Table 3.4). After 2–5 years of such successful treatment (cessation of epileptic fits), the treatment can be withdrawn in 60–70% of cases. The remainder have to continue on medication for the rest of their lives, but providing

Table 3.4 Effectiveness of interventions for epilepsy

Intervention	% seizure free after 1 year
Placebo	Not available
Carbamazepine	52
Phenobarbitone	54-73
Phenytoin	56

Sources:
Feksi AT et al. (1991). Comprehensive primary health care antiepileptic drug treatment programme in rural and semi-urban Kenya. *The Lancet*, 337(8738): 406–409.

Pal DK et al. (1998). Randomised controlled trial to assess acceptability of phenobarbital for epilepsy in rural India. *The Lancet*, 351(9095): 19–23.

they take the medication regularly, many are likely to remain free of seizures, while in others the frequency or severity of seizures can be much reduced. For some patients with intractable epilepsy, neurosurgical treatment may be successful. Psychological and social support are also valuable (ILAE/IBE/WHO 2000).

Phenobarbitone has become the front-line anti-epileptic drug in developing countries, perhaps because other drugs cost 5–20 times as much. A study in rural India found that 65% of those who received phenobarbitone were successfully treated, with the same proportion responding to phenytoin; adverse events were similar in both groups (Mani et al. 2001). A study in Indonesia concluded that, despite some disadvantages, phenobarbitone should still be used as the first-line drug in epilepsy treatment in developing countries. Studies in Ecuador and Kenya compared phenobarbitone to carbamazepine and found that there were no significant differences between them in terms of efficacy and safety (Scott et al. 2001). In most countries, the cost of treatment with phenobarbitone can be as low as US$ 5 per patient per year.

ALZHEIMER'S DISEASE

Primary prevention of Alzheimer's disease is not possible at present. The goals of care are to maintain the functioning of the individual; reduce disability due to lost mental functions; reorganize routines so as to maximize use of the retained functions; minimize disturbing functions, such as psychotic symptoms (for example, suspiciousness), agitation and depression; and provide support to families.

A central goal in research into treatment for Alzheimer's disease is the identification of agents that defer the onset, slow the progression, or improve the symptoms of the disease. Cholinergic receptor agonists (AChEs) have generally been beneficial in ameliorating global cognitive dysfunction and are most effective in improving attention. Amelioration of learning and memory impairments, the most prominent cognitive deficits in Alzheimer's disease, has been found less consistently. Treatment with these AChE inhibitors also appears to benefit non-cognitive symptoms in Alzheimer's disease, such as delusions and behavioural symptoms.

Treatment of depression in Alzheimer's disease patients has the potential to improve

---

Box 3.7 Caring for tomorrow's grandparents

The significant worldwide increase in the elderly population that is now being witnessed is the result not only of sociodemographic changes but also of an extended life span achieved during the 20th century, largely through improvements in sanitation and public health. This achievement, however, also poses one of the greatest challenges in the coming decades: managing the well-being of elderly people who, by the year 2025, will make up more than 20% of the total world population.

The greying of the population is likely to be accompanied by major changes in the frequency and distribution of somatic and mental disorders, and the inter-relationship between these two types of disorder.

Mental health problems among elderly people are frequent, and can be severe and diverse. In addition to Alzheimer's disease, seen almost exclusively in this age group, many other problems such as depression, anxiety and psychotic disorders also have a high prevalence. Suicide rates reach their peaks particularly among elderly men. Substance misuse, including alcohol and medication, is also highly prevalent, though largely ignored.

These problems create a high level of suffering not only to the elderly people themselves, but also to their relatives. In many instances family members have to sacrifice much of their personal life to dedicate themselves fully to the ill relative. The burden this creates for families and communities is high, and more often than not, inadequate health care resources leave patients and their families without the necessary support.

Many of these problems could be dealt with efficiently, but most countries have no policies, programmes or services prepared to meet these needs. A prevailing double stigma – attached to mental disorders in general and to the end of life in particular – does not help in facilitating access to necessary assistance.

The right to life and the right to quality of life calls for profound modifications in how societies see their elders, and for breaking associated taboos. The way societies organize themselves to care for the elderly is a good indicator of the importance they give to the dignity of the human being.

functional ability. Of the behavioural symptoms experienced by patients with Alzheimer's disease, depression and anxiety occur most frequently during the early stages, with psychotic symptoms and aggressive behaviour occurring later. In view of the increasing numbers of elderly people, managing their well-being is a challenge for the future (Box 3.7).

Psychosocial interventions are extremely important in Alzheimer's disease, both for patients and family caregivers, who themselves are at risk of depression, anxiety and somatic problems. These include psycho-education, support, cognitive behavioural techniques, self-help, and respite care. One psychosocial intervention – individual and family counselling plus support group participation – aimed at carer spouses has been shown in a study to delay institutionalization of patients with dementia by almost a year (Mittleman et al. 1996).

MENTAL RETARDATION

Because of the severity of mental retardation, and the heavy burden that it imposes on affected individuals, their families and the health services, prevention is extremely important. In view of the variety of different etiologies of mental retardation, preventive action must be targeted to specific causative factors. Examples include the iodization of water or salt to prevent iodine-deficiency mental retardation (cretinism) (Mubbashar 1999), abstinence from alcohol by pregnant women to avoid fetal alcohol syndrome, dietary control to prevent mental retardation in people with phenylketonuria, genetic counselling to prevent certain forms of mental retardation (such as Down's syndrome), adequate prenatal and postnatal care, and environmental control to prevent mental retardation due to intoxication from heavy metals, such as lead.

The goals of treatment are early recognition and optimal utilization of the intellectual capacities of the individual by training, behaviour modification, family education and support, vocational training and opportunities for work in protected settings.

Early intervention comprises planned efforts to promote development through a series of manipulations of environmental or experimental factors, and is initiated during the first five years of life. The objectives are to accelerate the rate of acquisition and development of new behaviours and skills, to enhance independent functioning, and to minimize the impact of impairment. Typically, a child is given sensory motor training within an infant stimulation programme, along with supportive psychosocial interventions.

The training of parents to act as trainers in the skills of daily living has become central to the care of persons with mental retardation, especially in developing countries. This means that parents have to be aware of learning principles and to be educated in behaviour modification and vocational training techniques. In addition, parents can support each other through self-help groups.

The majority of children with mental retardation experience difficulties in regular school curricula. They need additional help, and some need to attend special schools where the emphasis is on daily activities such as feeding, dressing, social skills, and the concept of numbers and letters. Behaviour modification techniques play an important role in developing many of these skills, as well as in increasing desirable behaviours while reducing undesirable behaviours.

Vocational training in sheltered settings and using behavioural skills has led to a large number of people with mental retardation leading active lives.

HYPERKINETIC DISORDERS

The precise etiology of the hyperkinetic disorders – hyperactivity in children, often with involuntary muscular spasms – is unknown, thus primary prevention is currently not possible. It is possible, however, to prevent the onset of symptoms that are often misdiagnosed as hyperkinetic disorders through preventive interventions with families and schools.

The treatment of hyperkinetic disorders cannot be considered without first addressing the adequacy and appropriateness of diagnosis. All too often, hyperkinetic disorders are diagnosed even though the patient does not meet the objective diagnostic criteria. Failure to make an appropriate diagnosis leads to difficulties in establishing the patient's response to therapeutic interventions. Hyperkinetic symptoms can be seen in a range of disorders for which there are specific treatments that are more appropriate than the treatment for hyperkinetic disorder. For instance, some children and adolescents with symptoms of hyperkinetic disorder are suffering from psychosis, or may be manifesting obsessive–compulsive disorder. Others may have specific learning disorders. Still others may be within the normal range of behaviour but are seen in environments with a reduced tolerance for the behaviours that are reported. Some children manifest hyperkinetic symptoms as a response to acute stress in the school or home. A thorough diagnostic process is thus essential, for which specialist help is often needed.

While treatment with amphetamine-like stimulants is now common, there is support for the use of behavioural therapy and environmental manipulation to reduce hyperkinetic symptoms. Therapies should be evaluated for their appropriateness as first-line treatments, especially where the diagnosis of hyperkinetic disorder is subject to question. In the absence of universally accepted guidelines for the use of psychostimulants in children and adolescents, it is important to start with low dosages and only gradually increase to an appropriate dose of psychostimulants, under continuous observation. Sustained-action medications are now available, but the same caution regarding appropriate dosage applies. Tricyclic antidepressants and other medications have been reported to be of use, but are not currently seen as first-line medications.

The diagnosis of hyperkinetic disorder is often not made until children reach school age, when they may benefit from an increase in structure in the school environment, or more

---

Box 3.8 Two national approaches to suicide prevention

Finland. Between 1950 and 1980 suicide rates in Finland increased by almost 50% among men, to 41.6 per 100 000, and doubled among women to 10.8 per 100 000. The Finnish Government responded by launching, in 1986, an innovative and comprehensive suicide prevention campaign. By 1996, an overall reduction in suicide rates of 17.5% had been achieved in relation to the peak year of 1990.

The internal process evaluation and the field survey[1] showed that running the programme from the very beginning as a common enterprise was decisive for its good progress. According to an evalua-tion survey, around 100 000 professionals had participated in prevention. This involved some 2000 working units, or 43% of all "human service units".

Although there is no definitive analysis available to explain the decrease, the set of interventions organized as part of the national project is believed to have played a major role. Specific factors probably related to the decrease are a reduction in alcohol consumption (due to the economic recession), and an increase in the consumption of antidepressant medication.

India. Over 95 000 Indians killed themselves in 1997, equal to one suicide every six minutes. One in every three was in the 15–29-year age group. Between 1987 and 1997, the suicide rate rose from 7.5 to 10.03 per 100 000 population. Of India's four major cities, Chennai's suicide rate of 17.23 is the highest. India has no national policy or programme for suicide prevention, and for a population of a billion there are only 3500 psychiatrists. The enormity of the problem combined with the paucity of services led to the formation of Sneha, a voluntary charitable organization for suicide prevention, affiliated to Befrienders International, an organization which provides "listening therapy" with human contact and emotional support.[2]

Sneha functions from early morning to late evening every day of the year, and is entirely staffed by carefully selected and trained volunteers who are skilled in empathetic listening and effective intervention. So far, Sneha has received over 100 000 calls of distress. An estimated 40% of callers are regarded as at medium to high risk of suicide.

Sneha has helped establish 10 similar centres in various parts of India, providing them with training and support. Together these centres function as Befrienders India. Sneha is now helping to set up the first survivor support groups in India.

[1] Upanne M et al. (1999). *Can suicide be prevented? The suicide project in Finland 1992-1996: goals, implementation and evaluation.* Saarijävi, Stakes.
[2] Vijayakumar L (2001). Personal communication.

individualized instruction. In the home environment, parental support and the amelioration of unrealistic expectations or conflicts can facilitate a reduction in hyperkinetic symptoms. Once thought to be a disorder that children outgrew, it is now known that, for some
people, hyperkinetic disorder persists into adulthood. Recognition of this by the patient
can help him (rarely her) to find life situations that are better adapted to limiting the debilitating effects of the untreated disorder.

SUICIDE PREVENTION

There is compelling evidence indicating that adequate prevention and treatment of some
mental and behavioural disorders can reduce suicide rates, whether such interventions are
directed towards individuals, families, schools or other sections of the general community
(Box 3.8). The early recognition and treatment of depression, alcohol dependence and schizophrenia are important strategies in the primary prevention of suicide. Educational programmes to train practitioners and primary care personnel in the diagnosis and treatment
of depressed patients are particularly important. In one study of such a programme on the
island of Gotland, Sweden (Rutz et al. 1995), the suicide rate, particularly of women, dropped
significantly in the year after an educational programme for general practitioners was introduced, but increased once the programme was discontinued.

The ingestion of toxic substances, such as pesticides, herbicides or medication, is the
preferred method for committing suicide in many places, particularly in rural areas of developing countries. For example, in Western Samoa in 1982, the ingestion of paraquat, a
herbicide, had become the predominant method of suicide. Reducing the availability of
paraquat to the general population achieved significant reductions in total suicide, without
a corresponding increase in suicide by other methods (Bowles 1995). Similar successful
examples relate to the control of other toxic substances and the detoxification of domestic
gas and of car exhausts. In many places, the lack of easily accessible emergency care makes
the ingestion of toxic substances – which in most industrialized countries would be a suicide attempt – another fatality.

In the Russian Federation, as well as in other neighbouring countries, alcohol consumption has increased precipitously in recent years, and has been linked to an increase in rates
of suicide and alcohol poisoning (Vroublevsky & Harwin 1998), and to a decline in male life
expectancy (Notzon et al. 1998; Leon & Shkolnikov 1998).

Several studies have shown an association between the possession of handguns at home
and suicide rates (Kellerman et al. 1992; Lester & Murrell 1980). Legislation restricting
access to handguns may have a beneficial effect. This is suggested by studies in the United
States, where the restriction of the selling and purchasing of handguns was associated with
lower firearm suicide rates. States with the strictest handgun control laws had the lowest
firearm suicide rates, and there was no switching to an alternative method of suicide (Lester
1995).

As well as interventions that involve restricting access to common methods of suicide,
school-based interventions involving crisis management, enhancement of self-esteem, and
the development of coping skills and healthy decision-making have been shown to lower
the risk of suicide among young people (Mishara & Ystgaard 2000).

The media can assist in prevention by limiting graphic and unnecessary depictions of
suicide and by deglamorizing news reports of suicides. In a number of countries, a decrease
in suicide rates coincided with the media's consent to minimize the reporting of suicides
and to follow proposed guidelines. Glamorizing suicide may lead to imitation.

CHAPTER FOUR

Mental Health Policy and Service Provision

Governments, as the ultimate stewards of mental health, need to set policies – within the context of general health systems and financing arrangements – that will protect and improve the mental health of the population. In terms of financing, people should be protected from catastrophic financial risk; the healthy should subsidize the sick; and the well-off should subsidize the poor. Mental health policy should be reinforced by coherent alcohol and drug policies, as well as social welfare services such as housing. Policies should be drawn up with the involvement of all stakeholders and should be based on reliable information. Policies should ensure the respect of human rights and take account of the needs of vulnerable groups. Care should shift away from large psychiatric hospitals to community services that are integrated into general health services. Psychotropic drugs need to be available, and the required health workers need to be trained. The mass media and public awareness campaigns can be effective in reducing stigma and discrimination. Nongovernmental organizations and consumer groups should also be supported, as they can be instrumental in improving service quality and public attitudes. Further research is needed to improve policy and services, in particular to take account of cultural differences.

4

MENTAL HEALTH POLICY
AND SERVICE PROVISION

DEVELOPING POLICY

*T*o protect and improve the mental health of the population is a complex task involving multiple decisions. It requires priorities to be set among mental health needs, conditions, services, treatments, and prevention and promotion strategies, and choices to be made about their funding. Mental health services and strategies must be well coordinated among themselves and with other services, such as social security, education, employment and housing. Mental health outcomes must be monitored and analysed so that decisions can be continually adjusted to meet existing challenges.

Governments, as the ultimate stewards of mental health, need to assume the responsibility for ensuring that these complex activities are carried out. One critical role in stewardship is to develop and implement policy. Policy identifies the major issues and objectives, defines the respective roles of the public and private sectors in financing and provision, identifies policy instruments and organizational arrangements required in the public and possibly in the private sectors to meet mental health objectives, sets the agenda for capacity building and organizational development, and provides guidance for prioritizing expenditure, thus linking analysis of problems to decisions about resource allocation.

The stewardship function for mental health is poorly developed in many countries. The WHO Project Atlas (see Box 4.1) collected basic information on mental health resources from 181 countries. According to these data, which are used to illustrate the main points in this chapter, one-third of countries do not report a specific mental health budget, although they presumably devote some resources to mental health. Half the rest allocate less than 1% of their public health budget to mental health, even though neuropsychiatric problems represent 12% of the total global burden of disease. A non-existent or limited budget for mental health is a significant barrier to providing treatment and care.

Related to this budgetary problem is the fact that approximately four out of ten countries have no explicit mental health policy and approximately one-third have no drug and alcohol policy. The lack of policy related specifically to children and adolescents is even more dramatic (Graham & Orley 1998). It may be argued that a policy is neither necessary nor sufficient for good results, and that for those countries without a mental health policy it would suffice to have a defined mental health programme or plan. But one-third of countries have no programme and a quarter have neither a policy nor a programme. These findings indicate the lack of expressed commitment to address mental health problems and the absence of requirements to undertake national level planning, coordination and evaluation of mental health strategies, services and capacity (see Figure 4.1).

Box 4.1 Project Atlas

The WHO Project Atlas of Mental Health Resources is one of the most recent to examine the current status of mental health systems in countries.[1] It involves 181 of WHO's Member States, thus covering 98.7% of the world population. The information was obtained during the period October 2000 to March 2001 from ministries of health, using a short questionnaire, and was partially validated on the basis of reports from experts and from the published literature. While this information gives an indication of mental health resources in the world, some limitations need to be kept in mind. The first is that the information was based on self-reporting, and not all responses could be validated independently. Second, not all Member States responded, and this, together with other missing data on survey items, is likely to have biased the results. Finally, the results do not provide a comprehensive analysis of all mental health variables of relevance to countries, and therefore leave some questions unanswered.

[1] *Mental health resources in the world. Initial results of Project Atlas* (2001). Geneva, World Health Organization (Fact Sheet No. 260, April 2001).

HEALTH SYSTEM AND FINANCING ARRANGEMENTS

Mental health policy and service provision occur within the context of general health systems and financing arrangements. The implications of these arrangements for the delivery of mental health services need to be considered in policy formulation and implementation.

Over the past thirty years, health systems in developed countries have evolved from a highly centralized system of care to a decentralized system in which responsibility for policy implementation and service provision has been transferred from central to local structures. This process has also influenced the shape of systems in many developing countries. There are typically two main features of decentralization: reforms aimed at cost-containment and efficiency (discussed in this section); and the use of contracts with private and public service providers (discussed below in connection with providing mental health services).

The characteristics of good financing for mental health services are no different from what makes for good financing for health services in general (WHO 2000c, Chapter 5). There are three principal desiderata. First, people should be protected from catastrophic financial risk, which means minimizing out-of-pocket payments and particularly requiring such payments only for small expenses on affordable goods or services. All forms of prepayment, whether via general taxation, mandatory social insurance or voluntary private insurance, are preferable in this respect, because they pool risks and allow the use of services to be at least partly separated from payment for them. Mental problems are often chronic, so what matters is not only the cost of an individual treatment or service but the likelihood of its being repeated over long intervals. What an individual or a household can afford once, in a crisis, may be unaffordable in the long term, just as with certain other chronic noncommunicable problems such as diabetes.

Second, the healthy should subsidize the sick. Any prepayment mechanism will do this in general – as out-of-pocket payment will not – but whether subsidies flow in the right direction for mental health depends on whether prepayment covers the specific needs of the mentally ill. A financing system could be adequate in this respect for many services but still not transfer resources from the healthy to the sick where mental or behavioural problems are concerned, simply because those problems are not covered. The effect of a particular financing arrangement on mental health therefore depends on the choice of interventions to finance.

Finally, a good financing system will also mean that the well-off subsidize the poor, at least to some extent. This is the hardest characteristic to assure, because it depends on the coverage and progressivity of the tax system and on who is covered by social or private insurance. Insurance makes the well-off subsidize the worse-off only if both groups are included, rather than insurance being limited to the well-off; and if contributions are at least partly income-related, rather than uniform or related only to risks. As always, the magnitude and direction of subsidy also depends on what services are covered.

Prepayment typically accounts for a larger share of total health spending in richer countries, and this has consequences for mental health financing. When a government provides 70–80% of all that is spent on health, as occurs in many OECD countries, decisions about the priority to give mental health can be directly implemented through the budget, probably with only minor offsetting effects on private spending. When a government provides only 20–30% of total financing, as in China, Cyprus, India, Lebanon, Myanmar, Nepal, Nigeria, Pakistan and Sudan (WHO 2000c, Annex Table 8), and there is also little insurance coverage, mental health is likely to suffer relative to other health problems because most spending must be out of pocket. Individuals with mental disorders, particularly in developing countries, are commonly poorer than the rest of the population, and often less able or willing to seek care owing to stigma, or previous negative experiences of services, so having to pay out of their or their families' pockets is even more of an obstacle than it is for many acute physical health problems. Finding ways to increase the share of prepayment, particularly for expensive or repeated procedures, as recommended in *The World Health Report 2000*, can therefore benefit mental health spending preferentially, provided enough of the additional prepayment is dedicated to mental and behavioural disorders. Movement in the other direction – from prepayment to more out-of-pocket spending, as has occurred with the economic transition in several countries of the former Soviet Union – is likely to diminish the resources for mental health.

In countries with a low share of prepayment and difficulties in raising tax revenues or extending social insurance because much of the population is rural and has no formal employment, community financing schemes may seem an attractive way to reduce the out-of-pocket burden. The evidence of their success is scanty and mixed so far, but it should be noted that unless such schemes receive substantial subsidies from governments, nongovernmental organizations or external donors, they are not likely to solve the chronic problems of an easily identified part of the beneficiary population. People who are willing to help their neighbours in acute health need will be much less willing to contribute far more perma-

Figure 4.1 Presence of mental health policies and legislation, percentage of Member States in WHO Regions, 2000

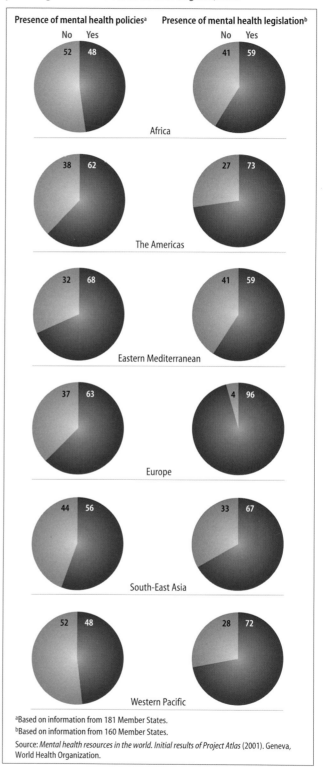

ᵃBased on information from 181 Member States.
ᵇBased on information from 160 Member States.
Source: *Mental health resources in the world. Initial results of Project Atlas* (2001). Geneva, World Health Organization.

nent support. They cannot therefore be counted on as a significant source of financing for mental health: community-based services should not imply or depend on community-based finance.

These same poor countries are sometimes heavily dependent on external donors to pay for health care. This is potentially a valuable source of funds for mental health, just as for other problems, but donors often have their own priorities which need not coincide with those of the government. In particular, currently they seldom give mental health a high priority over communicable diseases. In that case, governments have to decide whether to try to persuade donors to align aid more closely with the priorities of the country, or whether to use their own limited funds in areas neglected by donors, in particular by devoting a greater proportion of domestic resources to mental problems.

Formulating mental health policy

Within general health policy, special consideration needs to be given to mental health policy, as well as to alcohol and drug policies, not least because of the stigma and human rights violations suffered by many people with these mental and behavioural disorders, and the help a large portion of them need in finding suitable housing or income support.

The formulation of mental health, alcohol and drug policies must be undertaken within the context of a complex body of government health, welfare and general social policies. Social, political and economic realities must be recognized at local, regional and national levels. In drawing up these policies, a number of questions should be asked (see Box 4.2).

Alcohol and drug policies are a special issue as they need to include law enforcement and other controls over the supply of psychoactive substances, and a range of options to deal with the negative consequences of substance use that are a threat to public safety, in addition to covering education, prevention, treatment and rehabilitation (WHO 1998).

An important step in the development of a mental health policy is the identification, by the government, of those responsible for its formulation. The process of policy development must include the views of a wide array of stakeholders: patients (sometimes called consumers), family members, professionals, policy-makers and other interested parties. Some, such as employers and members of the criminal justice system, may not consider themselves to be stakeholders, but they need to be convinced of the importance of their participation. The policy should set priorities and outline approaches, based on identified needs and taking into account available resources.

Box 4.2 Formulating policy: the key questions

The successful formulation of a mental health policy depends on ensuring that it responds affirmatively to the following questions.

- Does the policy promote the development of community-based care?
- Are services comprehensive and integrated into primary health care?
- Does the policy encourage partnerships between individuals, families and health professionals?
- Does the policy promote the empowerment of individuals, families and communities?
- Does the policy create a system that respects, protects and fulfils the human rights of people with mental disorders?
- Are evidence-based practices utilized wherever possible?
- Is there an adequate supply of appropriately trained service providers to ensure that the policy can be implemented?

- Are the special needs of women, children and adolescents recognized?
- Is there parity between mental health services and other health services?
- Does the policy require the continuous monitoring and evaluation of services?
- Does the policy create a system that is responsive to the needs of underserved and vulnerable populations?
- Is adequate attention paid to strategies for prevention and promotion?
- Does the policy foster intersectoral links between the mental health and other sectors?

Box 4.3 Mental health reform in Uganda

Mental health services in Uganda were decentralized in the 1960s, and mental health units were built at regional referral hospitals. These units resembled prisons and were manned by psychiatric clinical officers. Services were plagued by low staff morale, a chronic shortage of drugs and no funds for any community activities. Most people had little understanding of mental disorders or did not know that effective treatments and services were available. Up to 80% of patients went to traditional healers before reporting to the health system.[1]

In 1996, encouraged by WHO, the health ministry began to strengthen mental health services and integrate them into primary health care. Standards and guidelines were developed for the care of epilepsy and for the mental health of children and adults, from community level to tertiary institutions. Health workers were trained to recognize and manage or refer common mental and neurological disorders. A new referral system was established along with a supervisory support network. Linkages were set up with other programmes such as those on AIDS, adolescent and reproductive health, and health education. Efforts were made to raise awareness of mental health in the general population. The Mental Health Act was revised and integrated into a Health Services Bill. Mental and neurological drugs have been included in the essential drugs list.

Mental health has been included as a component of the national minimum health care package. Mental health is now part of the health ministry budget. Mental health units are to be built at 6 of the 10 regional referral hospitals, and the capacity of the 900-bed national psychiatric hospital is to be reduced by half.

[1] Baingana F (1990). Personal communication.

In some countries, mental health is being integrated into primary health care but fundamental reforms to psychiatric hospitals and in relation to community-based options are not being carried out. Major reforms of the health sectors in many countries are opportunities to strengthen the position of mental health in those sectors, and to begin the integration process at policy, health service and community levels. In Uganda (Box 4.3) for example, mental health was until recently given low priority.

ESTABLISHING AN INFORMATION BASE

The formulation of policy must be based upon up-to-date and reliable information concerning the community, mental health indicators, effective treatments, prevention and promotion strategies, and mental health resources. The policy will need to be reviewed periodically to allow for the modification or updating of programmes.

An important task is to collect and analyse epidemiological information to identify the broad psychosocial determinants of mental problems, as well as to provide quantitative information on the extent and type of problems in the community. Another important task is to carry out a comprehensive survey of existing resources and structures within communities and regions, along with a critical analysis of the extent to which they are fulfilling the defined needs. In this respect, it is helpful to use a "mixed economy matrix" to map out different provider sectors, how they are provided with resources, and the ways in which these sectors and resources are linked together. Mental health and associated services, such as social welfare support and housing, could be provided by public (state), private (for-profit), voluntary (non-profit), or informal (family or community) organizations or groups. The reality for most people is that they will receive only a few formal services, alongside informal support from family, friends and community. These services are likely to be funded by a mix of five basic revenue collection modes: out of pocket, private insurance schemes, social insurance, general taxation, and donations by charitable bodies (nongovernmental organizations). After the matrix has been established, a more systematic analysis can be undertaken of the types and quality of services, the main providers, and the questions of access and equity.

Both the formulation and evaluation of policy require the existence of a well-functioning and coordinated information system for measuring a minimum number of mental health indicators. Currently around a third of countries have no system for the annual reporting of mental health data. Those which have such a system often lack sufficiently detailed information to allow for the evaluation of policy, services and treatment effectiveness. About half the countries have no facilities for the collection of epidemiological or service data at the national level.

Governments need to invest resources in developing information monitoring systems which incorporate indicators for the major demographic and socioeconomic determinants of mental health, the mental health status of the general population and those in treatment (including specific diagnostic categories by age and sex), and health systems. Indicators for the latter might include, for example, the number of psychiatric and general hospital beds, the number of hospital admissions and re-admissions, the length of stay, duration of illness at first contact, treatment utilization patterns, recovery rates, the number of outpatient visits, the frequency of primary care visits, the frequency and dosage of medication, and the number of staff and training facilities.

Methods of measurement could include population surveys, systematic data collection of patients treated at tertiary, secondary and primary levels of care, and the use of mortality data. The system set-up in countries must enable the information collected at local and regional levels to be collated and analysed systematically at the national level.

HIGHLIGHTING VULNERABLE GROUPS AND SPECIAL PROBLEMS

Policy should highlight vulnerable groups which have special mental health needs. Within most countries, these groups would include children, elderly people, and abused women. There are also likely to be vulnerable groups specific to the sociopolitical environment within countries, for example, refugees and displaced persons in regions experiencing civil wars or internal conflicts.

For *children*, policies should aim to prevent child mental disability through adequate nutrition, prenatal and perinatal care, avoidance of alcohol and drug consumption during pregnancy, immunization, iodization of salt, child safety measures, treatment of common childhood disorders such as epilepsy, early detection through primary care, early identification, and health promotion through schools. The latter is feasible, as shown by experience in Alexandria, Egypt, where child counsellors were trained to work in schools to detect and treat childhood mental and behavioural disorders (El-Din et al. 1996). The United Nations Convention on the Rights of the Child recognizes that children and adolescents have the right to appropriate services (UN 1989). Youth services, which should be coordinated with schools and primary health care, can tackle mental and physical health in an integrated and comprehensive way, covering such problems as early and unwanted pregnancies; tobacco, alcohol and other substance use; violent behaviour; attempted suicide; and the prevention of HIV and sexually transmitted diseases.

For the *elderly*, policies should support and improve the care already provided to elderly people by their families, incorporate mental health assessment and management into general health services, and provide respite care for family members who often are the principal caregivers.

For *women*, policies must overcome discrimination in access to mental health services, treatment, and community services. Services need to be created in the community and at primary and secondary care levels to support women who have experienced sexual, domestic or other forms of violence, as well as for those who themselves have problems of alcohol and substance use.

For *internally displaced groups and refugees*, policies must deal with housing, employment, shelter, clothing and food, as well as the psychological and emotional effects of experiencing war, dislocation and loss of loved ones. Community intervention should be the basis for policy action.

In view of the specificities of *suicidal behaviour*, policies must reduce environmental factors, particularly access to the means most commonly used to commit suicide in a given place. Policies must ensure care for at-risk individuals, particularly those with mental disorders, and survivors of suicide attempts.

Alcohol-related problems are not limited to alcohol-dependent people. Public health action should be directed at the whole drinking population, rather than to the users who are alcohol-dependent. Political feasibility, the capacity of the country in question to respond, public acceptance and likelihood of impact have to be considered when policies are being determined. The most effective alcohol control policies involve increasing the real price of, and taxes on, alcoholic beverages; restricting their consumption by controlling their availability, including the use of minimum drinking age legislation, and restricting the number, types and opening hours of outlets serving or selling alcohol; drink-drive laws; and server interventions (through policies and training leading to a refusal to serve alcohol to intoxicated persons). Also important are the control of alcohol advertising, particularly that which is targeted to young people; providing public education on the negative consequences of drinking alcohol (for example, through mass media and social marketing campaigns); warning labels; strict controls on product safety; and implementing measures against the illicit production and sale of alcoholic beverages. Finally, the provision of treatment for persons with alcohol-related problems should be part of society's health and social care responsibilities (Jernigan et al. 2000).

Policies concerning *illicit drug use* should aim to control the supply of illicit drugs; reduce demand, by prevention and other means; reduce the negative consequences of drug dependence; and provide treatment. These policies should target the general population and various risk groups. The development of effective programmes and services requires an understanding of the extent of drug use and related problems, and how they change over time according to patterns of substance use. Information dissemination needs to be accurate and appropriate for the target group. It should avoid sensationalism, promote psychosocial competence through life skills, and empower individuals to make healthier choices regarding their substance use. As substance use is intertwined with a number of social problems and exclusion, prevention efforts are likely to be more successful if they are integrated with strategies that aim to improve the lives of people and communities, including access to education and health care.

RESPECTING HUMAN RIGHTS

Mental health policies and programmes should promote the following rights: equality and non-discrimination; the right to privacy; individual autonomy; physical integrity; the right to information and participation; and freedom of religion, assembly and movement.

Human rights instruments also demand that any planning or development of mental health policies or programmes should involve vulnerable groups (such as indigenous and tribal populations; national, ethnic, religious and linguistic minorities; migrant workers; refugees and stateless persons; children and adolescents; and elderly people) in the planning and development of mental health policies and programmes.

Beyond the legally binding *International Covenant on Civil and Political Rights* and the *International Covenant on Economic, Social and Cultural Rights*, which are applicable to the human rights of those suffering from mental and behavioural disorders, the most significant and serious international effort to protect the rights of the mentally ill is the United

Nations General Assembly Resolution 46/119 on the *Protection of Persons with Mental Illness and the Improvement of Mental Health Care*, adopted in 1991 (UN 1991). Although not legally binding, the resolution brings together a set of basic rights which the international community regards as inviolable either in the community or when mentally ill persons receive treatment from the health care system. There are 25 principles which fall into two general categories: civil rights and procedures, and access to and quality of care. Principles include statements of the fundamental freedoms and basic rights of mentally ill persons, criteria for the determination of mental illness, protection of confidentiality, standards of care and treatment including involuntary admission and consent to treatment, rights of mentally ill persons in mental health facilities, provision of resources for mental health facilities, provision of review mechanisms, providing for protection of the rights of mentally ill offenders, and procedural safeguards to protect the rights of mentally ill persons.

The United Nations *Convention on the Rights of the Child* (1989) provides guidance for policy development specifically relevant to children and adolescents. It covers protection from all forms of physical and mental abuse; non-discrimination; the right to life, survival and development; the best interests of the child; and respect for the views of the child.

There are also a number of regional instruments to protect the rights of the mentally ill, including the *European Convention for Protection of Human Rights and Fundamental Freedoms*, backed by the European Court of Human Rights; *Recommendation 1235 (1994) on Psychiatry and Human Rights* adopted by the Parliamentary Assembly of the Council of Europe; the *American Convention on Human Rights*, 1978; and the *Declaration of Caracas* adopted by the Regional Conference on Restructuring Psychiatric care in Latin America in 1990 (see Box 3.3).

The human rights treaty monitoring bodies represent one example of an underutilized means to enhance the accountability of governments as regards mental health and to shape international law to address mental health matters. Nongovernmental organizations and the medical and public health professions should be encouraged to make use of these existing mechanisms to prompt governments to provide the resources to fulfil their obligations towards the health care of persons with mental disorders, protecting them from discrimination in society, and safeguarding other relevant human rights.

MENTAL HEALTH LEGISLATION

Mental health legislation should codify and consolidate the fundamental principles, values, goals, and objectives of mental health policy. Such legislation is essential to guarantee that the dignity of patients is preserved and that their fundamental human rights are protected.

Of 160 countries providing information on legislation (WHO 2001), nearly a quarter have no legislation on mental health (Figure 4.1). About half of the existing legislation was formulated in the past decade, but nearly one-fifth dates back over 40 years to a period before most of the current treatment methods became available.

Governments need to develop up-to-date national legislation for mental health which is consistent with international human rights obligations and which applies the important principles mentioned above, including those in United Nations General Assembly Resolution 46/119.

PROVIDING SERVICES

Many barriers limit the dissemination of effective interventions for mental and behavioural disorders (Figure 4.2). Specific health system barriers vary across countries but there are some commonalities relating to the sheer lack of mental health services, the poor quality of treatment and services, and issues related to access and equity.

While many countries have undertaken reform or are in the process of reforming their mental health systems, the extent and types of reform also vary tremendously. No country has managed to achieve the full spectrum of reform required to overcome all the barriers. Italy has successfully reformed its psychiatric services, but has left its primary care services untouched (Box 4.4). In Australia, (Box 4.5) health spending on mental health has increased and there has been a shift towards community care. There have also been attempts to integrate mental health into primary care and to increase consumer participation in decision-making. But community care, particularly regarding housing, has been extremely poor in some places.

Although psychiatric institutions with a large number of beds are not recommended for mental health care, a certain number of beds in general hospitals for acute care are essential. There is a wide variation in the number of beds available for mental health care (Figure 4.3). The median number for the world population is 1.5 per 10 000 population, ranging from 0.33 in the WHO South-East Asia Region to 9.3 in the European Region. Nearly two-thirds of the global population has access to fewer than one bed per 10 000 population, and more than half of all the beds are still in psychiatric institutions which often provide custodial care rather than mental health care.

Figure 4.2 Barriers to implementation of effective intervention for mental disorders

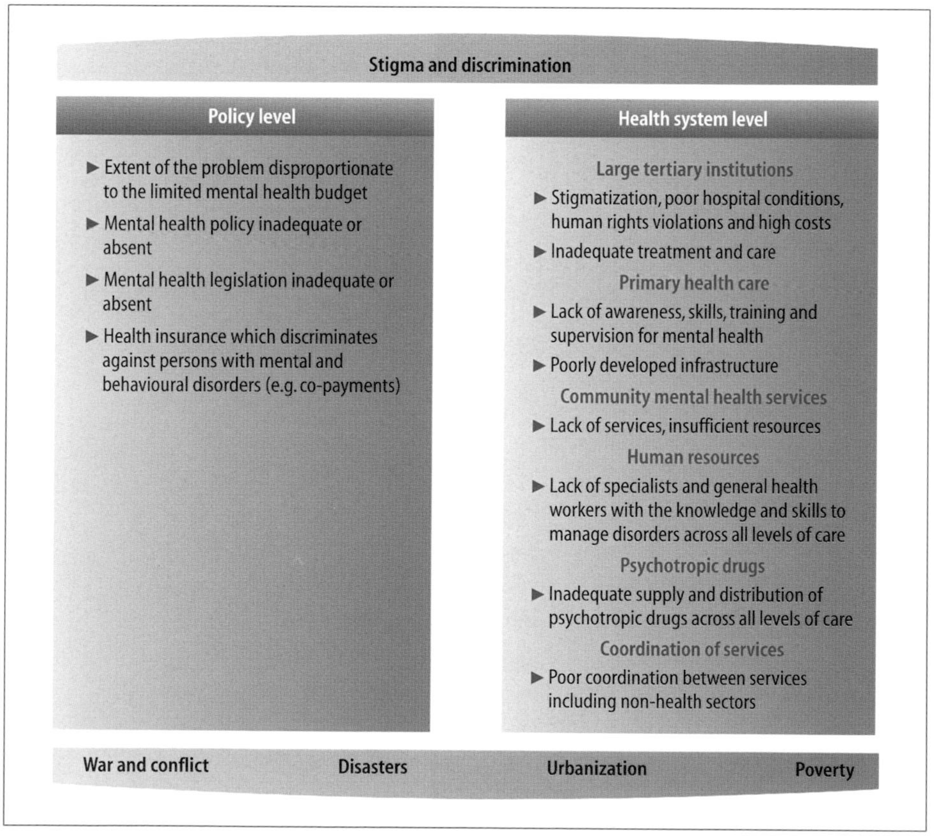

Stigma and discrimination

Policy level

▶ Extent of the problem disproportionate to the limited mental health budget
▶ Mental health policy inadequate or absent
▶ Mental health legislation inadequate or absent
▶ Health insurance which discriminates against persons with mental and behavioural disorders (e.g. co-payments)

Health system level

Large tertiary institutions
▶ Stigmatization, poor hospital conditions, human rights violations and high costs
▶ Inadequate treatment and care

Primary health care
▶ Lack of awareness, skills, training and supervision for mental health
▶ Poorly developed infrastructure

Community mental health services
▶ Lack of services, insufficient resources

Human resources
▶ Lack of specialists and general health workers with the knowledge and skills to manage disorders across all levels of care

Psychotropic drugs
▶ Inadequate supply and distribution of psychotropic drugs across all levels of care

Coordination of services
▶ Poor coordination between services including non-health sectors

War and conflict   Disasters   Urbanization   Poverty

Figure 4.3 Psychiatric beds per 10 000 population by WHO Region, 2000[a]

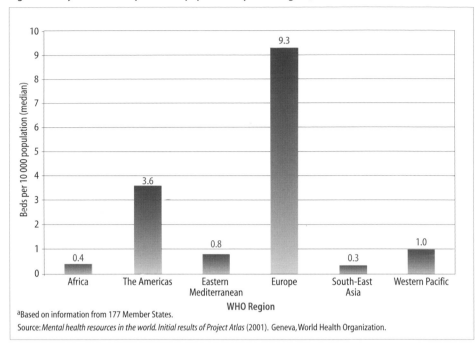

[a]Based on information from 177 Member States.

Source: *Mental health resources in the world. Initial results of Project Atlas* (2001). Geneva, World Health Organization.

Box 4.4 Mental health reform in Italy

Twenty years ago the Italian Parliament passed "Law 180" which aimed to bring about a radical change in psychiatric care throughout the country. The law comprised framework legislation (*legge quadro*), entrusting regions with the tasks of drafting and implementing detailed norms, methods, and timetables for the translation of the law's general principles into specific action. For the management of psychiatric illness, three alternatives to mental hospitals have been set up: psychiatric beds in general hospitals; residential, non-hospital facilities, with full-time or part-time staff; and non-residential, outpatient facilities, which include day hospitals, day centres, and outpatient clinics.[1]

In the first 10 years following approval of the law, the number of mental hospital residents dropped by 53%. The total number discharged over the past two decades is, however, not known precisely. Compulsory admissions, as a percentage of total psychiatric admissions, have steadily declined from about 50% in 1975 to about 20% in 1984 and 11.8% in 1994. The "revolving door" phenomenon – discharged patients who are readmitted – is evident only in areas that lack well-organized, effective, community-based services.

Even in the context of the new services, recent surveys show that psychiatric patients are unlikely to receive optimum pharmacotherapy, and evidence-based psychosocial modes of treatment are unevenly distributed across mental health services. For example, although psycho-educational intervention is widely regarded as essential in the care of patients suffering from schizophrenia, only 8% of families received some form of such treatment. The scant data available seem to show that families have informally taken on some of the care for the ill relative, which was previously a responsibility of the mental hospital. At least some of the advantages to patients appear to be attributable more to everyday family support than to the services provided.

The following lessons may be drawn. First, the transition from a predominantly hospital-based service to a predominantly community-based service cannot be accomplished simply by closing the psychiatric institutions: appropriate alternative structures must be provided, as was the case in Italy. Second, political and administrative commitment is necessary if community care is to be effective. Investments have to be made in buildings, staff, training, and the provision of backup facilities. Third, monitoring and evaluation are important aspects of change: planning and evaluation should go hand in hand, and evaluation should, wherever possible, have an epidemiological basis. Last, a reform law should not only provide guidelines (as in Italy), but should be prescriptive: minimum standards need to be determined in terms of care, and in establishing reliable monitoring systems; compulsory timetables need to be set for implementing the envisaged facilities; and central mechanisms are required for the verification, control and comparison of the quality of services.

[1]de Girolomo G, Cozza M (2000). The Italian psychiatric reform: a 20-year perspective. *International Journal of Law and Psychiatry*, 23(3–4): 197–214.

The fact remains that, in many countries, large tertiary institutions with both acute and long-term facilities are still the predominant means of providing treatment and care. Such facilities are associated with poor outcomes and human rights violations. The fact that the public mental health budget in many countries is directed towards maintaining institutional care means that few or no resources are available for more effective services in general hospitals and in the community. Data indicate that community-based services are not available in 38% of countries. Even in countries that promote community care, coverage is far from complete. Within countries there are large variations between regions and between rural and urban areas (see Box 4.6).

In most countries, services for mental health need to be assessed, re-evaluated and reformed to provide the best available treatment and care. There are ways of improving how services are organized, even with limited resources, so that those who need them can make full use of them. The first is to shift care away from mental hospitals; the second is to develop community mental health services; and the third is to integrate mental health services into general health care. The degree of collaboration between mental health services and other non-health services, the availability of essential psychotropic drugs, methods for selecting mental health interventions, and the roles of the public and private sectors in delivering interventions are also crucial issues for service reorganization, as discussed below.

SHIFTING CARE AWAY FROM LARGE PSYCHIATRIC HOSPITALS

The ultimate goal is community-based treatment and care. This implies closing down large psychiatric hospitals (see Table 4.1). It may not be realistic to do this immediately. As a short-term measure, that is, until all patients can be discharged into the community with adequate community support, psychiatric hospitals need to be downsized, the living conditions of patients need to be improved, staff need to be trained, procedures need to be set up to protect patients against unnecessary involuntary admissions and treatments, and independent bodies need to be created to monitor and review hospital conditions. Furthermore, hospitals need to be converted into centres for active treatment and rehabilitation.

Box 4.5 Mental health reform in Australia

In Australia, where depression is ranked as the fourth most common cause of the total disease burden, and is the most common cause of disability,[1] the country's first national mental health strategy was adopted in 1992 by the Federal government and the health ministers of all states. A collaborative framework was established to pursue the agreed priority areas over a five-year period (1993–98).

This five-year programme has demonstrated the changes that can be achieved in national mental health reform. National spending on mental health care increased by 30% in real terms, while spending on community-based services grew by 87%. By 1998, the amount of mental health spending dedicated to caring for people in the community increased from 29% to 46%. Resources released through institutional downsizing funded

48% of the growth in community-based and general hospital services. The number of clinical staff providing community care rose by 68%, in parallel with increased spending.

Stand-alone psychiatric institutions, which had accounted for 49% of total mental health resources, were reduced to 29% of those resources and the number of beds in institutions fell by 42%. At the same time, the number of acute psychiatric beds in general hospitals rose by

34%. Formal mechanisms for consumer and carer participation were established by 61% of public mental health organizations. The nongovernmental sector increased its overall share of mental health funding from 2% to 5%, and funds allocated to nongovernmental organizations to provide community support to people with psychiatric disability grew by 200%.

[1] Whiteford H et al. (2000). The Australian mental health system. *International Journal of Law and Psychiatry*, 23(3–4):403–417.

Developing community mental health services

Community mental health services need to provide comprehensive and locally based treatment and care which is readily accessible to patients and their families. Services should be comprehensive in that they provide a range of facilities to meet the mental health needs of the population at large as well as of special groups, such as children, adolescents, women and elderly people. Ideally, services should include: nutrition; provision for acute admissions to general hospitals; outpatient care; community centres; outreach services; residential homes; respite for families and carers; occupational, vocational and rehabilitation supports; and basic necessities such as shelter and clothing (see Table 4.1). If de-institutionalization is being pursued, community services must be developed in tandem. All the positive functions of the institution should be reproduced in the community without perpetuating the negative aspects.

Three key financing recommendations should be considered. The first is to release resources for the development of community services through partial hospital closure. The second is to use transitional funding for initial investment in new services, to facilitate movement from hospitals to the community. The third is to maintain parallel funding in order to continue the financing of a certain level of institutional care even after community-based services have been established.

Countries face problems in their attempts to create comprehensive mental health care because of the scarcity of funds. Although, in some countries, funds may be redirected or reinvested in community care as a result of de-institutionalization, this is rarely sufficient on its own. In other countries, it may be difficult to divert funds. For example, in South Africa, where budgets are integrated within the various levels of primary, secondary and

---

Box 4.6 Mental health services: the urban–rural imbalance

The province of Neuquen in **Argentina** provides mental health care to both urban and remote rural communities, but the balance of specialized human mental health resources is still located in the urban centres. Cities have primary care clinics, secondary level psychiatric units in general hospitals and tertiary mental health centres, whereas resident community health workers, fortnightly visits from general practitioners, and local primary health care clinics serve remote rural communities.[1] Similarly, a community-based rehabilitation programme for severely mentally ill patients in the capital city has no counterpart in the rural areas of the province.[2] In **Nigeria**, urban hospitals have more medical personnel and their support facilities function more efficiently in comparison with government hospitals in the country.[3] In **Costa Rica**, most mental health care workers are still concentrated in towns and cities, and the rural regions remain understaffed.[4] Among **Arab countries**, community mental health care facilities are usually found only in the large cities,[5] although **Saudi Arabia** has psychiatric clinics within some of the general hospitals in rural areas.[6] In **India** too, despite the emphasis on developing rural services, most mental health professionals reside in urban areas.[7] In **China**, community service provision is an urban/suburban model, despite the majority of the population being predominantly rural. Community care services in cities are run by neighbourhood and factory committees.[8] In the countries of the **former USSR,** mental health services are still organized by central planning bureaucracies and are clearly demarcated in terms of local and central administration of services. Authority resides at the centre – meaning the urban centres, whereas remote rural areas are obliged to supply services conceived and financed by the central bureaucracy.[9] In **Turkey**, private and public specialist mental health services are available in town and cities, whereas in rural and semi-rural areas patients have to rely on the primary health centre for local mental health services.[10]

[1] Collins PY et al. (1999a). Using local resources in Patagonia: primary care and mental health in Neuquen, Argentina. *International Journal of Mental Health*, 28**:** 3–16.

[2] Collins PY et al. (1999b). Using local resources in Patagonia: a model of community-based rehabilitation. *International Journal of Mental Health*, 28: 17–24.

[3] Gureje O et al. (1995). Results from the Ibadan centre. In: Üstün TB, Sartorius N, eds. *Mental illness in general health care: an international study.* Chichester, John Wiley & Sons: 157–173.

[4] Gallegos A, Montero F (1999). Issues in community-based rehabilitation for persons with mental illness in Costa Rica. *International Journal of Mental Health*, 28: 25–30.

[5] Okasha A, Karam E (1998). Mental health services and research in the Arab world. *Acta Psychiatrica Scandinavica*, 98: 406–413.

[6] Al-Subaie AS et al. (1997). Psychiatric emergencies in a university hospital in Riyadh, Saudi Arabia. *International Journal of Mental Health*, 25: 59–68.

[7] Srinivasa Murthy R (2000). Reaching the unreached. *The Lancet Perspective*, 356: 39.

[8] Pearson V (1992). Community and culture: a Chinese model of community care for the mentally ill. *International Journal of Social Psychiatry*, 38: 163–178.

[9] Tomov T (1999). Central and Eastern European countries. In: Thornicroft G, Tansella G, eds. *The mental health matrix: a manual to improve services.* Cambridge, Cambridge University Press: 216–227.

[10] Rezaki MS et al. (1995). Results from the Ankara centre. In: Üstün TB, Sartorius N, eds. *Mental illness in general health care: an international study.* Chichester, John Wiley & Sons: 39–55.

Table 4.1 Effects of transferring functions of the traditional mental hospital to community care

Functions of traditional mental hospital	Effects of transfer to community care
Physical assessment and treatment	May be better transferred to primary care or general health services
Active treatment for short-term and intermediate stays	Treatment maintained or improved, but results may not be generalizable
Long-term custody	Usually improved in residential homes for those who need long-term high support
Protection from exploitation	Some patients continue to be vulnerable to physical, sexual and financial exploitation
Day care and out-patient services	May be improved if local, accessible services are developed or may deteriorate if they are not; renegotiation of responsibilities is often necessary between health and social care agencies
Occupational, vocational and rehabilitation services	Improved in normal settings
Shelter, clothing, nutrition and basic income	At risk, so responsibilities and coordination must be clarified
Respite for family and carers	Usually unchanged: place of treatment at home, offset by potential for increased professional support to family
Research and training	New opportunities arise through decentralization

Source: Thornicroft G, Tansella M (2000). *Balancing community-based and hospital-based mental health care: the new agenda.* Geneva, World Health Organization (unpublished document).

tertiary care, even though a policy of de-institutionalization has been adopted it is difficult to move the money spent on hospital care to the primary care or community care level. Even if the money can be shifted out of the hospital budget, there is little guarantee that it will in fact be utilized for mental health programmes at the community level. Because of budgetary restrictions it is clear that comprehensive community care is unlikely to be a viable option without the support of primary and secondary care services.

INTEGRATING MENTAL HEALTH CARE INTO GENERAL HEALTH SERVICES

The integration of mental health care into general health services, particularly at the primary health care level, has many advantages. These include: less stigmatization of patients and staff, as mental and behavioural disorders are being seen and managed alongside physical health problems; improved screening and treatment, in particular improved detection rates for patients presenting with vague somatic complaints which are related to mental and behavioural disorders; the potential for improved treatment of the physical problems of those suffering from mental illness, and vice versa; and better treatment of mental aspects associated with "physical" problems. For the administrator, advantages include a shared infrastructure leading to cost-efficiency savings, the potential to provide universal coverage of mental health care, and the use of community resources which can partly offset the limited availability of mental health personnel.

Integration requires a careful analysis of what is and what is not possible for the treatment and care of mental problems at different levels of care. For example, early intervention strategies for alcohol are more effectively implemented at the primary care level, but acute psychosis might be better managed at a higher level to benefit from the availability of greater expertise, investigatory facilities and specialized drugs. Patients should then be referred back to the primary level for ongoing management, as primary health care workers are best placed to provide continuous support to patients and their families.

The specific ways in which mental health should be integrated into general health care will to a great extent depend on the current function and status of primary, secondary and tertiary care levels within countries' health systems. Box 4.7 summarizes experiences of integration of services in Cambodia, India and the Islamic Republic of Iran. For integration to be successful, policy-makers need to consider the following.

- General health staff must have the knowledge, skills and motivation to treat and manage patients suffering from mental disorders.
- There need to be sufficient numbers of staff with the knowledge and authority to prescribe psychotropic drugs at primary and secondary levels.
- Basic psychotropic drugs must be available at primary and secondary care levels.
- Mental health specialists are required to provide support to and monitor general health care personnel.
- Effective referral links between primary, secondary and tertiary levels of care need to be in place.
- Funds must be redistributed from tertiary to secondary and primary levels of care or new funds must be made available.
- Recording systems need to be set up to allow for continuous monitoring, evaluation and updating of integrated activities.

While it is clear that mental health should be financed from the same sources and with the same objectives for distributing the financial burden as health care in general, it is less clear what is the best way to direct funds to mental and behavioural disorders. Once funds have been raised and pooled, the issue arises of how rigidly to separate mental health from other items to be financed out of the same budget, or whether to provide a global budget for some constellation of institutions or services and allow the share used for mental health

---

Box 4.7 Integration of mental health into primary health care

Organization of mental health services in developing countries began comparatively recently. WHO supported the movement to dispense mental care within general health services in developing countries,[1] and conducted a seven-year feasibility study of integration with primary health care in Brazil, Colombia, Egypt, India, the Philippines, Senegal and Sudan.

A number of countries have used this approach to organize essential mental health services. In developing countries with limited resources, this has meant a new beginning of care for people with mental disorders. **India** started training primary health care workers in 1975, forming the basis of the National Mental Health Programme formulated in 1982. Currently the government sup-

ports 25 district level programmes in 22 states.[2] In **Cambodia**, the ministry of health trained a core group of personnel in community mental health, who in turn trained selected general medical staff at district hospitals.[3] In the **Islamic Republic of Iran**, efforts to integrate mental health care started in the late 1980s and the programme has since been extended to the whole country, with

services now covering about 20 million people.[4] Similar approaches have been adopted by countries such as Afghanistan, Malaysia, Morocco, Nepal, Pakistan,[5] Saudi Arabia, South Africa, the United Republic of Tanzania, and Zimbabwe. Some studies have been carried out to evaluate the impact of integration, but more are urgently needed.

[1] World Health Organization (1975). *Organization of mental health services in developing countries. Sixteenth report of the WHO Expert Committee on Mental Health, December 1974.* Geneva, World Health Organization (WHO Technical Report Series, No. 564).

[2] Srinivasa Murthy R (2000). Reaching the unreached. *The Lancet Perspective,* 356: 39.

[3] Somasundaram DJ et al. (1999). Starting mental health services in Cambodia. *Social Science and Medicine,* 48(8): 1029–1046.

[4] Mohit A et al. (1999). Mental health manpower development in Afghanistan: a report on a training course for primary health care physicians. *Eastern Mediterranean Health Journal,* 5: 231–240.

[5] Mubbashar MH (1999). Mental health services in rural Pakistan. In: Tansella M, Thornicroft G, eds. *Common mental disorders in primary care.* London, Routledge.

to be determined by demand, local decisions or other factors (bearing in mind that out-of-pocket spending is not pooled and is directed only by the consumer). At one extreme, line-item budgets which specify expenditure on every input for every service or programme are overly rigid and leave no discretion to administrators, so they almost guarantee inefficiency. They cannot readily be used to contract with private providers. Even within public facilities, they can lead to imbalance among inputs and make it hard to respond to changes in demand or need.

In spite of the lack of evidence, it is fair to say that these problems could probably be minimized by assigning global budgets, either to purchasing agencies which can contract out or to individual facilities. The advantages of such budgets include administrative simplicity, the encouragement of multi-agency decision-making, the encouragement of innovation via financial flexibility, and incentives for primary health care providers to collaborate with mental health care providers and to provide care at the primary care level.

However, if there is no budgeting according to end-use and no specific protection for particular services, the share going to mental health may continue to be very low, because of low apparent priority and the false impression that mental health is not important. This is a particular risk when the intention is to reform and expand mental health services relative to more established or better-funded services. To reduce that risk, a specific amount may be allocated to mental health, which cannot easily be diverted to other uses, while still allowing the managers of health facilities some flexibility in setting priorities among problems and treatments. "Ring-fencing" mental health resources in this way may be used to ensure their protection and stability over time. In particular, for countries with minimal current investment in mental health services, ring-fencing may be pertinent for indicating the priority accorded to mental health and for kick-starting a mental health programme. This need not imply a retreat from service organization, nor should it prevent mental health departments sharing in any additional funds that become available for health.

ENSURING THE AVAILABILITY OF PSYCHOTROPIC DRUGS

WHO recommends a limited set of essential drugs for the treatment and management of mental and behavioural disorders through its essential drugs list. However, it is common to find that many of these drugs are not available in developing countries. Data from the Atlas project suggest that about 25% of countries do not have commonly prescribed antipsychotic, antidepressant and antiepileptic drugs available at the primary care level.

Governments need to ensure that sufficient funds are allocated to purchase the basic essential psychotropic drugs and distribute them amongst the different levels of care, in accordance with the policy adopted. Where there is a policy of community care and integration into general health services, then not only must essential drugs be available at these levels, but also health workers need to be authorized to administer the drugs at these levels. Even where a primary care approach is adopted for the management of mental problems, a quarter of countries do not have the three essential drugs for the treatment of epilepsy, depression and schizophrenia available at the primary level. Drugs may be purchased under generic names from non-profit organizations, such as ECHO (Equipment for Charitable Hospitals Overseas) and the UNICEF Supply Division in Copenhagen, which supply drugs of good quality at low prices. In addition, WHO and Management Sciences for Health (2001) issue an annual drug price indicator guide of essential drugs, which includes addresses and prices of several reputable suppliers of different psychotropic drugs, at non-profit world-market wholesale prices.

CREATING INTERSECTORAL LINKS

Many mental disorders require psychosocial solutions. Thus links need to be established between mental health services and various community agencies at the local level so that appropriate housing, income support, disability benefits, employment, and other social service supports are mobilized on behalf of patients and in order that prevention and rehabilitation strategies can be more effectively implemented. In many poor countries, cooperation between sectors is often visible at the primary care level. In Zimbabwe, coordination between academics, public service providers and local community representatives at the primary care level led to the development of a culturally relevant community-based programme to detect, counsel and treat women suffering from depression. In the United Republic of Tanzania, an intersectoral strategy resulted in an innovative agricultural programme to rehabilitate persons suffering from mental and behavioural disorders (see Box 4.8).

CHOOSING MENTAL HEALTH STRATEGIES

Regardless of a country's economic situation, there will always seem to be too few resources to fund activities, services and treatments. For mental health, as for health generally, choices must be made among a large number of services and a wide range of prevention and promotion strategies. These choices will, of course, have different effects on different mental health conditions and different population groups in need. But it is important to recognize that choices have ultimately to be made among key strategies, rather than among specific disorders.

What is known about the costs and results of different interventions, particularly in poor countries, is still quite limited. Where evidence does exist, great care must be taken in applying conclusions to settings other than the one that generated the evidence: costs can differ greatly, and so may outcomes, depending on the capacity of the health system to deliver the intervention. Even if more were known, there is no simple formula for deciding which interventions to emphasize, much less for determining how much to spend on each of them. Private out-of-pocket spending is under no one's control but that of the consumers, and private prepayment for mental health care is quite low in all but a few countries.

The crucial decision for governments is how to use public funds. Cost-effectiveness is an important consideration in several circumstances, but is never the only criterion that matters. Public funding also should take account of whether an intervention is a public or partly public good, meaning that it confers costs or benefits on people other than those receiving the service. Although maximizing efficiency in the allocation of resources is desir-

---

Box 4.8 Intersectoral links for mental health

In the United Republic of Tanzania, psychiatric agricultural rehabilitation villages encapsulate an intersectoral response by local communities, the mental health sector, and the traditional healing sector to the treatment and rehabilitation of people with severe mental illness in rural areas.[1] Pa-tients and relatives live within an existing village population of farmers, fishermen and craftsmen, and are treated by both the medical and traditional healing sectors. Mental health nurses, nursing assistants, and local artisans supervise therapeutic activities; a psychiatrist and a medical social worker provide weekly assistance and consultation; and the involvement of traditional healers depends on the expressed needs of individual patients and relatives. There are also plans for a more formal collaboration between traditional and mental health sectors, including regular meetings and seminars. Traditional healers have participated in community mental health training programmes and shared their knowledge and skills in treating patients; they could play an increased role in managing stress-related disorders in the community.

[1] Kilonzo GP, Simmons N (1998). Development of mental health services in Tanzania: a reappraisal for the future. *Social Science and Medicine*, 47: 419–428.

able, governments will need to trade some efficiency gains to reallocate resources in the pursuit of equity.

While, in general, mental health services should be evaluated and decisions made about public spending on the same basis as for other health services, there appear to be certain significant features that distinguish at least some of the possible interventions. One is that there can be large benefits to controlling some mental disorders. In contrast to the benefits that arise from control of communicable diseases, where treating one case may prevent others and immunization of most of the susceptible population also protects the non-immunized, the benefits arising from mental health care often appear in non-health forms, such as reduced accidents and injuries in the case of alcohol use or lower cost of some social services. These cannot be captured in a cost-effectiveness analysis but require some judgement of the overall social benefit from both health and non-health gains.

Another possibly significant difference derives from the chronic nature of some mental disorders. This makes them – like some chronic physical conditions and unlike acute, un-predictable medical needs – difficult to cover via private insurance and therefore especially appropriate for public insurance, whether explicit (as in social security) or implicit (via gen-eral taxation). Finally, while many health problems contribute to poverty, long-term mental disorders are particularly associated with inability to work and therefore with poverty, so that attention to the poor should be emphasized in budgets for mental health services.

Difficult as it may be to work out priorities from the variety of relevant criteria, any rational consideration of the issues just mentioned offers the opportunity to improve on arbitrary or merely historical allocation of resources. This is especially true if mental health care is to get substantially more public resources: expansion in equal proportions of what-ever is currently financed is unlikely to be either efficient or equitable. Needs-based alloca-tion is a more equitable means for distributing resources, but it presupposes agreement on a definition of "need". Moreover, needs by themselves are not priorities, because not every need corresponds to an effective intervention – apart from the fact that what people need, and what they want or demand, may not coincide. This is a problem even for physical health problems when the consumer is competent to express his or her demand; it be-comes more complicated when some mental disorder limits that competence.

As emphasized above, financing intended for mental health has actually to be devoted to services, and whether this occurs may depend on how funds are organized through budgets or purchasing agreements. One technique for making that connection is to specify some mental health services, chosen on the basis of the criteria just described, as part of an overall package of basic or essential interventions which the public sector in effect promises to finance, whether or not the budget specifies the amount to be devoted to each such service. The same approach can in principle be used in the regulation of private insurance, requiring insurers to include certain mental health services in the basic package that all clients' policies will cover. Because insurers have a strong incentive to select clients on the basis of risk (and potential clients have a strong incentive to hide their known risks and purchase insurance against them), it is much harder to enforce such a package in the pri-vate than in the public sector. Nonetheless some countries – Brazil and Chile are examples among middle-income countries – require private insurers to offer the same services that are guaranteed by public finance. Whether such a course is feasible in much poorer coun-tries is doubtful because of the much lower coverage of private insurance and the lower regulatory capacity of governments. Deciding how far to try to impose public priorities on private payers or providers is always a complex question, perhaps more so for mental health than for physical problems. Data from Atlas show that insurance as a primary source of funding for mental health care is present only in about one-fifth of countries.

PURCHASING VERSUS PROVIDING: PUBLIC AND PRIVATE ROLES

The foregoing discussion emphasizes the financial role of the public sector, even when it accounts for only a small share of total health spending, because that is where the desirable reforms in mental health seem easiest to undertake and because some features of mental health services are particularly suited to public funding. But there is no necessary connection between public money and public provision, although traditionally most governments have spent most or all of their health funds on their own providing institutions. Both because of the move towards decentralization and because giving public facilities a monopoly on public resources removes any competitive stimulus to efficiency or more responsive service, there is an increasing split in some countries between purchasing and provision of services, (WHO 2000c, Chapter 3).

While the theoretical benefits of introducing more competition and regulation as substitutes for direct public provision are clear, evidence on the success of such arrangements is still scanty. Developing countries often lack the resources and experience to regulate contractual arrangements between health care purchasers and providers, and to enforce the delivery of the services agreed upon in the contract when these services are perceived to be a low priority by the provider. Without such controls there is great potential for waste and even fraud. If this is the case for contracts with service providers for general health services, mental health services may be still more difficult to contract effectively because of the greater difficulty of measuring outcomes. In countries where mental health services have been previously unavailable or were only provided directly by the health department, a separate detailed contract for mental health services may be necessary. For all these reasons, separating funding from providing should be approached cautiously where mental health services are concerned. Nonetheless it is worth considering whenever there are nongovernmental or local government providers able to take over provision and there is enough capacity to supervise them. In many countries, public health outpatient facilities offer no mental health services because of a funding emphasis on hospital inpatient care. Separation of funding and provision may therefore be especially valuable as a way to promote the desirable shift from public psychiatric hospitals to care provided in the community. Shifting the public budget priority without involving nongovernmental providers may even be essentially impossible because of internal resistance to innovation and lack of the required skills and experience.

Where substantial private provision exists and is paid for privately without public funding or regulation, several problems arise that call for the exercise of stewardship. There is likely to be inadequate referral between unregulated mental health service providers such as traditional healers and outpatient mental health services located in primary care and district hospitals. The poor may consume large amounts of low-quality mental health care from unregulated private mental health care providers such as drug sellers, traditional healers, and unqualified therapists. The inability of government health departments to enforce the regulation of private outpatient services leaves users vulnerable to financial exploitation and ineffective treatment procedures for mental ailments that are not addressed by the public health system. Contracts for primary and secondary providers, guidelines for mental health service items and costs, and accreditation of the different ambulatory mental health care providers are potential responses to these problems that do not require governments to expand spending massively or take on all the responsibility for provision.

Governments should also consider regulating specific provider groups within the informal health sector, such as traditional healers. Such regulation might include the introduction of practice registration to protect patients from harmful interventions and to prevent fraud and financial exploitation. Considerable progress in integrating traditional medicine into general health policy is being made in China, Viet Nam and Malaysia (Bodekar 2001).

Managed care, an important health care delivery system in the United States, combines the role of purchasing and financing health care for a defined population. A major concern is that managed care concentrates more on cost reduction than on service quality, and that it shifts the costs of care, for those who cannot afford insurance, from the public health system to families or charitable institutions (Hoge et al. 1998; Gittelman 1998). For mental and behavioural disorders, managed care efforts to date have often failed to provide an adequate response to the need for medical treatment combined with a long-term social support and rehabilitation strategy, although there have been some notable exceptions. Furthermore, the expertise, skills, and comprehensiveness of services required by a managed care system are beyond the current capabilities of most developing countries (Talbott 1999).

DEVELOPING HUMAN RESOURCES

In developing countries, the lack of specialists and health workers with the knowledge and skills to manage mental and behavioural disorders is an important barrier to providing treatment and care.

If health systems are to advance, time and energy need to be invested in assessing the numbers and types of professionals and workers required in the years to come. The ratio of mental health specialists to general health workers will vary according to existing resources and approaches to care. With the integration of mental health care into the general health system, the demand for generalists with training in mental health will increase and that for specialists will decrease, although a critical mass of mental health specialists will always be required to effectively treat and prevent these disorders.

There is a wide disparity in the type and numbers of the mental health workforce throughout the world. The median number of psychiatrists varies from 0.06 per 100 000 population in low income countries to 9 per 100 000 in high income countries (Figure 4.4). For psychiatric nurses, the median ranges from 0.1 per 100 000 in low income countries to 33.5 per 100 000 in high income countries (Figure 4.5). In almost half the world, there is fewer than one neurologist per million people. The situation for providers of care for children and adolescents is far worse.

The health workforce likely to be involved with mental health consists of general physicians, neurologists and psychiatrists, community and primary health care workers, allied mental health professionals (such as nurses, occupational therapists, psychologists and social workers), as well as other groups such as the clergy and traditional healers. Traditional healers are the main source of assistance for at least 80% of rural inhabitants in developing countries. They can be active case finders, and can facilitate referral and provide counselling, monitoring and follow-up care. The adoption of a system of integrated community-based care will require a redefinition of the roles of many health providers. A general health care worker may now have the additional responsibility of identifying and managing mental and behavioural disorders in the community, including screening and early intervention for tobacco, alcohol and other drug use, and a psychiatrist previously working in an institution may need to provide more training and supervision when moved to a community setting.

Figure 4.4 Number of psychiatrists per 100 000 population, 2000[a]

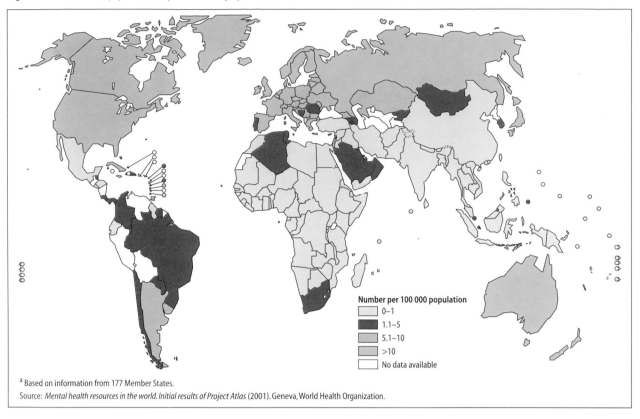

Number per 100 000 population
- 0–1
- 1.1–5
- 5.1–10
- >10
- No data available

[a] Based on information from 177 Member States.

Source: *Mental health resources in the world. Initial results of Project Atlas* (2001). Geneva, World Health Organization.

Decentralization of mental health services is also likely to have an impact on roles and responsibilities through the transfer of management and administration responsibilities to the local level. Redefinition of roles needs to be explicit, in order to ensure that new responsibilities are adopted more readily. Training is also required to provide the skills necessary to carry out new roles and responsibilities. Undoubtedly, the changing of roles will bring issues of power and control to the forefront, and these will act as barriers to change. For example, psychiatrists perceive and resist their own loss of power when other less experienced health workers are given the authority to manage mental disorders.

In developed and developing countries alike, undergraduate medical curricula need to be updated to ensure that graduating physicians are skilled in diagnosing and treating persons suffering from mental disorders. Recently Sri Lanka expanded the duration of training in psychiatry and included it as an examination subject in undergraduate medical education. Allied health professionals, such as nurses and social workers, require training to understand mental and behavioural disorders and the range of treatment options available, focusing on those areas most relevant to their work in the field. All courses should incorporate the application of evidence-based psychosocial strategies, and skill-building in the areas of administration and management, policy development and research methods. In developing countries, higher level educational opportunities are not always available; instead training is often undertaken in other countries. This has not always led to satisfactory outcomes: many trainees sent abroad do not return to their own countries and consequently their expertise is lost to the developing society. This needs to be addressed in the long term, through the setting up of centres of excellence for training and education within countries.

Figure 4.5 Number of psychiatric nurses per 100 000 population, 2000[a]

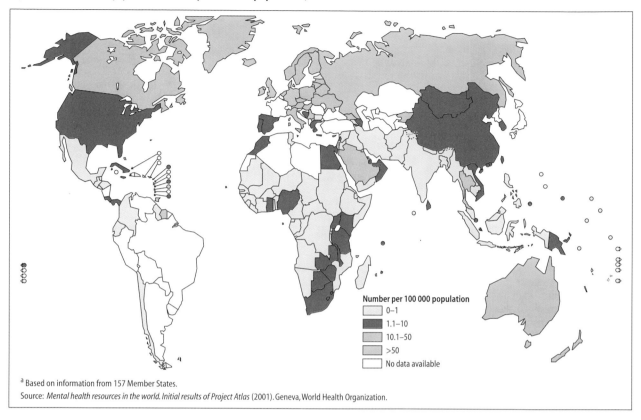

Number per 100 000 population
- 0–1
- 1.1–10
- 10.1–50
- >50
- No data available

[a] Based on information from 157 Member States.

Source: *Mental health resources in the world. Initial results of Project Atlas* (2001). Geneva, World Health Organization.

One promising approach is the use of the Internet to provide training and quick feedback by specialists on clinical diagnosis and management matters. Internet access is increasing rapidly in developing countries. Three years ago, only 12 countries in Africa had Internet access; now it is available in all African capital cities. Training must now include the use of information technology (Fraser et al. 2000).

PROMOTING MENTAL HEALTH

A wide range of strategies is available to improve mental health and prevent mental disorders. These strategies can also contribute to the reduction of other problems such as youth delinquency, child abuse, school dropout and work days lost to illness.

The most appropriate entry point for mental health promotion will depend both on needs and on the social and cultural context. The scope and level of activities will vary from local through to national levels as will the specific types of public health action taken (development of services, policy, dissemination of information, advocacy and so on). Examples are provided below of different entry points for intervention.

Interventions targeting factors determining or maintaining ill-health. Psychosocial and cognitive development of babies and infants depend upon their interaction with their parents. Programmes that enhance the quality of these relations can substantially improve the emotional, social, cognitive and physical development of children. For example, the USA programme Steps Towards Effective Enjoyable Parenting (STEEP) targeted first-time mothers and others with parenting problems, particularly in families with a low educational level (Erickson 1989). There was evidence of reductions in anxiety and depression in mothers, better-organized family life, and the creation of more stimulating environments for children.

Interventions targeting population groups. By 2025, there will be 1.2 billion people in the world who are over 60 years of age, close to three-quarters of them in the developing world. But if ageing is to be a positive experience it must be accompanied by improvements in the quality of life of those who have reached old age.

Interventions targeting particular settings. Schools are crucial in preparing children for life, but they need to be more involved in fostering healthy social and emotional development. Teaching life-skills such as problem-solving, critical thinking, communication, interpersonal relations, empathy, and methods to cope with emotions will enable children and adolescents to develop sound and positive mental health (Mishara & Ystgaard 2000).

A child-friendly school policy which encourages tolerance and equality between boys and girls and different ethnic, religious and social groups will promote a sound psychosocial environment (WHO 1990). It promotes active involvement and cooperation, avoids the use of physical punishment, and does not tolerate bullying. It helps to establish connections between school and family life, encourages creativity as well as academic abilities, and promotes the self-esteem and self-confidence of children.

Raising public awareness

The single most important barrier to overcome in the community is the stigma and associated discrimination towards persons suffering from mental and behavioural disorders.

Tackling stigma and discrimination requires a multilevel approach involving education of health professionals and workers, the closing down of psychiatric institutions which serve to maintain and reinforce stigma, the provision of mental health services in the community, and the implementation of legislation to protect the rights of the mentally ill. Fighting stigma also requires public information campaigns to educate and inform the community about the nature, extent and impact of mental disorders in order to dispel common myths and encourage more positive attitudes and behaviours.

Role of the mass media

The various forms of the mass media can be used to foster more positive community attitudes and behaviours towards people with mental disorders. Action can be taken to monitor, remove or prevent the use of images, messages or stories in the media that potentially would have negative consequences for persons suffering from mental and behavioural disorders. The media can also be used to inform the public, to persuade or motivate individual attitude and behaviour change, and to advocate for change in social, structural and economic factors that influence mental and behavioural disorders. Advertising, although expensive, is useful for increasing awareness of issues and events and for neutralizing misperceptions. Publicity is a relatively cheaper way to create news to attract the attention of the public and to frame issues and actions to achieve advocacy. The placement of educational health or social messages in the entertainment media (so-called "edutainment"), is useful for promoting change in attitudes, beliefs and behaviours.

Examples of public information campaigns which have used the media to overcome stigma include "Changing minds – every family in the land" by the Royal College of Psychiatrists in the UK and the World Psychiatric Association's campaign "Open the doors" (see Box 4.9).

The Internet is a powerful tool for communication and accessing mental health information. It is increasingly being used as a means to inform and educate patients, students, health professionals, consumer groups, nongovernmental organizations and the population at large about mental health; to host self-help and discussion groups; and to provide clinical care. With the Internet as source of information, the community will be more knowledgeable and as a consequence will have greater expectations regarding the treatment and care they receive from providers. On the negative side, they will have to analyse and understand a vast amount of complex literature, of varying degrees of accuracy (Griffiths & Christensen 2000). Increasingly, Internet users will expect to receive easy access to treatment and consultation from health professionals, including mental health care providers, ranging from simple inquiries to more sophisticated video-based consultations or telemedicine.

Major challenges are to use this information technology to benefit mental health in developing countries. This requires improved access to the Internet (fewer than one million people of a total of 700 million have access to it in Africa) and the availability of mental health information in a variety of languages.

USING COMMUNITY RESOURCES TO STIMULATE CHANGE

Although stigma and discrimination have their origin in the community, it should not be forgotten that the community can also be an important resource and setting for tackling their causes and effects and, more generally, for improving the treatment and care provided to persons suffering from mental and behavioural disorders.

The role of the community can range from the provision of self-help and mutual aid to lobbying for changes in mental health care and resources, carrying out educational activities, participating in the monitoring and evaluation of care, and advocacy to change attitudes and reduce stigma.

Nongovernmental organizations are also a valuable community resource for mental health. They are often more sensitive to local realities than are centrally driven programmes,

---

Box 4.9 Fighting stigma

"Open the doors" is the first-ever global programme against stigma and discrimination associated with schizophrenia. Launched by the World Psychiatric Association in 1999,[1,2] the goals are to increase awareness and knowledge about the nature of schizophrenia and treatment options; to improve public attitudes to people who have or have had schizophrenia and their families; and to generate action to eliminate stigma, discrimination and prejudice.

The Association has produced a step-by-step guide to developing an anti-stigma programme, and reports on the experience of countries that have undertaken the programme, as well as collecting information from around the world on other anti-stigma efforts. The materials have been put to trial use in Austria, Canada, China, Egypt, Germany, Greece, India, Italy and Spain, and other sites are starting to work on the programme as well. In each of the sites, a programme group has been established involving repre-

sentatives of government and nongovernmental organizations, journalists, health care professionals, members of patient and family organizations, and others committed to fighting stigma and discrimination. The results of programmes from different countries are added to the global database, so that future efforts benefit from previous experience. In addition, the Association has produced a compendium of the latest information available on the diagnosis and treatment of schizophrenia, and strategies for re-

integration of affected individuals into the community.

The stigma attached to schizophrenia creates a vicious cycle of alienation and discrimination – leading to social isolation, inability to work, alcohol or drug abuse, homelessness, or excessive institutionalization – which decreases the chance of recovery and normal life. "Open the doors" will allow people with schizophrenia to return to their families and to school or the workplace, and to face the future with hope.

[1] Sartorius N (1997). Fighting schizophrenia and its stigma. A new World Psychiatric Association educational programme. *British Journal of Psychiatry*, 170: 297.
[2] Sartorius N (1998a). Stigma: what can psychiatrists do about it? *The Lancet*, 352(9133): 1058–1059.

and are usually strongly committed to innovation and change. International nongovernmental organizations help in the exchange of experiences and function as pressure groups, while nongovernmental organizations in countries are responsible for many of the innovative programmes and solutions at the local level. They often play an extremely important role in the absence of a formal or well-functioning mental health system, filling the gap between community needs and available community services and strategies (see Box 4.10).

Consumer groups have emerged as a powerful, vocal and active force, often dissatisfied with the established provision of care and treatment. These groups have been instrumental in reforming mental health (WHO 1989). There now exist in many parts of the world a large number of consumer associations with interests, commitments and involvement in the mental health area. They range from informal loose groupings to fully fledged constitutionally and legally created organizations. Although they have differing aims and objectives, they all strongly advocate the consumer's viewpoint.

Authorities responsible for delivering services, treatment and care are accountable to the consumers of the system. One important step towards achieving accountability is to involve consumers in the creation of services, in reviewing hospital standards, and in the development and implementation of policy and legislation.

In many developing countries, families play a key role in caring for the mentally ill and in many ways they are the primary care providers. With the gradual closure of mental hospitals in countries with developed systems of care, responsibilities are also shifting to families. Families can have a positive or negative impact by virtue of their understanding, knowledge, skills and ability to care for the person affected by mental disorders. For these reasons, an important community-based strategy is to help families to understand the illness, encourage medication compliance, recognize early signs of relapse, and ensure swift

---

Box 4.10 The Geneva Initiative

The Geneva Initiative on Psychiatry was founded in 1980 to combat the political abuse of psychiatry as a tool of repression. Despite its name, the international Initiative is based in the Netherlands.

The All-Union Society of Psychiatrists and Neuropathologists (AUSPN) of the former USSR withdrew from the World Psychiatric Association (WPA) in early 1983 in response to pressure from campaigns by the Geneva Initiative, and in 1989 the WPA Congress set strict conditions for its return. The Russian Federation acknowledged that psychiatry had been abused for political purposes and invited

the WPA to send a team of observers to Russia. At the same time, increasing numbers of psychiatrists contacted the Geneva Initiative to assist them in reforming mental health care. By then, the situation was changing dramatically: in the preceding two years, virtually all political prisoners had been released from prisons, camps, exile and psychiatric hospitals.

Between 1989 and 1993 the Initiative concentrated on a few Eastern European countries, particularly Romania and Ukraine. It became clear that a new approach to the mental health reform movement was needed. Though many reforms had been undertaken throughout

the region and many people had acquired new skills and knowledge, no links existed among the reformers, and there was a lack of trust and unity. With financial support from the Soros Foundation, the first meeting of Reformers in Psychiatry was organized in Bratislava, Slovakia, in September 1993. Since then, over 20 similar network meetings have taken place.

Today, the Network of Reformers unites some 500 mental health reformers in 29 countries of Central and Eastern Europe and the newly independent states, and has links with over 100 nongovernmental mental health organizations. Its members are psychiatrists, psy-

chologists, psychiatric nurses, social workers, sociologists, lawyers, relatives of people with mental disorders, and a growing number of consumers of mental health services. Mostly through this Network, the Geneva Initiative now operates in over 20 countries, where it manages about 150 projects.

The Geneva Initiative strives for structural improvement, and thus concentrates on programmes concerned with reform of policy, institutional care and education. It aims to combat inertia and to achieve sustainability and maintain funding. Last year, the Initiative was awarded the Geneva Prize for Human Rights in Psychiatry.

More information about the Initiative can be found on the web site http://www.geneva-initiative.org/geneva/index.htm

resolution of crisis. This will lead to better recovery, and reduce social and personal disability. Visiting community nurses and other health workers can provide an important supportive role, as can networks of self-help groups for families and direct financial support.

A couple of cautionary notes are warranted. First, the erosion of the extended family in developing countries, coupled with migration to cities, presents a challenge to planners to utilize this resource for the care of patients. Second, when the family environment is not conducive to good quality care and support, and in fact may be damaging, a family solution may not be a viable option.

INVOLVING OTHER SECTORS

War, conflict, disasters, unplanned urbanization, and poverty are not only important determinants of mental ill-health but are also significant barriers to reducing the treatment gap. For example, war and conflict can destroy national economies and health and welfare systems, and can traumatize entire populations. With poverty comes an increased need for health and community services but a limited budget to develop comprehensive mental health services at the national level and a reduced ability to pay for these services at the individual level.

Mental health policy can partially address the effects of environmental determinants by meeting the special needs of vulnerable groups and ensuring that strategies are in place to prevent exclusion. But because many of the macro-determinants of mental health cut across almost all government departments, the extent of improvement in mental health of a population is also in part determined by the policies of other government departments. In other words, other government departments are responsible for some of the factors involved in mental and behavioural disorders, and should take responsibility for some of the solutions.

Intersectoral collaboration between government departments is fundamental in order for mental health policies to benefit from mainstream government programmes (see Table 4.2). In addition, mental health input is required to ensure that all government activities and policies contribute to and do not detract from mental health. Policies should be analysed for their mental health implications before being implemented, and all government policies should address the specific needs and issues of persons suffering from mental disorders. Some examples are provided below.

LABOUR AND EMPLOYMENT

The work environment should be free from all forms of discrimination as well as sexual harassment. Acceptable working conditions have to be defined and mental health services provided, either directly or indirectly through employee assistance programmes. Policies should maximize employment opportunities for the population as a whole, and retain people in the workforce, particularly because of the association between job loss and the increased risk of mental disorders and suicide. Work should be used as a mechanism to reintegrate persons with mental disorders into the community. People with severe mental disorders have higher unemployment rates than people with physical disabilities. Government policy can be instrumental in providing incentives for employers to employ persons with severe mental disorders and enforcing anti-discrimination policy. In some countries, employers are obliged to hire a certain percentage of disabled persons as part of their workforce. If they fail to do so, a fine can be imposed.

Table 4.2 Intersectoral collaboration for mental health

Government sector	Opportunities for improving mental health
Labour and employment	• Create a positive work environment free from discrimination, with acceptable working conditions and employee assistance programmes • Integrate people with severe mental illness into the workforce • Adopt policies that encourage high levels of employment, maintain people within the workforce, and assist the unemployed
Commerce	• Adopt policies of economic reform which reduce relative poverty as well as absolute poverty • Analyse and correct any potentially negative impact of economic reform on unemployment rates
Education	• Implement policies to prevent attrition before completion of secondary school education • Introduce anti-discrimination policies in schools • Incorporate life skills into the curriculum, to ensure child-friendly schools • Address the requirements of children with special needs, e.g. those with learning disabilities
Housing	• Give priority to housing people with mental disorders • Establish housing facilities (such as halfway houses) • Prevent discrimination in location of housing • Prevent geographical segregation
Social welfare services	• Consider the presence and severity of mental illness as priority factors for the receipt of social welfare benefits • Make benefits available to family members when they are the main carers • Train the staff of social welfare services
Criminal justice system	• Prevent the inappropriate imprisonment of people with mental disorders • Make treatment for mental and behavioural disorders available within prisons • Reduce the mental health consequences of confinement • Train staff throughout the criminal justice system

COMMERCE AND ECONOMICS

Some economic policies may negatively affect the poor, or lead to increased rates of mental disorders and suicide. Many of the economic reforms under way in countries have as a major goal the reduction of poverty. Given the association between poverty and mental health, it might be expected that these reforms would reduce mental problems. However, mental disorders are not only related to absolute poverty levels but also to relative poverty. The mental health imperatives are clear: inequalities must be reduced as part of strategies to increase absolute levels of income.

A second challenge is the potential adverse consequences of economic reform on unemployment rates. In many countries undergoing major economic restructuring, for example, Hungary (Kopp et al. 2000) and Thailand (Tangchararoensathien et al. 2000), reform has led to high job losses and an associated increase in the rates of mental disorders and suicides. Any economic policy involving restructuring must be evaluated in terms of its potential impact on employment rates. If there are potentially adverse consequences, then these policies need to be reconsidered or strategies need to be put in place to minimize the impact.

EDUCATION

An important determinant of mental health is education. While current efforts focus on increasing the numbers of children attending and completing primary school, the main risk for mental health is more likely to result from a lack of secondary-school education (10–12 years of schooling) (Patel 2001). Strategies for education therefore need to prevent attrition prior to the completion of secondary school. The relevance of the type of education offered, freedom from discrimination at school, and the needs of special groups, for example children with learning disabilities, also need to be considered.

HOUSING

Housing policy can support mental health policy by giving priority to mentally ill people in state housing schemes, providing subsidized housing schemes and, where practical, mandating local authorities to establish a range of housing facilities such as halfway homes and long-stay supported homes. Most importantly, housing legislation must include provisions to prevent the geographical segregation of mentally ill people. This requires specific provisions to prevent discrimination in siting and allocation of housing as well as health facilities for persons with mental disorders.

OTHER SOCIAL WELFARE SERVICES

The type, range and extent of other social welfare services varies across and within countries and is partly dependent on levels of income and the general attitude of the community towards groups in need.

Policies for social welfare benefits and services should incorporate a number of strategies. First, the disability resulting from mental illness should be one of the factors taken into account in setting priorities among groups receiving social welfare benefits and services. Second, under some circumstances, social welfare benefits should also be available to families that provide the care and support to family members suffering from mental and behavioural disorders. Third, staff working in the various social services need to be equipped with the knowledge and skills to recognize and assist people with mental disorders as part of their daily work. In particular they should be able to evaluate when and how to refer the more severe problems to specialized services. Fourth, welfare benefits and services need to be mobilized for groups likely to be adversely affected by the implementation of economic policy.

CRIMINAL JUSTICE SYSTEM

People with mental disorders often come into contact with the criminal justice system. In general, there is an over-representation of people with mental disorders and vulnerable groups in prisons, in a number of cases because of lack of services, because their behaviour is seen as disorderly and because of other factors such as drug-related crime and driving under the influence of alcohol. Policies should be put in place to prevent the inappropriate imprisonment of the mentally ill and to facilitate their referral or transfer to treatment centres instead. Furthermore, treatment and care for mental and behavioural disorders should be routinely available within prisons, even when imprisonment is appropriate. International standards with regard to the treatment of prisoners are set out in the Standard Minimum Rules for the Treatment of Prisoners which provide that the services of at least one qualified medical officer "who should have some knowledge of psychiatry" shall be available at every institution (adopted by the First United Nations Congress on the Prevention of Crime and the Treatment of Prisoners in 1955 and approved by the Economic and Social Council in 1957 and 1977).

Policy concerning the confinement of vulnerable groups needs to be examined in relation to the increased risk of suicide, and there needs to be a training strategy to improve the knowledge and skills of staff in the criminal justice system to enable them to manage mental and behavioural disorders.

PROMOTING RESEARCH

Although knowledge of mental and behavioural disorders has increased over the years, there still remain many unknown variables which contribute to the development of mental disorders, their course and their effective treatment. Alliances between public health agencies and research institutions in different countries will facilitate the generation of knowledge to help in understanding better the epidemiology of mental disorders, and the efficacy, effectiveness and cost-effectiveness of treatments, services and policies.

EPIDEMIOLOGICAL RESEARCH

Epidemiological data are essential for setting priorities within health and within mental health, and for designing and evaluating public health interventions. Yet there is a paucity of information on prevalence and the burden of major mental and behavioural disorders in all countries, particularly in developing countries. Similarly, longitudinal studies examining the course of major mental and behavioural disorders and their relationship with psychosocial, genetic, economic and other environmental determinants are lacking. Epidemiology, amongst other things, is also an important tool for advocacy, but the fact remains that many countries lack data to support advocacy for mental health.

TREATMENT, PREVENTION AND PROMOTION OUTCOME RESEARCH

The burden of mental and behavioural disorders will only be reduced if effective interventions are developed and disseminated. Research is needed to develop more effective drugs which are specific in their action and which have fewer adverse side-effects, more effective psychological and behavioural treatments, and more effective prevention and promotion programmes. Research is also needed on their cost-effectiveness. More knowledge is required to understand what treatment, either singly or in combination, works best and for whom. Adherence to a treatment, prevention or promotion programme can directly affect outcomes, and research is also needed to help understand those factors affecting adherence. This would include examination of factors related to: the beliefs, attitudes and behaviours of patients and providers; the mental and behavioural disorder itself; the complexity of the treatment regime; the service delivery system, including access and treatment affordability; and some of the broad determinants of mental health and ill-health, for example, poverty.

There remains a knowledge gap concerning the efficacy and effectiveness of a range of pharmacological, psychological and psychosocial interventions. While *efficacy research* refers to the examination of an intervention's effect under highly controlled experimental conditions, *effectiveness research* examines the effects of interventions in those settings or conditions in which the intervention will ultimately be delivered. Where there is an established knowledge base concerning the efficacy of treatments, as is the case for a number of psychotropic drugs, there needs to be a shift in research emphasis towards the conduct of effectiveness research. In addition, there is an urgent need to carry out *implementation or dissemination research* into those factors likely to enhance the uptake and utilization of effective interventions in the community.

POLICY AND SERVICE RESEARCH

Mental health systems are undergoing major reforms in many countries, including de-institutionalization, the development of community-based services, and integration into the overall health system. Interestingly, these reforms were initially stimulated by ideology, the development of new pharmacological and psychotherapeutic treatment models, and the belief that alternative forms of community treatment would be more cost-effective. Fortunately there is now an evidence base, derived from a number of controlled studies, demonstrating the effectiveness of these policy objectives. Most of the research to date has, however, been generated in industrialized countries and it is questionable whether results can be generalized to developing countries. Research is therefore needed to guide reform activities in developing countries.

Given the critical importance of human resources for administering treatments and delivering services, research needs to examine the training requirements for mental health providers. In particular, there is a need for controlled research on the longer term impact of training strategies, and the differential effectiveness of training strategies for different health providers working at different levels of the health system.

Research is also needed to understand better the important role played by the informal sector and if, how and in what ways the involvement of the traditional healers can either enhance or adversely affect treatment outcomes. For example, how can primary health care staff better collaborate with traditional healers in order to improve access, identification and successful treatment of persons suffering from mental and behavioural disorders? More research is required to understand better the effects of different types of policy decisions on access, equity and treatment outcomes, both overall and for the most disadvantaged groups. Examples of research areas include the type of contracting arrangement between purchasers and providers that would lead to better mental health service delivery and patient outcomes, the impact of different methods of provider reimbursement schemes on access and use of mental health services, and the impact of integrating budgets for mental health into general health financing systems.

ECONOMIC RESEARCH

Economic evaluations of treatment, prevention and promotion strategies will provide useful information to support rational planning and choice of interventions. Although there have been some economic evaluations of interventions for mental and behavioural disorders (for example, schizophrenia, depressive disorders and dementia), economic evaluations of interventions in general tend to be scarce. Again the overwhelming majority come from industrialized countries.

In all countries, there is a need for more research on the costs of mental illness and for economic evaluations of treatment, prevention and promotion programmes.

RESEARCH IN DEVELOPING COUNTRIES AND CROSS-CULTURAL COMPARISONS

In many developing countries there is a notable lack of scientific research on mental health epidemiology, services, treatment, prevention and promotion, and policy. Without such research, there is no rational basis to guide advocacy, planning and intervention (Sartorius 1998b, Okasha & Karam 1998).

Despite many similarities of mental problems and services across countries, the cultural context in which they occur can differ substantially. Just as programmes need to be culturally informed, so does research. Research tools and methods should not be imported from one country to another without careful analysis of the influence and effect of cultural factors on their reliability and validity.

WHO has developed a number of transcultural research tools and methods including the Present State Examination (PSE), Schedule for Comprehensive Assessment in Neuropsychiatry (SCAN), Composite International Diagnostic Interview (CIDI), Self Reporting Questionnaire (SRQ), International Personality Disorder Examination (IPDE), Diagnostic Criteria for Research (ICD-10DCR), World Health Organization Quality of Life Instrument (WHOQOL), and World Health Organization Disability Assessment Schedule (WHODAS) (Sartorius & Janca 1996). These and other scientific tools need to be further developed to allow valid international comparisons that will help in understanding the commonalities and differences in the nature of mental disorders and their management across different cultures.

One lesson of the past 50 years is that tackling mental disorders involves not only public health but also science and politics. What can be achieved by good public health policy and science can be destroyed by politics. If the political environment is supportive of mental health, science is still needed to advance understanding of the complex causes of mental disorders, and to improve their treatment.

CHAPTER FIVE

The Way Forward

Governments have a responsibility to give priority to mental health. In addition, international support is essential for many countries to initiate mental health programmes. The actions to be taken in each country will depend on the resources available and the current status of mental health care. In general, the report recommends: providing treatment for mental disorders within primary care; ensuring that psychotropic drugs are available; replacing large custodial mental hospitals by community care facilities backed by general hospital psychiatric beds and home care support; launching public awareness campaigns to overcome stigma and discrimination; involving communities, families and consumers in decision-making on policies and services; establishing national policies, programmes and legislation; training mental health professionals; linking mental health with other social sectors; monitoring mental health; and supporting research.

5

THE WAY FORWARD

PROVIDING EFFECTIVE SOLUTIONS

*T*his report has shown that there have been major advances in the understanding of mental health and its inseparable relationship with physical health. This new understanding makes a public health approach to mental health not only desirable, but feasible.

This report has also described the magnitude and burden of mental disorders, establishing that they are common – affecting at least a quarter of all people at some time during their lives – and occur in all societies. Notably, it has shown that mental disorders are even more common among the poor, the elderly, people affected by conflicts and disasters, and those who are physically ill. The burden on these people, and their families, in terms of human suffering, disability and economic costs, is massive.

Effective solutions for mental disorders are available. Advances in medical and psychosocial treatment mean that most individuals and families can be helped. Some mental disorders can be prevented, while most can be treated. Enlightened mental health policy and legislation – supported by training of professionals and adequate and sustainable financing – can help deliver appropriate services to those who need them at all levels of health care.

Only a few countries have adequate mental health resources. Some have almost none. The already large inequalities between and within countries in terms of overall health care are even greater for mental health care. Urban populations, and in particular the rich, have the greatest access, leaving essential services beyond the reach of vast populations. And for the mentally ill, human rights violations are commonplace.

There is a clear need for global and national initiatives to address these issues.

The recommendations for action contained here are based on two levels of evidence. The first is the cumulative experience of developing mental health care across many countries at various resource levels. Some of this experience has been illustrated earlier in Chapters 3 and 4, and includes the observation of successes and failures of initiatives, many of them supported by WHO, in a wide variety of settings.

The second level of evidence comes from scientific research available in the international and national literature. Though operational research in mental health service development is in its infancy, some initial evidence is available on the benefits of mental health programme development. Most of the available research is from high income countries, though some studies have been done in low income countries during recent years.

Actions can have benefits at many levels. These include direct benefits of services in alleviating the symptoms associated with mental disorders, decreasing the overall burden of these diseases by reducing mortality (for example, from suicide) and disability, and in improving the functioning and quality of life of sufferers and their families. There is also the possibility of economic benefits (through enhanced productivity) by providing timely services, though the evidence for this is still scanty.

Countries have the responsibility to give priority to mental health in their health planning and to implement the recommendations given below. In addition, international support is essential for many countries to initiate mental health programmes. This support from development agencies should include technical assistance as well as funding.

OVERALL RECOMMENDATIONS

This report makes ten overall recommendations.

1. PROVIDE TREATMENT IN PRIMARY CARE

The management and treatment of mental disorders in primary care is a fundamental step which enables the largest number of people to get easier and faster access to services – it needs to be recognized that many are already seeking help at this level. This not only gives better care; it cuts wastage resulting from unnecessary investigations and inappropriate and non-specific treatments. For this to happen, however, general health personnel need to be trained in the essential skills of mental health care. Such training ensures the best use of available knowledge for the largest number of people and makes possible the immediate application of interventions. Mental health should therefore be included in training curricula, with refresher courses to improve the effectiveness of the management of mental disorders in general health services.

2. MAKE PSYCHOTROPIC DRUGS AVAILABLE

Essential psychotropic drugs should be provided and made constantly available at all levels of health care. These medicines should be included in every country's essential drugs list, and the best drugs to treat conditions should be made available whenever possible. In some countries, this may require enabling legislation changes. These drugs can ameliorate symptoms, reduce disability, shorten the course of many disorders, and prevent relapse. They often provide the first-line treatment, especially in situations where psychosocial interventions and highly skilled professionals are unavailable.

3. GIVE CARE IN THE COMMUNITY

Community care has a better effect than institutional treatment on the outcome and quality of life of individuals with chronic mental disorders. Shifting patients from mental hospitals to care in the community is also cost-effective and respects human rights. Mental health services should therefore be provided in the community, with the use of all available resources. Community-based services can lead to early intervention and limit the stigma of taking treatment. Large custodial mental hospitals should be replaced by community care facilities, backed by general hospital psychiatric beds and home care support, which meet all the needs of the ill that were the responsibility of those hospitals. This shift towards community care requires health workers and rehabilitation services to be available at community level, along with the provision of crisis support, protected housing, and sheltered employment.

4. EDUCATE THE PUBLIC

Public education and awareness campaigns on mental health should be launched in all countries. The main goal is to reduce barriers to treatment and care by increasing awareness of the frequency of mental disorders, their treatability, the recovery process and the human rights of people with mental disorders. The care choices available and their benefits should be widely disseminated so that responses from the general population, professionals, media, policy-makers and politicians reflect the best available knowledge. This is already a priority for a number of countries, and national and international organizations. Well-planned public awareness and education campaigns can reduce stigma and discrimination, increase the use of mental health services, and bring mental and physical health care closer to each other.

5. INVOLVE COMMUNITIES, FAMILIES AND CONSUMERS

Communities, families and consumers should be included in the development and decision-making of policies, programmes and services. This should lead to services being better tailored to people's needs and better used. In addition, interventions should take account of age, sex, culture and social conditions, so as to meet the needs of people with mental disorders and their families.

6. ESTABLISH NATIONAL POLICIES, PROGRAMMES AND LEGISLATION

Mental health policy, programmes and legislation are necessary steps for significant and sustained action. These should be based on current knowledge and human rights considerations. Most countries need to increase their budgets for mental health programmes from existing low levels. Some countries that have recently developed or revised their policy and legislation have made progress in implementing their mental health care programmes. Mental health reforms should be part of the larger health system reforms. Health insurance schemes should not discriminate against persons with mental disorders, in order to give wider access to treatment and to reduce burdens of care.

7. DEVELOP HUMAN RESOURCES

Most developing countries need to increase and improve training of mental health professionals, who will provide specialized care as well as support the primary health care programmes. Most developing countries lack an adequate number of such specialists to staff mental health services. Once trained, these professionals should be encouraged to remain in their country in positions that make the best use of their skills. This human resource development is especially necessary for countries with few resources at present. Though primary care provides the most useful setting for initial care, specialists are needed to provide a wider range of services. Specialist mental health care teams ideally should include medical and non-medical professionals, such as psychiatrists, clinical psychologists, psychiatric nurses, psychiatric social workers and occupational therapists, who can work together towards the total care and integration of patients in the community.

8. Link with other sectors

Sectors other than health, such as education, labour, welfare, and law, and nongovernmental organizations should be involved in improving the mental health of communities. Nongovernmental organizations should be much more proactive, with better-defined roles, and should be encouraged to give greater support to local initiatives.

9. Monitor community mental health

The mental health of communities should be monitored by including mental health indicators in health information and reporting systems. The indices should include both the numbers of individuals with mental disorders and the quality of their care, as well as some more general measures of the mental health of communities. Such monitoring helps to determine trends and to detect mental health changes resulting from external events, such as disasters. Monitoring is necessary to assess the effectiveness of mental health prevention and treatment programmes, and it also strengthens arguments for the provision of more resources. New indicators for the mental health of communities are necessary.

10. Support more research

More research into biological and psychosocial aspects of mental health is needed in order to increase the understanding of mental disorders and to develop more effective interventions. Such research should be carried out on a wide international basis to understand variations across communities and to learn more about factors that influence the cause, course and outcome of mental disorders. Building research capacity in developing countries is an urgent need.

Action based on resource realities

While they are generally applicable, most of the above recommendations may appear to be far beyond the resources of many countries. But there is something here for everyone. With this in mind, three separate scenarios are provided to help guide developing countries in particular towards what is possible within their resource limitations. The scenarios can be used to identify specific actions. As well as being relevant to individual countries, they are also intended to be relevant to different population groups within those countries. This recognizes that there are disadvantaged areas or groups in all countries, even those which have the best resources and services.

Scenario A (Low level of resources)

This scenario refers mostly to low income countries where mental health resources are completely absent or very limited. Such countries have no mental health policy, programmes or appropriate legislation; or, if they exist, they are outdated and not implemented effectively. Governmental finances available to mental health are tiny, often less than 0.1% of the total health budget. There are no psychiatrists or psychiatric nurses, or very few of them for large populations. Specialized inpatient care facilities, if they exist, do so as centralized mental hospitals, which serve more for custodial care than mental health care, and often have less than one place per 10 000 population. There are no mental health services in primary or community care, and essential psychotropic drugs are seldom available. Mental health is not a part of epidemiological and health reporting systems.

While this scenario applies mostly to low income countries, in many high income countries essential mental health services remain beyond the reach of rural populations, indigenous groups and others. In brief, scenario A is characterized by low awareness and low availability of services.

What can be done in such circumstances? Even with very limited resources, countries can immediately recognize mental health as an integral part of general health, and begin to organize the basic mental health services as a part of primary health care. This need not be a costly exercise, and it would be greatly enhanced by the provision of essential neuropsychiatric drugs and in-service training of all general health personnel.

Scenario B (Medium level of resources)

In countries in this scenario, some resources are available for mental health, such as centres for treatment in big cities or pilot programmes for community care. But these resources do not provide even essential mental health services to the total population. These countries are likely to have mental health policies, programmes and legislation, but they are often not fully implemented. The government budget for mental health is less than 1% of the total health budget. There are inadequate numbers of mental health specialists, such as psychiatrists and psychiatric nurses, to serve the population. Primary care providers are largely untrained in mental health care. Specialized care facilities have fewer than five places per 10 000 population, and most of these are in large and centralized mental hospitals. Availability of psychotropic drugs and treatment for major mental disorders in primary care is limited and community mental health programmes are scarce. Admission and discharge records from mental hospitals provide the only information available in health reporting systems. To summarize, scenario B is characterized by medium awareness and medium access to mental health care.

For these countries the immediate action should be to enlarge mental health services to cover the total population. This can be done by extending training to all health personnel on essential mental health care, providing neuropsychiatric drugs in all health facilities, and bringing all of these activities under a mental health policy. A start should be made on closing down custodial hospitals and building community care facilities. Mental health care can be introduced in workplaces and schools.

Scenario C (High level of resources)

This scenario relates mostly to industrialized countries with a relatively high level of resources for mental health. Mental health policies, programmes and legislation are implemented reasonably effectively. The proportion of the total health budget allocated to mental health is 1% or more, and there are adequate numbers of specialized mental health professionals. Most primary care providers are trained in mental health care. Efforts are made to identify and treat major mental disorders in primary care, though effectiveness and coverage may be inadequate. Specialized care facilities are more comprehensive, but most may still be located in mental hospitals. Psychotropic drugs are readily available and community-based services are generally available. Mental health forms a part of health information systems, although only a few indicators may be included.

Even in these countries there are many barriers to the utilization of the available services. People with mental disorders and their families experience stigma and discrimination. Insurance policies fail to provide cover for the care of people with mental disorders to the same extent as for those with physical illness.

Table 5.1 Minimum actions required for mental health care, based on overall recommendations

Ten overall recommendations	Scenario A: Low level of resources	Scenario B: Medium level of resources	Scenario C: High level of resources
1. Provide treatment in primary care	• Recognize mental health as a component of primary health care • Include the recognition and treatment of common mental disorders in training curricula of all health personnel • Provide refresher training to primary care physicians (at least 50% coverage in 5 years)	• Develop locally relevant training materials • Provide refresher training to primary care physicians (100% coverage in 5 years)	• Improve effectiveness of management of mental disorders in primary health care • Improve referral patterns
2. Make psychotropic drugs available	• Ensure availability of 5 essential drugs in all health care settings	• Ensure availability of all essential psychotropic drugs in all health care settings	• Provide easier access to newer psychotropic drugs under public or private treatment plans
3. Give care in the community	• Move people with mental disorders out of prisons • Downsize mental hospitals and improve care within them • Develop general hospital psychiatric units • Provide community care facilities (at least 20% coverage)	• Close down custodial mental hospitals • Initiate pilot projects on integration of mental health care with general health care • Provide community care facilities (at least 50% coverage)	• Close down remaining custodial mental hospitals • Develop alternative residential facilities • Provide community care facilities (100% coverage) • Give individualized care in the community to people with serious mental disorders
4. Educate the public	• Promote public campaigns against stigma and discrimination • Support nongovernmental organizations in public education	• Use the mass media to promote mental health, foster positive attitudes, and help prevent disorders	• Launch public campaigns for the recognition and treatment of common mental disorders
5. Involve communities, families and consumers	• Support the formation of self-help groups • Fund schemes for nongovernmental organizations and mental health initiatives	• Ensure representation of communities, families, and consumers in services and policy-making	• Foster advocacy initiatives
6. Establish national policies, programmes and legislation	• Revise legislation based on current knowledge and human rights considerations • Formulate mental health programmes and policy • Increase the budget for mental health care	• Create drug and alcohol policies at national and subnational levels • Increase the budget for mental health care	• Ensure fairness in health care financing, including insurance
7. Develop human resources	• Train psychiatrists and psychiatric nurses	• Create national training centres for psychiatrists, psychiatric nurses, psychologists and psychiatric social workers	• Train specialists in advanced treatment skills
8. Link with other sectors	• Initiate school and workplace mental health programmes • Encourage the activities of nongovernmental organizations	• Strengthen school and workplace mental health programmes	• Provide special facilities in schools and the workplace for mentally disordered people • Initiate evidence-based mental health promotion programmes in collaboration with other sectors
9. Monitor community mental health	• Include mental disorders in basic health information systems • Survey high-risk population groups	• Institute surveillance for specific disorders in the community (e.g. depression)	• Develop advanced mental health monitoring systems • Monitor effectiveness of preventive programmes
10. Support more research	• Conduct studies in primary health care settings on the prevalence, course, outcome and impact of mental disorders in the community	• Institute effectiveness and cost-effectiveness studies for management of common mental disorders in primary health care	• Extend research on the causes of mental disorders • Carry out research on service delivery • Investigate evidence on the prevention of mental disorders

The first immediate action required is to increase public awareness, aimed principally at decreasing stigma and discrimination. Second, the newer medicines and psychosocial interventions should be made available as part of routine mental health care. Third, mental health information systems should be developed. Fourth, research on cost-effectiveness, evidence on prevention of mental disorders, and basic research on causes of mental disorders should be initiated or extended.

The recommended minimum actions required for mental health care in the three scenarios are summarized in Table 5.1. The table assumes that the actions recommended for countries in scenario A have already been taken by countries in scenarios B and C, and that there is an accumulation of actions in countries with high levels of resources.

This report recognizes that, in all scenarios, the time lag between initiation of actions and their resultant benefits can be long. But this is an added reason to encourage all countries to take immediate steps towards improving the mental health of their populations. For the poorest countries, these first steps may be small, but they are nonetheless worth taking. For rich and poor alike, mental well-being is as important as physical health. For all who suffer from mental disorders, there is hope; it is the responsibility of all governments to turn that hope into reality.

References

Abas MA, Broadhead JC (1997). Depression and anxiety among women in an urban setting in Zimbabwe. *Psychological Medicine*, 27: 59–71.

Al-Subaie AS, Marwa MKH, Hamari RA, Abdul-Rahim F-A (1997). Psychiatric emergencies in a university hospital in Riyadh, Saudi Arabia. *International Journal of Mental Health*, **25**: 59–68.

Almeida-Filho N, Mari J de J, Coutinho E, Franca JF, Fernandes J, Andreoli SB, Busnello ED (1997). Brazilian multicentric study of psychiatric morbidity. Methodological features and prevalence estimates. *British Journal of Psychiatry*, 171: 524–529.

American Psychiatric Association (APA) (1994). *Diagnostic and statistical manual of mental disorders, 4th edition (DSM-IV)*. Washington DC, American Psychiatric Association.

Andrews G, Henderson S, Wayne Hall W (2001). Prevalence, comorbidity, disability and service utilisation: overview of the Australian National Mental Health Survey. *British Journal of Psychiatry*, **178**: 145–153.

Andrews G, Peters L, Guzman A-M, Bird K (1995). A comparison of two structured diagnostic interviews: CIDI and SCAN. *Australian and New Zealand Journal of Psychiatry*, **29**: 124–132.

Artaud A (1935). Lettre ouverte aux médecins-chefs des asiles de fous [Open letter to medical directors of madhouses]. Paris, *La Révolution Surréaliste*, No. 3.

Awas M, Kebede D, Alem A (1999). Major mental disorders in Butajira, southern Ethiopia. *Acta Psychiatrica Scandinavica*, **100**(Suppl 397): 56–64.

Baingana F (1990). Personal communication.

Batra A (2000). Tobacco use and smoking cessation in the psychiatric patient. *Fortschritte der Neurologie-Psychiatrie*, **68**: 80–92.

Baxter LR, Schwartz JM, Bergman KS, Szuba MP, Guzem BH, Mazziotta JC, Alazraki A, Selin CE, Ferng HK, Munford P (1992). Caudate glucose metabolic rate changes with both drug and behavior therapy for obsessive–compulsive disorder. *Archives of General Psychiatry*, **49**(9): 681–689.

Beers C (1908). *A mind that found itself: an autobiography*. New York, Longmans Green.

Berke J, Hyman SE (2000). Addiction, dopamine and the molecular mechanisms of memory. *Neuron*, **25**: 515–532.

Bijl RV, Ravelli A, van Zessen G (1998). Prevalence of psychiatric disorder in the general population: results of the Netherlands Mental Health Survey and Incidence Study (NEMESIS). *Social Psychiatry and Psychiatric Epidemiology*, **33**: 587–595.

Bodekar G (2001). Lessons on integration from the developing world's experience. *British Medical Journal*, **322**(7279): 164–167.

Bower P, Byford S, Sibbald B, Ward E, King M, Lloyd M, Gabbay M (2000). Randomised controlled trial of non-directive counselling cognitive behaviour therapy, and usual general practitioner care for patients with depression. II: Cost-effectiveness. *British Medical Journal*, **321**: 1389–1392.

Bowles JR (1995). Suicide in Western Samoa: an example of a suicide prevention program in a developing country. In: Diekstra RFW, Gulbinat W, Kienhorst I, De Leo D. *Preventive strategies on suicide*. Lieden, Brill: 173–206.

Brookmeyer R, Gray S (2000). Methods for projecting the incidence and prevalence of chronic diseases in aging populations: application to Alzheimer's disease. *Statistics in Medicine*, **19**(11–12): 1481–1493.

Brown GW, Birley JLT, Wing JK (1972). Influence of family life on the course of schizophrenic disorder: a replication. *British Journal of Psychiatry*, **121**: 241–258.

Butcher J (2000). A Nobel pursuit. *Lancet*, **356**(9328): 1331.

Butzlaff RL, Hooley JM (1998). Expressed emotion and psychiatric relapse: a meta-analysis. *Archives of General Psychiatry*, **55**(8): 547–552.

Caldwell CB, Gottesman II (1990). Schizophrenics kill themselves too: a review of risk factors for suicide. *Schizophrenia Bulletin*, **16**: 571–589.

Castellanos FX, Giedd JN, Eckburg P (1994). Quantitative morphology of the caudate nucleus in attention deficit hyperactity disorder. *American Journal of Psychiatry*, **151**(12): 1791–1796.

Chisholm D, Sekar K, Kumar K, Kishore K, Saeed K, James S, Mubbashar M, Murthy RS (2000). Integration of mental health care into primary care: demonstration cost-outcome study in India and Pakistan. *British Journal of Psychiatry*, **176**: 581–588.

Ciechanowski PS, Katon WJ, Russo JE (2000). Depression and diabetes: impact of depressive symptoms on adherence, function, and costs. *Archives of Internal Medicine*, **160**: 3278–3285.

Cohen S, Tyrell DAJ, Smith AP (1991). Psychological stress and susceptibility to the common cold. *New England Journal of Medicine*, **325**(9): 606–612.

Collins D, Lapsley G (1996). *The social costs of drug abuse in Australia in 1988 and 1992*. Canberra, Commonwealth Department of Human Services and Health, Australian Government Printing Service (Monograph No. 30).

Collins PY, Adler FW, Boero M, Susser E (1999a). Using local resources in Patagonia: primary care and mental health in Neuquen, Argentina. *International Journal of Mental Health*, **28:** 3–16.

Collins PY, Lumerman J, Conover S, Susser E (1999b). Using local resources in Patagonia: a model of community-based rehabilitation. *International Journal of Mental Health*, **28**: 17–24.

Conolly J (1856). *The treatment of the insane without mechanical restraints*. London, Smith, Elder & Co.

Cooper PJ, Murray L (1998). Postnatal depression. *British Medical Journal*, **316**: 1884–1886.

Costello EJ, Angold A, Burns BJ, Stangl D, Tweed D, Erkanli A, Worthman CM (1996). The Great Smoky Mountains Study of Youth: goals, design, methods, and the prevalence of DSM-III-R disorders. *Archives of General Psychiatry*, **53**: 1129–1136.

Cottraux J (1993). Behaviour therapy. In: Sartorius N, De Girilamo G, Andrews G, German A, Eisenberg L, eds. *Treatment of mental disorders: a review of effectiveness*. Geneva, World Health Organization: 199–235.

Cuajungco MP, Lees GJ (1997). Zinc and Alzheimer's disease: is there a direct link? *Brain Research*, **23**(3): 219–236.

Czerner TB (2001). *What makes you tick? The brain in plain English*. New York, John Wiley & Sons.

Delange F (2000). The role of iodine in brain development. *Proceedings of the Nutrition Society*, **59**(1): 75–79.

Desjarlais R, Eisenberg L, Good B, Kleinman A (1995). World mental health: problems and priorities in low-income countries. New York, Oxford University Press.

Dill E, Dill C (1998). Video game violence: a review of the empirical literature. *Aggression and Violent Behavior*, **3**(4): 407–428.

DiMatteo MR, Lepper HS, Croghan TW (2000). Depression is a risk factor for noncompliance with medical treatment: meta-analysis of the effects of anxiety and depression on patient adherence. *Archives of Internal Medicine*, **160:** 2101–2107.

Dixon L, Adams C, Lucksted A (2000). Update on family psycho-education for schizophrenia. *Schizophrenia Bulletin*, **26**: 5–20.

Dixon LB, Lehman AF (1995). Family interventions for schizophrenia. *Schizophrenia Bulletin*, **21**(4): 631–643.

Dixon LB, Lehman AF, Levine J (1995). Conventional antipsychotic medications for schizophrenia. *Schizophrenia Bulletin*, **21**(4): 567–577.

Drouet B, Pincon-Raymond M, Chambaz J, Pillot T (2000). Molecular basis of Alzheimer's disease. *Cellular and Molecular Life Sciences*, **57**(5): 705–715.

Edwards G, Marshall EJ, Cook CCH, eds (1997). *The treatment of drinking problems: a guide to helping professions*, 3rd edition. Cambridge, Cambridge University Press.

El-Din AS, Kamel FA, Randa M, Atta HY (1996) Evaluation of an educational programme for the development of trainers in child mental health in Alexandria. *Eastern Mediterranean Health Journal*, **2**: 482–493.

Ellsberg MC, Pena R, Herrera A, Winkvist A, Kullgren G (1999). Domestic violence and emotional distress among Nicaraguan women: results from a population-based study. *American Psychologist*, **54**: 30–36.

Erickson MF (1989). The STEEP Programme: helping young families alone at risk. *Family Resource Coalition Report*, **3**: 14–15.

Fadden G, Bebbington P, Kuipers L (1987). The burden of care: the impact of functional psychiatric illness on the patient's family. *British Journal of Psychiatry*, **150**: 285–292.

Feksi AT, Kaamugisha J, Sander JW, Gatiti S, Shorvon SD (1991). Comprehensive primary health care antiepileptic drug treatment programme in rural and semi-urban Kenya. *Lancet*, **337**(8738): 406–409.

Ferketich AK, Schwartbaum JA, Frid DJ, Moeschberger ML (2000). Depression as an antecedent to heart disease among women and men in the NHANES I study. *Archives of Internal Medicine*, **160**(9): 1261–1268.

Fraser SFH, McGrath, St Hjohn D (2000). Information technology and telemedicine in sub-Saharan Africa (editorial). *British Medical Journal*, **321**: 465–466.

Gallagher SK, Mechanic D (1996). Living with the mentally ill: effects on the health and functioning of other members. *Social Science and Medicine*, **42**(12): 1691–1701.

Gallegos A, Montero F (1999). Issues in community-based rehabilitation for persons with mental illness in Costa Rica. *International Journal of Mental Health*, **28**: 25–30.

Geerlings SW, Beekman ATF, Deeg DJH, Van Tilburg W (2000). Physical health and the onset and persistence of depression in older adults: an eight-wave prospective community-based study. *Psychological Medicine*, **30**(2): 369–380.

Girolomo G de, Cozza M (2000). The Italian psychiatric reform: a 20-year perspective. *International Journal of Law and Psychiatry*, **23**(3–4): 197–214.

Gittelman M (1998). Public and private managed care. *International Journal of Mental Health*, **27**: 3–17.

Goff DC, Henderson DC, Amico D (1992). Cigarette smoking in schizophrenia: relationship to psychopathology and medication side-effects. *American Journal of Psychiatry*, **149**: 1189–1194.

Gold JH (1998). Gender differences in psychiatric illness and treatments: a critical review. *Journal of Nervous and Mental Diseases*, **186**(12): 769–775.

Goldberg DP, Lecrubier Y (1995). Form and frequency of mental disorders across centres. In: Üstün TB, Sartorius N, eds. *Mental illness in general health care: an international study*. Chichester, John Wiley & Sons on behalf of the World Health Organization: 323–334.

Gomel MK, Wutzke SE, Hardcastle DM, Lapsley H, Reznik RB (1995). Cost-effectiveness of strategies to market and train primary healthcare physicians in brief intervention techniques for hazardous alcohol use. *Social Science and Medicine*, **47**: 203–211.

Gomez-Beneyto M, Bonet A, Catala MA, Puche E, Vila V (1994). Prevalence of mental disorders among children in Valencia, Spain. *Acta Psychiatrica Scandinavica*, **89**: 352–357.

Goodman E, Capitman J (2000). Depressive symptoms and cigarette smoking among teens. *Pediatrics*, **106**(4): 748–755.

Goodwin FK, Jamison KR (1990). Suicide, in manic-depressive illness. New York, Oxford University Press: 227–244.

Gossop M, Stewart MS, Lehman P, Edwards C, Wilson A, Segar G (1998). Substance use, health and social problems of service users at 54 drug treatment agencies. *British Journal of Psychiatry*, **173**: 166–171.

Graham P, Orley J (1998). WHO and the mental health of children. *World Health Forum*, **19**: 268–272.

Griffiths K, Christensen H (2000). Quality of web-based information on treatment of depression: cross-sectional survey. *British Medical Journal*, **321**: 1511–1515.

Gureje O, Odejide AO, Olatawura MO, Ikuesan BA, Acha RA, Bamidele RW, Raji OS (1995). Results from the Ibadan centre. In: Ustun TB, Sartorius N, eds. *Mental illness in general health care: an international study*. Chichester, John Wiley & Sons on behalf of the World Health Organization: 157–173.

Gureje O, Von Korff M, Simon GE, Gater R (1998). Persistent pain and well-being: a World Health Organization study in primary care. *Journal of the American Medical Association*, **280**(2): 147–151.

Hakimi M, Hayati EN, Marlinawati VU, Winkvist A, Ellsberg M (2001). *Silence for the sake of harmony: domestic violence and women's health in Central Java*. Yogyakarta, Indonesia, Program for Appropriate Technology in Health.

Harnois G, Gabriel P (2000). *Mental health and work: impact, issues and good practices*. Geneva, World Health Organization and International Labour Office (WHO/MSD/MPS/00.2).

Harpham T, Blue I, eds (1995). *Urbanization and mental health in developing countries*. Aldershot, UK, Avebury.

Harris J, Best D, Man L, Welch S, Gossop M, Strang J (2000). Changes in cigarette smoking among alcohol and drug misusers during inpatient detoxification. *Addiction Biology*, **5**: 443–450.

Harwood H, Fountain D, Livermore G (1998). *The economic costs of alcohol and drug abuse in the United States, 1992. Report prepared for the National Institute on Drug Abuse and the National Institute on Alcohol Abuse and Alcoholism*. Rockville, MD, National Institute on Drug Abuse (NIH Publication No. 98-4327).

Hauenstein EJ, Boyd MR (1994). Depressive symptoms in young women of the Piedmont: prevalence in rural women. *Women and Health*, **21**(2/3): 105–123.

Heather N (1995). *Treatment approaches to alcohol problems: European Alcohol Action Plan*. Copenhagen, WHO Regional Office for Europe (WHO Regional Publications, European Series, No. 65).

Heim C, Newport DJ, Heit S, Graham YP, Wilcox M, Bonsall R, Miller AH, Nemeroff CB (2000). Pituitary-adrenal and autonomic responses to stress in women after sexual and physical abuse in childhood. *Journal of the American Medical Association*, **284**(5): 592–597.

Hoge MA, Davidson L, Griffith EEH, Jacobs S (1998). The crisis of managed care in the public sector. *International Journal of Mental Health*, **27**: 52–71.

Hughes JR,, Hatsukami DK, Mitchell JE, Dahlgren LA (1986). Prevalence of smoking among psychiatric outpatients. *Americal Journal of Psychiatry*, **143**: 993–997.

Hyman SE (2000). Mental illness: genetically complex disorders of neural circuitry and neural communication. *Neuron*, **28**: 321–323.

ILAE/IBE/WHO (2000). *Global campaign against epilepsy*. Geneva, World Health Organization.

Indian Council of Medical Research (ICMR) (2001). *Epidemiological study of child and adolescent psychiatric disorders in urban and rural areas*. New Delhi, Indian Council of Medical Research (unpublished data).

International Federation of Red Cross and Red Crescent Societies (IFRC) (2000). *World disasters report*. Geneva, International Federation of Red Cross and Red Crescent Societies.

International Network of Clinical Epidemiologists (INCLEN) (2001). *World Studies of Abuse in Family Environments (WorldSAFE)*. Manila, International Network of Clinical Epidemiologists.

Jablensky A, Sartorius N, Ernberg G, Anker M, Korten A, Cooper JE, Day R, Bertelsen A (1992). Schizophrenia: manifestations, incidence and course in different cultures: a World Health Organization ten-country study. *Psychological Medicine Monograph*, **20** (Suppl).

Jaffe JH (1995). *Encyclopedia of drugs and alcohol, Volume 1*. New York, Simon and Schuster.

Jernigan DH, Monteiro M, Room R, Saxena S (2000). Towards a global alcohol policy: alcohol, public health and the role of WHO. *Bulletin of the World Health Organization*, **78**: 491–499.

Katona C, Livingston G (2000). Impact of screening old people with physical illness for depression. *Lancet*, **356**: 91.

Kellerman AL, Rivara FP, Somes G, Reay DT, Francisco J, Benton JG, Prodzinski J, Fligner C, Hackman BB (1992). Suicide in the home in relation to gun ownership. *New England Journal of Medicine*, **327**: 467–472.

Kessler RC, McGonagle KA, Zhao S, Nelson CB, Hughes M, Eshleman S, Wittchen HU, Kendler KS (1994). Lifetime and 12-month prevalence of DSM-III-R psychiatric disorders in the United States. Results from the National Comorbidity Survey. *Archives of General Psychiatry*, **51: 8–19**.

Kielcot-Glaser JK, Page GG, Marucha PT, MacCallum RC, Glaser R (1999). Psychological influences on surgical recovery: perspectives from psychoneuroimmunology. *American Psychologist*, **53**(11): 1209–1218.

Kilonzo GP, Simmons N (1998). Development of mental health services in Tanzania: a reappraisal for the future. *Social Science and Medicine*, **47**: 419-428.

Klein N (1999). *No logo: taking on the brand bullies*. New York, Picador.

Kohn R, Dohrenwend BP, Mirotznik J (1998). Epidemiological findings on selected psychiatric disorders in the general population. In: Dohrenwend BP, ed. *Adversity, stress, and psychopathology*. Oxford, Oxford University Press: 235–284.

Kopp MS, Skrabski A, Szedmark S (2000). Psychosocial risk factors, inequality and self-rated morbidity in a changing society. *Social Science and Medicine*, **51**: 1351–1361.

Kuipers L, Bebbington PE (1990). *Working partnership: clinicians and carers in the management of longstanding mental illness*. Oxford, Heinemann Medical.

Kulhara P, Wig NN (1978). The chronicity of schizophrenia in North-West India. Results of a follow-up study. *British Journal of Psychiatry*, **132**: 186–190.

Lasser K, Wesley Boyd J, Woolhandler S, Himmelstein DU, McCormick D, Bor DH (2000). Smoking and mental illness: a population-based prevalence study. *Journal of the American Medical Association*, **284**: 2606–2610.

Leavell HR, Clark HG (1965). *Preventive medicine for the doctor in his community: an epidemiological approach*, 3rd edition. New York, McGraw-Hill Book Co.

Leff J, Gamble C (1995). Training of community psychiatric nurses in family work for schizophrenia. *International Journal of Mental Health*, **24**: 76–88.

Leff J, Wig NN, Ghosh A, Bedi A, Menon DK, Kuipers L, Morten A, Ernberg G, Day R, Sartotius N, Jablensky A (1987). Expressed emotion and schizophrenia in north India. III: Influences of relatives' expressed emotion on the course of schizophrenia in Chandigarh. *British Journal of Psychiatry*, **151**: 166–173.

Lehman AF, Steinwachs DM and the co-investigators of the PORT Project (1998). At issue: translating research into practice. The Schizophrenia Patient Outcomes Research Team (PORT) treatment recommendations. *Schizophrenia Bulletin*, **24**(1): 1–10.

Leon DA, Shkolnikov VM (1998). Social stress and the Russian mortality crisis. *Journal of the American Medical Association*, **279**(10): 790–791.

Leonardis M de, Mauri D, Rotelli F (1994). *L'imresa sociale*. Milan, Anabasi.

Leshner AI (1997). Addiction is a brain disease, and it matters. *Science*, **278**(5335): 45–47.

Lester D (1995). Preventing suicide by restricting access to methods for suicide. In: Diekstra RFW, Gulbinat W, Kienhorst I, De Leo D, eds. *Preventive strategies on suicide.* Lieden, Brill: 163–172.

Lester D, Murrell ME (1980). The influence of gun control laws on suicidal behaviour. *American Journal of Psychiatry*, **137**: 121–122.

Levav I, Gonzalez VR (2000). Rights of persons with mental illness in Central America. *Acta Psychiatrica Scandinavica*, **101**: 83–86.

Lewinsohn PM, Hops H, Roberts RE, Seeley JR, Andrews JA (1993). Adolescent psychopathology. I: Prevalence and incidence of depression and other DSM-III-R disorders in high school students. *Journal of Abnormal Psychology*, **102**: 133–144 (erratum, **102**: 517).

Lewis DA, Lieberman JA (2000). Catching up on schizophrenia: natural history and neurobiology. *Neuron*, **28**: 325–334.

Lindeman S, Hämäläinen J, Isometsä E, Kaprio J, Poikolainin K, Heikkinen A, Aro H (2000). The 12-month prevalence and risk factors for major depressive episode in Finland: representative sample of 5993 adults. *Acta Psychiatrica Scandinavica*, **102**: 178–184.

Lustman PJ, Freedland KE, Griffith LS, Clouse RE (2000). Fluoxetine for depression in diabetes: a randomized double-blind placebo-controlled trial. *Diabetes Care*, **23**(5): 618–623.

Lustman PJ, Griffith LS, Clause RE, Freedland KE, Eisen SA, Rubin EH, Carney RM, McGill JB (1995). Effects of alprazolam on glucose regulation in diabetes: results of a double-blind, placebo-controlled trial. *Diabetes Care*, **18**(8): 1133–1139.

Lustman PJ, Griffith LS, Clause RE, Freedland KE, Eisen SA, Rubin EH, Carney RM, McGill JB (1997). Effects of nortriptyline on depression and glycemic control in diabetes: results of a double-blind placebo-controlled trial. *Psychosomatic Medicine*, **59**(3): 241–250.

McGorry PD (2000). Evaluating the importance of reducing the duration of untreated psychosis. *Australian and New Zealand Journal of Psychiatry*, **34** (suppl.): 145–149.

McLellan AT, Lewis DC, O'Brien CP, Kleber HD (2000). Drug dependence, a chronic medical illness: implications for treatment, insurance, and outcomes evaluation. *Journal of the American Medical Association*, **284**(13): 1689–1695.

Maj M, Janssen R, Starace F, Zaudig M, Satz P, Sughondhabirom B, Luabeya M, Riedel R, Ndetei D, Calil B, Bing EG, St Louis M, Sartorius N (1994a). WHO Neuropsychiatric AIDS Study, Cross-sectional Phase I: Study design and psychiatric findings. *Archives of General Psychiatry*, **51**(1): 39–49.

Maj M, Satz P, Janssen R, Zaudig M, Starace F, D'Elia L, Sughondhabirom B, Mussa M, Naber D, Dnetei D, Schulte G, Sartorius N (1994b). WHO Neuropsychiatric AIDS Study, Cross-sectional Phase II: Neuropsychological and neurological findings. *Archives of General Psychiatry*, **51**(1): 51–61.

Management Sciences for Health (from 2001, in collaboration with WHO). *International drug price indicator guide*. Arlington, VA, Management Sciences for Health.

Mani KS, Rangan G, Srinivas HV, Srindharan VS, Subbakrishna DK (2001). Epilepsy control with phenobarbital or phenytoin in rural south India: the Yelandur study. *Lancet*, **357**: 1316–1320.

Meerding WJ, Bonneux L, Polder JJ, Koopmanschap MA, Maas PJ van der (1998). Demographic and epidemiological determinants of healthcare costs in the Netherlands: cost of illness study. *British Medical Journal*, **317**: 111–115.

Mendlowicz MV, Stein MB (2000). Quality of life in individuals with anxiety disorders. *American Journal of Psychiatry*, **157**(5): 669–682.

Merkl PE (1993). Which are today's democracies? *International Social Science Journal*, **136**: 257–270.

Mishara BL, Ystgaard M (2000). Exploring the potential for primary prevention: evaluation of the Befrienders International Reaching Young People Pilot Programme in Denmark. *Crisis*, **21**(1): 4–7.

Mittelman MS, Ferris SH, Shulman E, Steinberg G, Levin B (1996). A family intervention to delay nursing home placement of patients with Alzheimer's disease. *Journal of the American Medical Association*, **276**(21): 1725–1731.

Mohit A (1999). Mental health in the Eastern Mediterranean Region of the World Health Organization with a view to future trends. *Eastern Mediterranean Health Journal*, **5**: 231–240.

Mohit A, Saeed K, Shahmohammadi D, Bolhari J, Bina M, Gater R, Mubbashar MH (1999). Mental health manpower development in Afghanistan: a report on a training course for primary health care physicians. *Eastern Mediterranean Health Journal*, **5**: 231–240.

Morita H, Suzuki M, Suzuki S, Kamoshita S (1993). Psychiatric disorders in Japanese secondary school children. *Journal of Child Psychology and Psychiatry*, **34**: 317–332.

Mubbashar MH (1999). Mental health services in rural Pakistan. In: Tansella M, Thornicroft G, eds. *Common mental disorders in primary care*. London, Routledge.

Murray CJL, Lopez AD, eds (1996a). *The global burden of disease: a comprehensive assessment of mortality and disability from diseases, injuries and risk factors in 1990 and projected to 2020*. Cambridge, MA, Harvard School of Public Health on behalf of the World Health Organization and the World Bank (Global Burden of Disease and Injury Series, Vol. I).

Murray CJL, Lopez AD (1996b). *Global health statistics*. Cambridge, MA, Harvard School of Public Health on behalf of the World Health Organization and the World Bank (Global Burden of Disease and Injury Series, Vol. II).

Murray CJL, Lopez AD (1997). Alternative projections of mortality and disability by cause 1990–2020: Global Burden of Disease Study. *Lancet*, **349**: 1498–1504.

Murray CJL, Lopez AD (2000). Progress and directions in refining the global burden of disease approach: a response to Williams. *Health Economics*, **9**: 69–82.

Mynors-Wallis L (1996). Problem-solving treatment: evidence for effectiveness and feasibility in primary care. *International Journal of Psychiatry Medicine*, **26**: 249–262.

Narayan D, Chambers R, Shah MK, Petesch P (2000). *Voices of the poor, crying out for change*. New York, Oxford University Press for the World Bank.

National Human Rights Commission (1999). *Quality assurance in mental health*. New Delhi, National Human Rights Commission of India.

New Mexico Department of Health (2001). *Alcohol-related hospital charges in New Mexico for 1998 estimated at $51 million*. New Mexico Department of Health (Press Release, 16 January 2001).

Newman SC, Bland RC, Orn HT (1998). The prevalence of mental disorders in the elderly in Edmonton: a community survey using GMS-AGECAT. *Canadian Journal of Psychiatry*, **43**: 910–914.

NIDA (2000). *Principles of drug addiction treatment: a research-based guide*. Bethesda, MD, National Institute on Drug Abuse (NIH Publication No.00-4180).

Notzon FC, Komarov YM, Ermakov SP, Sempos CT, Marks JS, Sempos EV (1998). Causes of declining life expectancy in Russia. *Journal of the American Medical Association*, **279**(10): 793–800.

O'Brien SJ, Menotti-Raymond M, Murphy WJ, Nash WG, Wienberg J, Stanyon R, Copeland NG, Jenkins NA, Womack JE, Marshall Graves JA (1999). The promise of comparative genomics in mammals. *Science*, **286**: 458–481.

Okasha A, Karam E (1998). Mental health services and research in the Arab world. *Acta Psychiatrica Scandinavica*, **98**: 406–413.

Orley J, Kuyken W (1994). *Quality of life assessment: international perspectives*. Basel, Springer-Verlag.

Orley J, Saxena S, Herrman H (1998). Quality of life and mental illness: reflections from the perspective of WHOQOL. *British Journal of Psychiatry*, **172**: 291–293.

PAHO (1991). Declaration of Caracas, 1990. *International Digest of Health Legislation*, **42**(2): 336–338.

Pai S, Kapur RL (1982). Impact on treatment intervention on the relationship between the dimensions of clinical psychopathology, social dysfunction and burden on families of schizophrenic patients. *Psychological Medicine*, **12**: 651–658.

Pal DK, Das T, Chaudhury G, Johnson AL, Neville B (1998). Randomised controlled trial to assess acceptability of phenobarbital for epilepsy in rural India. *Lancet*, **351**(9095): 19–23.

Patel A, Knapp MRJ (1998). Costs of mental illness in England. *Mental Health Research Review*, **5**: 4–10.

Patel V (2001). Poverty, inequality, and mental health in developing countries. In: Leon D, Walt G, eds. *Poverty, inequality and health: an international perspective*. Oxford, Oxford University Press: 247–261.

Patel V, Araya R, de Lima M, Ludermir A, Todd C (1999). Women, poverty and common mental disorders in four restructuring societies. *Social Science and Medicine*, **49**: 1461–1471.

Paykel ES (1994). Life events, social support and depression. *Acta Psychiatrica Scandinavica*, **377** (Suppl): 50–58.

Pearson V (1992). Community and culture: a Chinese model of community care for the mentally ill. *International Journal of Social Psychiatry*, **38**: 163–178.

Pearson V (1995). Goods on which one loses: women and mental health in China. *Social Science and Medicine*, **41**(8): 1159–1173.

Pharaoh FM, Marij J, Streiner D (2000). Family intervention for schizophrenia. *Cochrane Collaboration database of systematic reviews*, **1**: 1–36.

Pomerleau OF, Downey KK, Stelson FW, Polerleau CS (1995). Cigarette smoking in adult patients diagnosed with attention deficit hyperactivity disorder. *Journal of Substance Abuse*, **7**(3): 373–378.

Radomsky ED, Haas GL, Mann JJ, Sweeney JA (1999). Suicidal behavior in patients with schizophrenia and other psychotic disorders. *American Journal of Psychiatry*, **156**(10): 1590–1595.

Ranrakha S, Caspi A, Dickson N, Moffitt TE, Paul C (2000). Psychiatric disorders and risky sexual behaviours in young adulthood: cross sectional study in birth cohort. *British Medical Journal*, **321**(7256): 263–266.

Rashliesel J, Scott K, Dixon L (1999). Co-occurring severe mental illness and substance abuse disorders: a review of recent research. *Psychiatric Services*, **50**(11): 1427–1434.

Reed GM, Kemeny ME, Taylor SE, Wang HYJ, Vissher BR (1994). Realistic acceptance as a predictor of decreased survival time in gay men with AIDS. *Health Psychology*, **13**(4): 299–307.

Regier DA, Boyd JH, Burke JD, Rae DS, Myers JK, Kramer M, Robins LN, George LK, Karno M, Locke BZ (1988). One-month prevalence of mental disorders in the United States. Based on five Epidemiologic Catchment Area sites. *Archives of General Psychiatry* **45**: 977–986.

Rezaki MS, Ozgen G, Kaplan I, Gursoy BM, Sagduyu A, Ozturk OM (1995). Results from the Ankara centre. In: Ustun TB, Sartorius N, eds. *Mental illness in general health care: an international study.* Chichester, John Wiley & Sons on behalf of the World Health Organization: 39–55.

Rice DP, Fox PJ, Max W, Webber PA, Lindeman DA, Hauck WW, Segura E (1993). The economic burden of Alzheimer's disease care. *Health Affairs*, **12**(2): 164–176.

Rice DP, Kelman S, Miller LS (1991). Estimates of economic costs of alcohol and drug abuse and mental illness, 1985 and 1988. *Public Health Reports*, **106**(3): 280–292.

Rice DP, Kelman S, Miller LS, Dummeyer S (1990). *The economic costs of alcohol and drug abuse and mental illness: 1985*. Rockville, MD, Alcohol, Drug Abuse and Mental Health Administration (Publication No. (ADM) 90-1694).

Riley L, Marshall M, eds (1999). *Alcohol and public health in eight developing countries*. Geneva, World Health Organization (unpublished document WHO/HSC/SAB/99.9).

Rosenbaum JF, Hylan TR (1999). Costs of depressive disorders. In: Maj M, Sartorius N, eds. *Evidence and practice in psychiatry: depressive disorders*. New York, John Wiley & Sons: 401–449.

Rosenberg ML, Mercy JA, Potter LB (1999). Firearms and suicide. *New England Journal of Medicine*, **341**: 1609–1611.

Rossow I (2000). Suicide, violence and child abuse: a review of the impact of alcohol consumption on social problems. *Contemporary Drug Problems*, **27**(3): 397–334.

Rutz W, Knorring L, Walinder, J (1995). Long-term effects of an educational program for general practitioners given by the Swedish Committee for the Prevention and Treatment of Depression. *Acta Psychiatrica Scandinavica*, **85**: 83–88.

Saeed K, Rehman I, Mubbashar MH (2000). Prevalence of psychiatric morbidity among the attendees of a native faithhealer at Rawalpindi. *Journal of College of Physicians and Surgeons of Pakistan*, **10**: 7–9.

Sankar R, Pulger T, Rai B, Gomathi S, Gyatso TR, Pandav CS (1998). Epidemiology of endemic cretinism in Sikkim, India. *Indian Journal of Pediatrics*, **65**(2): 303–309.

Saraceno B, Barbui C (1997). Poverty and mental illness. *Canadian Journal of Psychiatry*, **42**: 285–290.

Sartorius N (1997). Fighting schizophrenia and its stigma. A new World Psychiatric Association educational programme. *British Journal of Psychiatry*, **170**: 297.

Sartorius N (1998a). Stigma: what can psychiatrists do about it? *Lancet*, **352**(9133): 1058–1059.

Sartorius N (1998b). Scientific work in the Third World Countries. *Acta Psychiatrica Scandinavica*, **98**: 345–347.

Sartorius N, Jablensky A, Korten A, Ernberg G, Anker M, Cooper JE, Day R (1986). Early manifestations and first-contact incidence of schizophrenia in different cultures. A preliminary report on the initial evaluation phase of the WHO Collaborative Study on determinants of outcome of severe mental disorders. *Psychological Medicine*, **16**: 909–928.

Sartorius N, Janca A (1996). Psychiatric assessment instruments developed by the World Health Organization. *Social Psychiatry and Psychiatric Epidemiology*, **31**(2): 55–69.

Schulberg HC, Block MR, Madonia MJ, Scott CP, Rodriguez E, Imber SD, Perel J, Lave J, Houck PR, Coulehan JL (1996). Treating major depression in primary care practice: eight-month clinical outcomes. *Archives of General Psychiatry*, **53**: 913–919.

Schulberg HC, Katon W, Simon GE, Rush J (1998). Treating major depression in primary care practice: an update of the Agency for Health Care Policy and Research Practice Guidelines. *Archives of General Psychiatry*, **55**: 1121–1127.

Scott RA, Lhatoo SD, Sander JWAS (2001). The treatment of epilepsy in developing countries: where do we go from here? *Bulletin of the World Health Organization*, **79**: 344–351.

Senanayake N, Román GC (1993). Epidemiology of epilepsy in developing countries. *Bulletin of the World Health Organization*, **71**: 247–258.

Shaffer D, Fisher P, Dulcan MK, Davies M, Piacentini J, Schwab-Stone ME, Lahey BB, Bourdon K, Jensen PS, Bird HR, Canino C, Regier DA (1996). The NIMH Diagnostic Interview Schedule for Children version 2.3 (DISC-2.3): description acceptability, prevalence rates, and performance in the MECA study. *Journal of the American Academy of Child and Adolescent Psychiatry*, **35**: 865–877.

Somasundaram DJ, van de Put WA, Eisenbach M, Jong JT de (1999). Starting mental health services in Cambodia. *Social Science and Medicine*, **48**(8): 1029–1046.

Spagna ME, Cantwell DP, Baker L (2000). Reading disorder. In: Sadock BJ, Sadock VA, etc. *Comprehensive textbook of psychiatry*. Philadelphia, Lippincott Williams & Wilkins: 2614–2619.

Spiegel D, Bloom JR, Kraemer HC, Gottheil E (1989). Effect of psychosocial treatment on survival of patients with metastatic breast cancer. *Lancet*, **2**(8668): 888–891.

Srinivasa Murthy R (2000). Reaching the unreached. *The Lancet Perspective*, **356**: 39.

Sriram TG, Chandrasekar CR, Issac MK, Srinivasa Murthy R, Shanmugam V (1990). Training primary care medical officers in mental health care: an evaluation using a multiple choice questionnaire. *Acta Psychiatrica Scandinavica*, **81**: 414–417.

Starace F, Baldassarre C, Biancolilli V, Fea M, Serpelloni G, Bartoli L, Maj M (1998). Early neuropsychological impairment in HIV-seropositive intravenous drug users: evidence from the Italian Multicentre Neuropsychological HIV Study. *Acta Psychiatrica Scandinavica*, **97**(2): 132–138.

Steinhausen HC, Winkler C, Metzke CW, Meier M, Kannenberg R (1998). Prevalence of child and adolescent psychiatric disorders: the Zurich Epidemiological Study. *Acta Psychiatrica Scandinavica*, **98**: 262–271.

Summerfield D (2001). The invention of post-traumatic stress disorder and the social usefulness of a psychiatric category. *British Medical Journal*, **322** (7278): 95–98.

Tadesse B, Kebede D, Tegegne T, Alem A (1999). Childhood behavioural disorders in Ambo district, Western Ethiopia: I. Prevalence estimates. *Acta Psychiatrica Scandinavica*, **100**(Suppl): 92–97.

Talbott, JA (1999). The American experience with managed care – how Europe can avoid it. In: Guimon J, Sartorius N, eds. *Manage or perish? The challenges of managed mental health in Europe*. New York, Khluwer.

Tangchararoensathien V, Harnvoravongchai P, Pitayarangsarit S, Kasemsup V (2000). Health aspects of rapid socioeconomic changes in Thailand. *Social Science and Medicine*, **51**: 789–807.

Tansella M, Thornicroft G, eds. (1999). *Common mental disorders in primary care.* London, Routledge.

Thara R, Eaton WW (1996). Outcome of schizophrenia: the Madras longitudinal study. *Australian and New Zealand Journal of Psychiatry,* **30**(4): 516–522.

Thara R, Henrietta M, Joseph A, Rajkumar S, Eaton WW (1994). Ten-year course of schizophrenia: the Madras longitudinal study. *Acta Psychiatrica Scandinavica,* **90**: 344–351.

Thornicroft G, Sartorius N (1993). The course and outcome of depression in different cultures: 10-year follow-up of the WHO Collaborative Study on the Assessment of Depressive Disorders. *Psychological Medicine,* **23**: 1023–1032.

Thornicroft G, Tansella M (2000). *Balancing community-based and hospital-based mental health care: the new agenda.* Geneva, World Health Organization (unpublished document).

Tomov T (1999). Central and Eastern European countries. In: Thornicroft G, Tansella G, eds. *The mental health matrix: a manual to improve services.* Cambridge, Cambridge University Press: 216–227.

True WR, Xian H, Scherrer JF, Madden PAF, Kathleen K, Health AC, Andrew C, Eisen SA, Lyons MJ, Goldberg J, Tsuang M (1999). Common genetic vulnerability for nicotine and alcohol dependence in men. *Archives of General Psychiatry,* **56**: 655–661.

UK700 Group (1999). Predictors of quality of life in people with severe mental illness. *British Journal of Psychiatry,* **175**: 426–432.

UNAIDS (Joint United Nations Programme on HIV/AIDS) (2000). *Report on the global HIV/AIDS epidemic.* Geneva, UNAIDS.

United Nations (1957; 1977). *Standard minimum rules for the treatment of prisoners.* New York, United Nations (ECOSOC resolution 663C (XXIV); ECOSOC resolution 2076 (LXII)).

United Nations (1989). *Convention on the Rights of the Child.* New York, United Nations (UNGA document A/RES/44/25) .

United Nations (1991). *The protection of persons with mental illness and the improvement of mental health care.* UN General Assembly resolution A/RES/46.119 (available at: http://www.un.org/ga/documents/ gadocs.htm).

Upanne M, Hakanen J, Rautava M (1999). *Can suicide be prevented? The suicide project in Finland 1992– 1996: goals, implementation and evaluation.* Saarijävi, Stakes.

US Department of Health and Human Services (DHHS) (1999). *Mental health: a report of the Surgeon General – Executive summary.* Rockville, MD, Department of Health and Human Services, US Public Health Service.

US Department of Health and Human Services (DHHS) (2001). *Report of the Surgeon General's Conference on Children's Mental Health: a national action agenda.* Rockville, MD, US Department of Health and Human Services.

Üstün TB, Rehm J, Chatterji S, Saxena S, Trotter R, Room R, Bickenbach J, and the WHO/NIH Joint Project CAR Study Group (1999). Multiple-informant ranking of the disabling effects of different health conditions in 14 countries. *Lancet,* **354**(9173): 111–115.

Üstün TB, Sartorius N (1995). *Mental illness in general health care: an international study.* Chichester, John Wiley & Sons on behalf of the World Health Organization.

Vijayakumar L (2001). Personal communication.

Von Korff M, Moore JE, Lorig K, Cherkin DC, Saunders K, Gonzalez VM, Laurent D, Rutter C, Comite F (1998). A randomized trial of a lay person-led self-management group intervention for back pain patients in primary care. *Spine,* **23**(23): 2608–2615.

Vos T, Mathers CD (2000). Burden of mental disorders: Australia and Global Burden of Disease studies. *Bulletin of the World Health Organization,* **78**: 427–438.

Vroublevsky A, Harwin J (1998). Russia. In: Grant M, ed. *Alcohol and emerging markets: patterns, problems and responses.* Philadelphia, Brunner Mazel: 203–223.

Wang X, Gao L, Zhang H, Zhao C, Shen Y, Shinfuku N (2000). Post-earthquake quality of life and psychological well being: longitudinal evaluation in a rural community sample in Northern China. *Psychiatry and Clinical Neurosciences,* **54**: 427–433.

Ward E, King M, Lloyd M, Bower P, Sibbald B, Farelly S, Gabbay M, Tarrier N, Addington-Hall J (2000). Randomised controlled trial of non-directive counselling, cognitive behaviour therapy and usual general practitioner care for patients with depression. I: clinical effectiveness. *British Medical Journal,* **321**: 1381–1388.

Wells JE, Bushnell JA, Hornblow AR, Joyce PR, Oakley-Browne MA (1989). Christchurch Psychiatric Epidemiology Study, part I: methodology and lifetime prevalence for specific psychiatric disorders. *Australian and New Zealand Journal of Psychiatry,* **23**: 315–326.

Weyerer S, Castell R, Biener A, Artner K, Dilling H (1988). Prevalence and treatment of psychiatric disorders in 3–14-year-old children: results of a representative field study in the small rural town region of Traunstein, Upper Bavaria. *Acta Psychiatrica Scandinavica,* **77**: 290–296.

Whiteford H, Thompson I, Casey D (2000). The Australian mental health system. *International Journal of Law and Psychiatry,* **23**(3–4): 403–417.

WHO International Consortium of Psychiatric Epidemiology (2000). Cross-national comparisons of mental disorders. *Bulletin of the World Health Organization,* **78**: 413–426.

WHO Multi-country Study on Women's Health and Domestic Violence (2001). Preliminary results. Geneva, World Health Organization.

Wilk AI, Jensen NM, Havighurst TC (1997). Meta-analysis of randomized control trials addressing brief interventions in heavy alcohol drinkers. *Journal of General Internal Medicine,* **12**: 274–283.

Williams DR, Williams-Morris, R (2000). Racism and mental health: the African American experience. *Ethnicity and Health,* **5**(3/4): 243–268.

Winefield HR, Harvey EJ (1994). Needs of family care-givers in chronic schizophrenia. *Schizophrenia Bulletin,* **20**(3): 557–566.

Wing JK, Cooper JE, Sartorius N (1974). *The measurement and classification of psychiatric symptoms.* London, Cambridge University Press.

Wintemute GJ, Parham CA, Beaumont JJ, Wright M, Drake C (1999). Mortality among recent purchasers of handguns. *New England Journal of Medicine,* **341**: 1583–1589.

Wittchen HU, Nelson CB, Lachner G (1998). Prevalence of mental disorders and psychosocial impairments in adolescents and young adults. *Psychological Medicine,* **28**: 109–126.

Wittchen HU, Robins LN, Cottler LB, Sartorius N, Burke JD, Regier D and Participants in the Multicentre WHO/ADAMHA Field Trials (1991). *British Journal of Psychiatry,* **159**: 645–653.

World Bank (1993). *World development report 1993: investing in health.* New York, Oxford University Press for the World Bank.

World Bank (1999). *Development in practice – Curbing the epidemic: governments and the economics of tobacco control.* Washington DC, World Bank.

World Health Organization (1975). *Organization of mental health services in developing countries. Sixteenth report of the WHO Expert Committee on Mental Health, December 1974.* Geneva, World Health Organization (WHO Technical Report Series, No. 564).

World Health Organization (1988). *Benzidiazepines and therapeutic counselling. Report from a WHO Collaborative Study.* Berlin, Springer-Verlag.

World Health Organization (1989). *Consumer involvement in mental health and rehabilitation services.* Geneva, World Health Organization (unpublished document WHO/MNH/MEP/89.7).

World Health Organization (1990). *WHO child care facility schedule.* Geneva, World Health Organization (unpublished document WHO/MNH/PSF/90.3).

World Health Organization (1992a). *International statistical classification of diseases and related health problems, Tenth revision 1992 (ICD-10). Vol. 1: Tabular list. Vol. 2: Instruction manual. Vol. 3: Alphabetical index.* Geneva, World Health Organization.

World Health Organization (1992b). *The ICD-10 classification of mental and behavioural disorders: clinical descriptions and diagnostic guidelines.* Geneva, World Health Organization.

World Health Organization (1993a). *The ICD-10 classification of mental and behavioural disorders: diagnostic criteria for research.* Geneva, World Health Organization.

World Health Organization (1993b). *Essential treatments in psychiatry.* Geneva, World Health Organization (unpublished document WHO/MNH/MND/93.26).

World Health Organization (1994). Cause-of-death statistics and vital rates, civil registration systems and alternative sources of information. *World Health Statistics Annual 1993,* Section A/B: China 11–17.

World Health Organization (1995). *Psychosocial rehabilitation: a consensus statement.* Geneva, World Health Organization (unpublished document WHO/MNH/MND/96.2).

World Health Organization (1996). WHO Brief Intervention Study Group: a cross-national trial of brief interventions with heavy drinkers. *American Journal of Public Health,* **86**: 948–955.

World Health Organization (1997a). *Violence against women.* Geneva, World Health Organization (unpublished document WHO/FRH/WHD/97.8).

World Health Organization (1997b). *An overview of a strategy to improve the mental health of underserved populations: Nations for Mental Health.* Geneva, World Health Organization (unpublished document WHO/MSA/NAM/97.3).

World Health Organization (1998). *WHO Expert Committee on Drug Dependence, thirtieth report.* Geneva, World Health Organization (WHO Technical Report Series, No. 873).

World Health Organization (1999). *Global status report on alcohol.* Geneva, World Health Organization (unpublished document WHO/HSC/SAB/99.11).

World Health Organization (2000a). *Gender and the use of medications: a systematic review.* Geneva, World Health Organization (unpublished working document WHO/GHW).

World Health Organization (2000b). *Women's mental health: an evidence-based review.* Geneva, World Health Organization (unpublished document WHO/MSD/MHP/00.1).

World Health Organization (2000c). *The World Health Report 2000 – Health systems: improving performance.* Geneva, World Health Organization.

World Health Organization (2001). *Mental health resources in the world. Initial results of Project Atlas.* Geneva, World Health Organization (Fact Sheet No. 260, April 2001).

Xu Huilan, Xiao Shuiyuan, Chen Jiping, Lui Lianzhong (2000). Epidemiological study on committed suicide among the elderly in some urban and rural areas of Hunan province, China. *Chinese Mental Health Journal,* **14**(2): 121–124.

Ziegelstein RC, Fauerbach JA, Stevens SS, Romanelli J, Richter DP, Bush DE (2000). Patients with depression are less likely to follow recommendations to reduce cardiac risk during recovery from a myocardial infarction. *Archives of Internal Medicine,* **160**: 1818–1823.

Zimmerman M, McDermut W, Mattia JI (2000). Frequency of anxiety disorders in psychiatric outpatients with major depressive disorder. *American Journal of Psychiatry,* **157**: 1337–1340.

Statistical Annex

The tables in this technical annex present updated information on the burden of disease and summary measures of population health in WHO Member States and Regions for the year 2000. The material in these tables will be presented on an annual basis in each World health report. As with any innovative approach, methods and data sources can be refined and improved. It is hoped that careful scrutiny and use of the results will lead to progressively better measurement of health attainment in the coming World health reports. All the main results are reported with uncertainty intervals in order to communicate to the user the plausible range of estimates for each country on each measure. Where data are presented by country, initial WHO estimates and technical explanations were sent to Member States for comment. Comments or data provided in response were discussed with them and incorporated where possible. The estimates reported here should still be interpreted as the best estimates of WHO rather than the official viewpoint of Member States.

STATISTICAL ANNEX

EXPLANATORY NOTES

The tables in this technical annex present updated information on the burden of disease and summary measures of population health in WHO Member States and Regions for the year 2000. The work leading to these annex tables was undertaken mostly by the WHO Global Programme on Evidence for Health Policy and the Department of Health Financing and Stewardship in collaboration with counterparts from the Regional Offices of WHO. The material in these tables will be presented on an annual basis in each *World health report*. Working papers have been prepared which provide details on the concepts, methods and results that are only briefly mentioned here. The footnotes to these technical notes include a complete listing of the detailed working papers.

As with any innovative approach, methods and data sources can be refined and improved. It is hoped that careful scrutiny and use of the results will lead to progressively better measurement of health attainment in the coming *World health reports*. All the main results are reported with uncertainty intervals in order to communicate to the user the plausible range of estimates for each country on each measure. Where data are presented by country, initial WHO estimates and technical explanations were sent to Member States for comment. Comments or data provided in response were discussed with them and incorporated where possible. The estimates reported here should still be interpreted as the best estimates of WHO rather than the official viewpoint of Member States.

ANNEX TABLE 1

To assess overall levels of health achievement, it is crucial to develop the best possible assessment of the life table for each country. New life tables have been developed for all 191 Member States starting with a systematic review of all available evidence from surveys, censuses, sample registration systems, population laboratories and vital registration on levels and trends in child mortality and adult mortality.[1] This review benefited greatly from the work undertaken on child mortality by UNICEF[2] and on general mortality by the United States Census Bureau[3] and the UN Population Division 2000 demographic assessment.[4] All estimates of population size and structure for 2000 are based on the 2000 demographic assessment prepared by the United nations Population Division.[4] These estimates refer to the de facto resident population, and not the de jure population in each Member State. To aid in demographic, cause of death and burden of disease analyses, the 191 Member States have been divided into 5 mortality strata on the basis of their level of child (5q0) and adult male mortality (45q15). The matrix defined by the six WHO Regions and the 5 mortality strata leads to 14 subregions, since not every mortality stratum is represented in every Region. These subregions are used in Tables 2 and 3 for presentation of results.

Because of increasing heterogeneity of patterns of adult and child mortality, WHO has developed a model life table system of two-parameter logit life tables using a global standard, and with additional age-specific parameters to correct for systematic biases in the application of a two-parameter system.[5] This system of model life tables has been used extensively in the development of life tables for those Member States without adequate vital registration and in projecting life tables to 2000 when the most recent data available are from earlier years. Details on the data, methods and results by country of this life table analysis are available in the corresponding technical paper.[1] The World Health Organization uses a standard method to estimate and project life tables for all Member States with comparable data. This may lead to minor differences compared with official life tables prepared by Member States.

To capture the uncertainty due to sampling, indirect estimation technique or projection to 2000, a total of 1000 life tables have been developed for each Member State. Uncertainty bounds are reported in Annex Table 1 by giving key life table values at the 10th percentile and the 90th percentile. This uncertainty analysis was facilitated by the development of new methods and software tools.[6] In countries with a substantial HIV epidemic, recent estimates of the level and uncertainty range of the magnitude of the HIV epidemic have been incorporated into the life table uncertainty analysis.[7]

ANNEX TABLES 2 AND 3

Causes of death for the 14 subregions and the world have been estimated based on data from national vital registration systems that capture about 17 million deaths annually. In addition, information from sample registration systems, population laboratories and epidemiological analyses of specific conditions has been used to improve estimates of the cause of death patterns.[6-8] WHO is intensifying efforts with Member States to obtain and verify recent vital registration data on causes of death.

Cause of death data have been carefully analysed to take into account incomplete coverage of vital registration in countries and the likely differences in cause of death patterns that would be expected in the uncovered and often poorer sub-populations. Techniques to undertake this analysis have been developed based on the global burden of disease study[9] and further refined using a much more extensive database and more robust modelling techniques.[10]

Special attention has been paid to problems of misattribution or miscoding of causes of death in cardiovascular diseases, cancer, injuries and general ill-defined categories. A correction algorithm for reclassifying ill-defined cardiovascular codes has been developed.[11] Cancer mortality by site has been evaluated using both vital registration data and population-based cancer incidence registries. The latter have been analysed using a complete age, period cohort model of cancer survival in each region.[8]

Annex Table 3 provides estimates of the burden of disease using disability-adjusted life years (DALYs) as a measure of the health gap in the world in 2000. DALYs along with healthy life expectancy are summary measures of population health.[12,13] One DALY can be thought of as one lost year of "healthy" life and the burden of disease as a measurement of the gap between the current health of a population and an ideal situation where everyone in the population lives into old age in full health. DALYs for a disease or health condition are calculated as the sum of the years of life lost due to premature mortality (YLL) in the population and the years lost due to disability (YLD) for incident cases of the health condition. For a review of the development of the DALY and recent advances in the measurement of the burden of disease, see Murray & Lopez.[14] For a more comprehensive review of the conceptual and other issues underlying summary measures of population health, see Murray et al.[13] DALYs for 2000 have been estimated based on cause of death information for each Region and regional assessments of the epidemiology of major disabling conditions. For this report, burden of disease estimates have been updated for many of the cause categories included in the Global Burden of Disease 2000 study, based on the wealth of data on major diseases and injuries available to WHO technical programmes and through collaboration with scientists worldwide.[15] Examples are the extensive data sets on tuberculosis, maternal conditions, injuries, diabetes, cancer, and sexually transmitted infections. These data, together with new and revised estimates of deaths by cause, age and sex, for all Member States, have been used to develop internally consistent estimates of incidence, prevalence, duration and DALYs for over 130 major causes, for 14 sub-regions of the world.

ANNEX TABLE 4

Annex Table 4 reports the average level of population health for WHO Member States in terms of healthy life expectancy. Based on more than 15 years of work, WHO introduced disability-adjusted life expectancy (DALE) as a summary measure of the level of health attained by populations in *The World Health Report 2000*.[16,17] To better reflect the inclusion of all states of health in the calculation of healthy life expectancy, the name of the indicator used to measure healthy life expectancy has been changed from disability-adjusted life expectancy (DALE) to health-adjusted life expectancy (HALE). HALE is based on life expectancy at birth (see Annex Table 1) but includes an adjustment for *time spent in poor health*. It is most easily understood as the equivalent number of years in full health that a newborn can expect to live based on current rates of ill-health and mortality.

The measurement of *time spent in poor health* is based on combining condition-specific estimates from the Global Burden of Disease 2000 study with estimates of the prevalence of different health states by age and sex derived from health surveys carried out by WHO.[18] Representative household surveys are being undertaken in approximately 70 countries using a new instrument based on the International Classification of Functioning, Disability and Health,[19] which seeks information from a representative sample of respondents on their current states of health according to 7 core domains.[20] These domains were identified from an extensive review of the currently available health status measurement instruments.

Analyses of over 50 national health surveys for the calculation of healthy life expectancy in *The World Health Report 2000* identified severe limitations in the comparability of self-reported health status data from different populations, even when identical survey instruments and methods are used.[17,21] To overcome this problem, the WHO survey instrument uses performance tests and vignettes to calibrate self-reported health on selected domains such as cognition, mobility and vision. WHO is developing several statistical methods for correcting biases in self-reported health using these data, based on the hierarchical ordered probit (HOPIT) model.[22] The calibrated responses are used to estimate the true prevalence of different states of health by age and sex.

The uncertainty ranges for healthy life expectancy given in Annex Table 4 are based on the 10th percentile and 90th percentile of the relevant uncertainty distributions.[23] The ranges thus define 80% uncertainty intervals around the estimates. HALE uncertainty is a function of the uncertainty in age-specific mortality measurement for each country, of the uncertainty in burden of disease based estimates of country-level disability prevalence, and of uncertainty in the health state prevalences derived from health surveys.

Healthy life expectancy estimates for Member States for the year 2000 are not directly comparable with those published in last year's World Health Report for 1999 as they incorporate new epidemiological information, new data from health surveys, and new information on mortality rates, as well as improvements in methods.

The new evidence from the WHO Multi-country Household Survey Study has resulted in an overall increase in severity-weighted prevalences, an increase for females relative to males, and hence to a reduction in HALE estimates. This has affected all Member States and at the global level, reduced HALE at birth from the previous estimate of 56.8 years in 1999 to the current estimate of 56.0 years for the year 2000. For some Member States, there have also been changes in HALE estimates due to new information provided on age-specific mortality rates.

ANNEX TABLE 5

National Health Accounts are designed to be a policy relevant, comprehensive, consistent, timely and standardized instrument that traces the levels and trends of consumption of health goods and services (the expenditure approach), the value added created by service and manufacturing industries producing these commodities (the production approach) and the incomes generated by this process as well as the taxes, mandatory contributions, premiums and direct payments that fund the system (the income approach). The current developmental stage of WHO's tentative summary National Health Accounts leans more towards a measurement of the financing flows.

The estimates shown are *measured* expenditure and order of magnitude only. All estimates are preliminary.

As in every systems accounting build-up, the "first round data" are likely to be substantially modified in subsequent stages of the accounting development process. The very first estimates for 1997 have been thoroughly revised in light of statistics and other data made accessible after the completion of *The World Health Report 2000*.

Public expenditure on health comprises the current and capital outlays of territorial government (central/federal authorities, regional/provincial/state authorities, and local/municipal authorities) plus social security schemes whose affiliation is compulsory for a sizeable share of the population and extrabudgetary funds earmarked for health services delivery or financing. They include grants and loans provided by international agencies, other national authorities and sometimes commercial banks.

Private expenditure on health comprises private insurance schemes and prepaid medical care plans, services delivered or financed by enterprises (other than contributions to social security and prepaid plans), mandated or not, outlays by nongovernmental organizations and non-profit institutions serving mainly households, out-of-pocket payments, and other privately funded schemes not elsewhere classified, including investment outlays.

The intended *Social security funding* of health expenditure is that of contributions by employers and employees at the exclusion of government transfer payments and subsidies to Social Security institutions which are tax funded flows; this netting-out has only been partly attained in the present state of health accounting.

The *External resources* contribution to health systems financing is mostly directed towards public programmes but includes transfers towards private programmes whose magnitude could not be documented. The ratios of traceable external resources below 0.05% of public expenditure on health, as well as a few entries known to be positive but without quantitative evidence, are shown as "…".

A share of *Tax-funded outlays* is directed in some countries towards the prepayment of loans contracted for health, which could not always be separated from direct expenditure on health services delivery and administration.

For the purpose of Annex Table 5, other private prepaid health plans that are not strictly based on risk-related contracts have been added to *Private insurance* as another form of risk pooling. Zeros in that column do not necessarily indicate the absence of such financial intermediaries and may only mean that, in the absence of data, this form of financing is lumped with out-of-pocket outlays. In cases of suspected positive entries without quantitative evidence, "…" has been used.

Out-of-pocket (OOP) disbursements include, to the extent possible, deductibles and co-payments under social security and other prepaid schemes, other costs incurred by households net of reimbursements under a private or public prepaid arrangement, and other private pre-paid plans.

When no information is available for *Private insurance, Nongovernmental organizations* (NGOs) and/or *Enterprise outlays on health service*, the lacunae inflate the OOPs. Private insurance and OOPs do not necessarily add up to Private expenditure on health.

Exchange rates are the average observed rates at which currencies are traded by the banking system, expressed in US dollars. International dollar estimates are derived by dividing local currency units by an estimate of their purchasing power parity (PPP) compared to US$. PPPs are the rates of currency conversion that equalise the purchasing power of different currencies by eliminating the differences in price levels between countries.

The GDP levels for the OECD countries follow the new Standard National Accounts (SNA93) and those originating from the United Nations and the IMF incorporate SNA93 time series whenever Member States' statistical agencies moved to the new concepts and definitions. For non-OECD countries, where there were differences between the United Nations, the IMF and the World Bank, the reported number reflects the most plausible trend.

For statistical purposes, the data for China do not include those for the Hong Kong Special Administrative Region and the Macao Special Administrative Region. For Jordan, data for territory under occupation since 1967 by Israel is excluded.

Sources of data

Health Expenditure (Public, Private, Social Security, Tax-funded, External, Private Insurance, Out-of-pocket): WHO NHA data files based on *OECD Health Data 2001*; National Health Expenditure accounts in several Member States; IMF *Government Financial Statistics*; United Nations *National Accounts,* Tables 2.1 and 2.5 extended through 1998; World Bank *Development Indicators*; national *Statistical Yearbooks* and other reports containing estimates consistent with the principles underlying the data lifted from the sources quoted; household surveys; WHO secretariat estimates and correspondence with officials in Member States.

GDP: United Nations *National Accounts*, IMF *International Financial Statistics*, World Bank *World Development Indicators*, OECD *National Accounts.*

General Government Expenditures: United Nations *National Accounts*, Table 1.4 extended to 1998; OECD *National Accounts*, vol. II tables 5 and 6; IMF *International Financial Statistics*, central government disbursements grossed up to include regional and local authorities where possible.

Exchange rates: IMF *International Financial Statistics.* Purchasing power parities (PPPs) were estimated using methods similar to those used by the World Bank. PPPs were based on price comparison studies for 1996 where they existed. For other countries they were estimated using the GDP per capita in US dollars, UN post adjustment multipliers, and other geographical dummy variables. Forward projections were made to 1998 using the real GDP growth rate with the adjustment for US inflation using the US GDP deflators.

[1] Lopez AD, Ahmad O, Guillot M, Inoue M, Ferguson B (2001). *Life tables for 191 countries for 2000: data, methods, results.* Geneva, World Health Organization (GPE Discussion Paper No. 40).

[2] Hill K, Rohini PO, Mahy M, Jones G (1999). *Trends in child mortality in the developing world: 1960 to 1996.* New York, UNICEF.

[3] United States Bureau of the Census: International database available at http://www.census.gov/ipc/www/idbnew.html

[4] *World population prospects: the 2000 revision* (2001). New York , United Nations.

[5] Murray CJL, Ferguson B, Lopez AD, Guillot M, Salomon JA, Ahmad O (2001). *Modified-logit life table system: principles, empirical validation and application.* Geneva, World Health Organization (GPE Discussion Paper No. 39).

[6] Murray CJL, Salomon JA (1998). Modeling the impact of global tuberculosis control strategies. *Proceedings of the National Academy of Science of the USA*, 95(23): 13881–13886.

[7] Salomon JA, Murray CJL (2001). Modelling HIV/AIDS epidemics in sub-Saharan Africa using seroprevalence data from antenatal clinics. *Bulletin of the World Health Organization* 79(7): 596–607.

[8] Mathers CD, Murray CJL, Lopez AD, Boschi-Pinto C (2001). *Cancer incidence, mortality and survival by site for 14 regions of the world.* Geneva, World Health Organization (GPE Discussion Paper No. 13).

[9] Murray CJL, Lopez AD, eds (1996). *The global burden of disease: a comprehensive assessment of mortality and disability from diseases, injuries and risk factors in 1990 and projected to 2020.* Cambridge, MA, Harvard School of Public Health on behalf of the World Health Organization and the World Bank (Global Burden of Disease and Injury Series, Vol. 1).

[10] Salomon JA, Murray CJL (2000). *The epidemiological transition revisited: new compositional models for mortality by age, sex and cause.* Geneva, World Health Organization (GPE Discussion Paper No. 11, revised edition).

[11] Lozano R, Murray CJL, Lopez AD, Satoh T (2001). *Miscoding and misclassification of ischaemic heart disease mortality.* Geneva, World Health Organization (GPE Discussion Paper No. 12).

[12] Murray CJL, Salomon JA, Mathers CD (2000). A critical examination of summary measures of population health. *Bulletin of the World Health Organization*, 78: 981–994.

[13] Murray CJL, Salomon JA, Mathers CD, Lopez AD, eds (forthcoming in 2002). *Summary measures of population health: concepts, ethics, measurement and applications.* Geneva, World Health Organization.

[14] Murray CJL, Lopez AD (2000). Progress and directions in refining the global burden of disease approach: response to Williams. *Health Economics*, 9: 69–82.

[15] Murray CJL, Lopez AD, Mathers CD, Stein C (2001). *The Global Burden of Disease 2000 project: aims, methods and data sources.* Geneva, World Health Organization (GPE Discussion Paper No. 36).

[16] World Health Organization (2000). *The World Health Report 2000 – Health systems: improving performance.* Geneva, World Health Organization.

[17] Mathers CD, Sadana R, Salomon JA, Murray CJL, Lopez AD (2001). Healthy life expectancy in 191 countries, 1999. *Lancet*, 357(9269): 1685–1691.

[18] Mathers CD, Murray CJL, Lopez AD, Salomon JA, Sadana R, Tandon A, Üstün TB, Chatterji S. (2001). *Estimates of healthy life expectancy for 191 countries in the year 2000: methods and results.* Geneva, World Health Organization (GPE discussion paper No. 38).

[19] World Health Organization (2001). *International classification of functioning, disability and health (ICF).* Geneva, World Health Organization.

[20] Üstün TB, Chatterji S, Villanueva M, Bendib L, Sadana R, Valentine N, Mathers CD, Ortiz J, Tandon A, Salomon J, Yang C, Xie Wan J, Murray CJL. *WHO Multi-country Household Survey Study on Health and Responsiveness, 2000-2001* (2001). Geneva, World Health Organization (GPE discussion paper No. 37).

[21] Sadana R, Mathers CD, Lopez AD, Murray CJL (2000). *Comparative analysis of more than 50 household surveys on health status.* Geneva, World Health Organization (GPE Discussion Paper No. 15).

[22] Murray CJL, Tandon A, Salomon JA, Mathers CD (2000). *Enhancing cross-population comparability of survey results.* Geneva, World Health Organization (GPE Discussion Paper No. 35).

[23] Salomon JA, Murray CJL, Mathers CD (2000). *Methods for life expectancy and healthy life expectancy uncertainty analysis.* Geneva, World Health Organization (GPE Discussion Paper No. 10).

Annex Table 1 Basic indicators for all Member States

	Member State	POPULATION ESTIMATES							
		Total population (000)	Annual growth rate (%)	Dependency ratio (per 100)		Percentage of population aged 60+ years		Total fertility rate	
		2000	1990–2000	1990	2000	1990	2000	1990	2000
1	Afghanistan	21 765	4.8	88	86	4.7	4.7	7.1	6.9
2	Albania	3 134	−0.5	62	56	7.8	9.0	3.0	2.4
3	Algeria	30 291	2.0	84	64	5.7	6.0	4.5	3.0
4	Andorra	86	5.0	35	37	14.4	15.6	1.4	1.2
5	Angola	13 134	3.2	100	104	4.7	4.5	7.2	7.2
6	Antigua and Barbuda	65	0.3	64	57	9.1	9.9	1.9	1.6
7	Argentina	37 032	1.3	65	60	12.9	13.3	2.9	2.5
8	Armenia	3 787	0.7	56	48	10.0	13.2	2.3	1.2
9	Australia	19 138	1.3	49	49	15.5	16 3	1.9	1.8
10	Austria	8 080	0.4	48	47	20.1	20.7	1.5	1.3
11	Azerbaijan	8 041	1.1	61	56	8.0	10.5	2.7	1.7
12	Bahamas	304	1.8	59	54	6.7	8.0	2.6	2.4
13	Bahrain	640	2.7	51	45	3.8	4.7	3.7	2.5
14	Bangladesh	137 439	2.2	82	72	4.8	4.9	4.6	3.7
15	Barbados	267	0.4	57	45	15.3	13.4	1.7	1.5
16	Belarus	10 187	−0.1	51	47	16.5	18.9	1.8	1.2
17	Belgium	10 249	0.3	49	52	20.5	22.1	1.6	1.5
18	Belize	226	2.0	94	74	6.1	6.0	4.4	3.2
19	Benin	6 272	3.0	106	96	4.8	4.2	6.7	5.9
20	Bhutan	2 085	2.1	85	89	6.0	6.5	5.8	5.3
21	Bolivia	8 329	2.4	81	77	5.8	6.2	4.9	4.1
22	Bosnia and Herzegovina	3 977	−0.8	43	41	10.4	14.9	1.7	1.3
23	Botswana	1 541	2.2	95	82	3.6	4.5	5.1	4.1
24	Brazil	170 406	1.4	64	51	6.7	7.8	2.7	2.2
25	Brunei Darussalam	328	2.5	59	54	4.1	5.1	3.2	2.7
26	Bulgaria	7 949	−0.9	50	47	19.1	21.7	1.7	1.1
27	Burkina Faso	11 535	2.5	108	108	5.2	4.8	7.3	6.8
28	Burundi	6 356	1.2	93	102	4.7	4.3	6.8	6.8
29	Cambodia	13 104	3.1	90	88	4.4	4.4	5.6	5.0
30	Cameroon	14 876	2.5	95	88	5.6	5.6	5.9	4.9
31	Canada	30 757	1.1	47	46	15.5	16.7	1.7	1.6
32	Cape Verde	427	2.3	93	78	7.0	6.5	4.3	3.4
33	Central African Republic	3 717	2.4	90	89	6.3	6.1	5.6	5.1
34	Chad	7 885	3.1	95	98	5.3	4.9	6.7	6.7
35	Chile	15 211	1.5	57	55	9.0	10.2	2.6	2.4
36	China	1 282 437	1.0	50	46	8.6	10.0	2.2	1.8
37	Colombia	42 105	1.9	68	60	6.3	6.9	3.1	2.7
38	Comoros	706	3.0	98	84	4.1	4.2	6.2	5.2
39	Congo	3 018	3.1	95	98	5.3	5.1	6.3	6.3
40	Cook Islands	20	0.7	70	65	5.7	6.8	4.2	3.3
41	Costa Rica	4 024	2.8	69	60	6.4	7.5	3.2	2.7
42	Côte d'Ivoire	16 013	2.4	96	83	4.2	5.0	6.3	4.9
43	Croatia	4 654	0.3	47	47	17.1	20.2	1.7	1.7
44	Cuba	11 199	0.5	46	44	11.7	13.7	1.7	1.6
45	Cyprus	784	1.4	58	53	14.8	15.7	2.4	2.0
46	Czech Republic	10 272	0.0	51	43	17.7	18.4	1.8	1.2
47	Democratic People's Republic of Korea	22 268	1.1	47	48	7.6	10.0	2.4	2.1
48	Democratic Republic of the Congo	50 948	3.3	100	107	4.6	4.5	6.7	6.7
49	Denmark	5 320	0.3	48	50	20.4	20.0	1.6	1.7
50	Djibouti	632	2.3	82	87	4.1	5.5	6.3	5.9
51	Dominica	71	−0.1	64	57	9.1	9.9	2.2	1.8
52	Dominican Republic	8 373	1.7	72	61	5.4	6.6	3.4	2.8
53	Ecuador	12 646	2.1	76	63	6.1	6.9	3.8	2.9
54	Egypt	67 884	1.9	78	65	6.0	6.3	4.2	3.1
55	El Salvador	6 278	2.1	82	68	6.4	7.2	3.7	3.0

	PROBABILITY OF DYING (per 1000)								LIFE EXPECTANCY AT BIRTH (years)			
	Under age 5 years				Between ages 15 and 59 years							
	Males		Females		Males		Females		Males		Females	
	2000	Uncertainty interval	2000	Uncertainty interval	2000	Uncertainty interval	2000	Uncertainty interval	2000	Uncertainty interval	2000	Uncertainty interval
1	252	202 – 301	249	199 – 299	437	341 – 529	376	280 – 473	44.2	38.5 – 50.1	45.1	39.2 – 51.7
2	47	37 – 57	40	31 – 50	209	191 – 227	95	85 – 107	64.3	62.8 – 65.7	72.9	71.6 – 74.1
3	54	44 – 63	47	38 – 56	155	141 – 168	119	106 – 132	68.1	66.9 – 69.4	71.2	69.9 – 72.4
4	5	3 – 7	4	2 – 6	105	71 – 137	41	21 – 61	77.2	74.4 – 81.7	83.8	80.2 – 89.5
5	217	192 – 242	198	175 – 220	492	412 – 565	386	317 – 452	44.3	40.8 – 47.9	48.3	44.9 – 52.0
6	25	20 – 30	22	17 – 27	183	165 – 200	133	118 – 147	71.8	70.5 – 73.1	76.6	75.4 – 77.9
7	24	22 – 27	20	19 – 23	184	178 – 190	92	88 – 96	70.2	69.8 – 70.6	77.8	77.3 – 78.3
8	56	50 – 62	38	32 – 44	223	213 – 233	106	96 – 118	64.4	63.8 – 65.0	71.2	70.2 – 72.2
9	7	6 – 8	5	4 – 6	100	95 – 103	54	51 – 58	76.6	76.3 – 77.1	82.1	81.7 – 82.5
10	6	5 – 7	5	4 – 5	125	118 – 133	60	57 – 63	74.9	74.4 – 75.4	81.4	81.0 – 81.8
11	101	82 – 121	88	71 – 106	261	231 – 290	153	134 – 172	61.7	59.2 – 64.2	68.9	66.6 – 71.3
12	14	10 – 20	12	9 – 18	267	252 – 281	161	149 – 173	68.0	67.1 – 68.9	74.8	73.9 – 75.6
13	11	7 – 15	8	5 – 12	120	110 – 130	93	83 – 103	72.7	71.9 – 73.9	74.7	73.7 – 75.8
14	91	81 – 101	93	83 – 103	262	235 – 290	252	227 – 276	60.4	58.6 – 62.3	60.8	59.1 – 62.6
15	13	9 – 16	13	10 – 16	180	161 – 200	122	110 – 134	71.6	70.4 – 72.8	77.7	76.6 – 78.9
16	17	13 – 21	12	9 – 15	381	362 – 401	133	123 – 143	62.0	61.0 – 62.9	74.0	73.2 – 74.9
17	8	7 – 9	6	5 – 7	128	124 – 132	67	62 – 70	74.6	74.2 – 75.0	80.9	80.5 – 81.3
18	37	30 – 40	32	28 – 35	200	185 – 216	124	120 – 132	69.1	68.0 – 70.3	74.7	74.0 – 75.2
19	162	153 – 168	151	143 – 158	384	356 – 408	328	297 – 350	51.7	50.4 – 53.0	53.8	52.5 – 55.8
20	93	72 – 112	92	73 – 113	268	213 – 325	222	173 – 271	60.4	57.0 – 64.4	62.5	58.9 – 66.3
21	88	81 – 96	80	66 – 80	264	239 – 292	219	189 – 236	60.9	59.1 – 62.4	63.6	62.7 – 65.9
22	21	17 – 26	16	13 – 22	200	166 – 224	93	80 – 108	68.7	67.4 – 70.7	74.7	73.3 – 76.0
23	85	70 – 100	83	73 – 102	703	660 – 738	669	637 – 696	44.6	42.4 – 47.1	44.4	42.3 – 46.5
24	49	41 – 58	42	35 – 49	259	240 – 282	136	120 – 155	64.5	63.0 – 65.7	71.9	70.2 – 73.5
25	12	10 – 15	7	6 – 10	144	128 – 163	97	85 – 110	73.4	72.1 – 74.8	78.7	77.3 – 80.3
26	22	20 – 24	17	16 – 19	239	235 – 249	103	98 – 106	67.4	66.8 – 67.6	74.9	74.6 – 75.4
27	217	212 – 222	206	201 – 211	559	544 – 573	507	493 – 520	42.6	42.0 – 43.4	43.6	42.9 – 44.4
28	196	172 – 221	183	158 – 208	648	586 – 700	603	538 – 657	40.6	37.7 – 43.7	41.3	38.2 – 45.5
29	136	131 – 141	120	114 – 124	373	361 – 384	264	252 – 273	53.4	52.7 – 54.2	58.5	57.9 – 59.5
30	149	142 – 157	140	133 – 148	488	460 – 513	440	413 – 464	49.0	47.6 – 50.4	50.4	48.9 – 51.9
31	6	5 – 6	5	4 – 5	101	96 – 105	57	53 – 60	76.0	75.6 – 76.5	81.5	81.1 – 81.9
32	56	45 – 70	40	30 – 54	210	191 – 239	121	111 – 133	66.5	64.4 – 67.9	72.3	71.1 – 73.3
33	199	192 – 206	185	177 – 192	620	588 – 652	573	536 – 605	41.6	40.3 – 43.1	42.5	41.1 – 44.4
34	192	182 – 202	171	161 – 181	449	429 – 471	361	340 – 381	47.4	46.1 – 48.7	51.1	49.7 – 52.6
35	12	10 – 14	10	8 – 11	151	132 – 157	67	60 – 71	72.5	72.0 – 73.8	79.5	78.8 – 80.4
36	38	31 – 41	44	38 – 49	161	150 – 170	110	100 – 120	68.9	68.2 – 69.7	73.0	72.0 – 74.2
37	29	25 – 34	21	17 – 24	238	225 – 250	115	108 – 122	67.2	66.3 – 68.1	75.1	74.3 – 75.8
38	107	99 – 114	95	88 – 102	381	345 – 415	325	294 – 356	55.3	53.6 – 57.1	58.1	56.3 – 59.8
39	134	124 – 154	122	103 – 142	475	413 – 537	406	344 – 465	50.1	46.8 – 52.7	52.9	49.5 – 56.4
40	23	16 – 28	20	14 – 24	175	163 – 190	152	140 – 164	68.7	67.8 – 69.4	72.1	71.2 – 73.0
41	18	15 – 20	15	12 – 17	131	118 – 139	78	71 – 82	73.4	72.7 – 74.5	78.8	78.1 – 79.8
42	152	142 – 162	138	130 – 146	553	507 – 588	494	451 – 527	46.4	44.9 – 48.5	48.4	46.8 – 50.6
43	10	9 – 12	7	7 – 9	178	173 – 183	74	70 – 79	69.8	69.5 – 70.1	77.7	77.3 – 78.1
44	9	9 – 10	8	7 – 9	143	139 – 147	94	91 – 99	73.7	73.3 – 74.0	77.5	77.1 – 77.8
45	9	8 – 9	7	6 – 8	116	107 – 122	59	52 – 64	74.8	74.3 – 75.6	79.0	78.3 – 79.8
46	6	6 – 7	6	5 – 6	174	171 – 177	75	72 – 76	71.5	71.3 – 71.7	78.2	78.0 – 78.6
47	54	31 – 80	52	30 – 79	238	215 – 264	192	167 – 217	64.5	62.0 – 66.3	67.2	64.6 – 69.2
48	218	170 – 247	205	169 – 229	571	512 – 631	493	451 – 535	41.6	38.6 – 45.8	44.0	41.2 – 47.5
49	7	6 – 7	5	5 – 6	129	126 – 133	82	76 – 85	74.2	73.8 – 74.5	78.5	78.2 – 79.0
50	184	153 – 212	168	139 – 195	590	497 – 667	541	461 – 618	43.5	39.9 – 48.2	44.7	40.1 – 49.3
51	14	10 – 18	13	9 – 16	183	173 – 197	105	95 – 115	72.6	71.5 – 73.6	78.3	77.0 – 79.7
52	55	50 – 60	45	41 – 50	234	222 – 246	146	136 – 158	65.5	64.5 – 66.4	71.6	70.5 – 72.6
53	41	36 – 44	33	30 – 36	199	189 – 208	120	114 – 127	68.2	67.5 – 68.9	74.2	73.6 – 74.8
54	51	46 – 54	49	45 – 53	210	201 – 219	147	140 – 153	65.4	64.8 – 66.0	69.1	68.5 – 69.7
55	40	36 – 44	33	28 – 36	250	238 – 262	148	135 – 158	66.3	65.4 – 67.1	73.3	72.4 – 74.4

Annex Table 1 Basic indicators for all Member States

	Member State	POPULATION ESTIMATES								
		Total population (000)	Annual growth rate (%)	Dependency ratio (per 100)		Percentage of population aged 60+ years		Total fertility rate	
		2000	1990–2000	1990	2000	1990	2000	1990	2000
56	Equatorial Guinea	457	2.6	87	91	6.4	6.0	5.9	5.9
57	Eritrea	3 659	1.7	88	88	4.4	4.7	6.2	5.5
58	Estonia	1 393	−1.2	51	47	17.2	20.2	1.9	1.2
59	Ethiopia	62 908	2.8	90	93	4.5	4.7	6.9	6.8
60	Fiji	814	1.2	69	58	4.9	5.7	3.4	3.1
61	Finland	5 172	0.4	49	49	18.5	19.9	1.7	1.6
62	France	59 238	0.4	52	53	19.1	20.5	1.8	1.8
63	Gabon	1 230	2.8	75	85	9.2	8.7	5.1	5.4
64	Gambia	1 303	3.4	81	77	4.8	5.2	5.9	5.0
65	Georgia	5 262	−0.4	51	50	15.0	18.7	2.1	1.5
66	Germany	82 017	0.3	45	47	20.4	23.2	1.4	1.3
67	Ghana	19 306	2.5	93	79	4.6	5.1	5.7	4.4
68	Greece	10 610	0.4	49	48	20.0	23.4	1.5	1.3
69	Grenada	94	0.3	64	57	9.1	9.9	4.2	3.5
70	Guatemala	11 385	2.7	97	89	5.1	5.3	5.6	4.7
71	Guinea	8 154	2.9	94	88	4.4	4.4	6.6	6.1
72	Guinea–Bissau	1 199	2.4	86	89	5.9	5.6	6.0	6.0
73	Guyana	761	0.4	70	55	6.7	6.9	2.6	2.4
74	Haiti	8 142	1.7	93	80	5.8	5.6	5.4	4.2
75	Honduras	6 417	2.8	93	82	4.5	5.1	5.1	4.0
76	Hungary	9 968	−0.4	51	46	19.0	19.7	1.8	1.3
77	Iceland	279	0.9	55	54	14.6	15.1	2.2	2.0
78	India	1 008 937	1.8	69	62	6.8	7.6	3.9	3.1
79	Indonesia	212 092	1.5	66	55	6.2	7.6	3.3	2.4
80	Iran, Islamic Republic of	70 330	1.9	89	69	4.7	5.2	5.0	3.0
81	Iraq	22 946	2.9	89	80	4.5	4.6	5.9	5.0
82	Ireland	3 803	0.8	63	49	15.1	15.2	2.1	2.0
83	Israel	6 040	3.0	68	62	12.4	13.2	3.0	2.8
84	Italy	57 530	0.1	45	48	21.1	24.1	1.3	1.2
85	Jamaica	2 576	0.8	74	63	10.0	9.6	2.8	2.4
86	Japan	127 096	0.3	44	47	17.4	23.2	1.6	1.4
87	Jordan	4 913	4.2	100	75	4.8	4.5	5.8	4.5
88	Kazakhstan	16 172	−0.3	60	51	9.6	11.2	2.7	2.0
89	Kenya	30 669	2.7	109	86	4.1	4.2	6.1	4.4
90	Kiribati	83	1.5	69	76	6.0	6.8	4.4	4.6
91	Kuwait	1 914	−1.1	61	50	2.1	4.4	3.6	2.8
92	Kyrgyzstan	4 921	1.1	74	67	8.3	9.0	3.7	2.6
93	Lao People's Democratic Republic	5 279	2.5	91	86	6.1	5.6	6.1	5.1
94	Latvia	2 421	−1.0	50	47	17.7	20.9	1.9	1.1
95	Lebanon	3 496	2.6	67	59	8.1	8.5	3.2	2.2
96	Lesotho	2 035	1.9	81	77	6.0	6.5	5.2	4.6
97	Liberia	2 913	3.1	118	84	5.1	4.5	6.8	6.8
98	Libyan Arab Jamahiriya	5 290	2.1	86	60	4.2	5.5	4.9	3.6
99	Lithuania	3 696	−0.1	50	49	16.1	18.6	1.9	1.3
100	Luxembourg	437	1.4	44	49	18.9	19.4	1.6	1.7
101	Madagascar	15 970	2.9	92	91	4.8	4.7	6.3	5.9
102	Malawi	11 308	1.8	99	97	4.3	4.6	7.3	6.5
103	Malaysia	22 218	2.2	67	62	5.8	6.6	3.8	3.1
104	Maldives	291	3.0	99	89	5.4	5.3	6.4	5.6
105	Mali	11 351	2.6	97	100	5.2	5.7	7.0	7.0
106	Malta	390	0.8	51	48	14.7	17.0	2.0	1.8
107	Marshall Islands	51	1.4	69	76	6.0	6.8	5.6	5.9
108	Mauritania	2 665	2.9	93	90	4.9	4.7	6.2	6.0
109	Mauritius	1 161	0.9	54	47	8.3	9.0	2.2	2.0
110	Mexico	98 872	1.7	74	61	5.9	6.9	3.4	2.6

	PROBABILITY OF DYING (per 1000)								LIFE EXPECTANCY AT BIRTH (years)			
	Under age 5 years				Between ages 15 and 59 years							
	Males		Females		Males		Females		Males		Females	
	2000	Uncertainty interval	2000	Uncertainty interval	2000	Uncertainty interval	2000	Uncertainty interval	2000	Uncertainty interval	2000	Uncertainty interval
56	156	137 – 185	143	127 – 167	339	270 – 414	280	224 – 338	53.5	49.0 – 57.0	56.2	52.4 – 59.6
57	142	129 – 153	130	119 – 142	493	422 – 554	441	375 – 499	49.1	46.6 – 52.6	51.0	48.3 – 54.6
58	14	12 – 16	9	8 – 12	316	302 – 328	114	100 – 122	65.4	64.8 – 66.1	76.5	75.6 – 77.8
59	187	155 – 215	171	142 – 197	594	485 – 684	535	431 – 624	42.8	39.0 – 48.3	44.7	40.5 – 50.5
60	27	20 – 34	24	18 – 30	240	221 – 262	180	160 – 199	66.9	65.7 – 68.1	71.2	69.9 – 72.3
61	6	5 – 6	5	4 – 5	144	141 – 147	61	58 – 64	73.7	73.5 – 74.0	80.9	80.5 – 81.3
62	8	8 – 9	6	5 – 6	144	139 – 148	61	56 – 64	75.2	74.8 – 75.5	83.1	82.5 – 83.8
63	118	105 – 145	109	99 – 134	380	299 – 460	330	268 – 408	54.6	50.3 – 59.0	56.9	51.9 – 60.2
64	101	85 – 115	90	77 – 102	373	305 – 440	320	261 – 381	55.9	52.4 – 59.4	58.7	55.2 – 62.2
65	30	22 – 38	19	15 – 25	250	213 – 282	133	107 – 155	65.7	64.0 – 67.7	71.8	70.3 – 74.2
66	6	6 – 7	5	4 – 6	127	122 – 131	60	58 – 63	74.3	74.0 – 74.8	80.6	80.3 – 80.9
67	112	104 – 119	98	89 – 104	379	344 – 410	326	295 – 357	55.0	53.7 – 56.8	57.9	56.0 – 59.8
68	7	6 – 8	6	5 – 7	114	110 – 118	47	44 – 52	75.4	75.0 – 75.7	80.8	80.1 – 81.5
69	25	18 – 30	22	15 – 27	202	187 – 222	159	146 – 171	70.9	69.5 – 72.1	73.2	72.1 – 74.6
70	54	50 – 59	52	47 – 56	286	260 – 308	182	157 – 200	63.5	62.2 – 65.2	68.6	67.2 – 70.6
71	174	163 – 183	156	144 – 164	432	392 – 468	366	331 – 398	49.0	47.4 – 51.1	52.0	50.4 – 54.1
72	215	205 – 220	197	188 – 203	495	467 – 521	427	401 – 451	44.5	43.4 – 46.0	46.9	45.7 – 48.5
73	77	62 – 91	66	50 – 80	299	275 – 335	209	176 – 235	61.5	59.2 – 63.2	67.0	64.9 – 69.8
74	111	84 – 134	96	70 – 119	524	387 – 563	373	278 – 430	49.7	47.0 – 56.9	56.1	52.4 – 62.2
75	45	40 – 50	42	38 – 48	221	200 – 249	157	140 – 178	66.3	64.5 – 67.9	71.0	69.2 – 72.5
76	11	10 – 12	8	8 – 9	295	291 – 299	123	120 – 126	66.3	66.1 – 66.5	75.2	74.9 – 75.5
77	5	3 – 8	5	3 – 6	85	75 – 95	51	43 – 59	77.1	75.7 – 78.6	81.8	80.5 – 83.9
78	90	83 – 97	99	90 – 108	287	251 – 310	213	179 – 236	59.8	58.5 – 62.0	62.7	60.8 – 65.6
79	61	54 – 68	49	43 – 55	250	232 – 266	191	177 – 205	63.4	62.4 – 64.6	67.4	66.4 – 68.5
80	44	35 – 50	47	38 – 53	170	159 – 179	139	128 – 147	68.1	67.4 – 69.0	69.9	69.2 – 70.8
81	80	64 – 94	73	60 – 90	258	229 – 289	208	178 – 236	61.7	59.7 – 64.0	64.7	62.2 – 67.0
82	6	6 – 7	5	5 – 6	108	103 – 114	62	60 – 65	74.1	73.6 – 74.5	79.7	79.3 – 80.0
83	8	7 – 8	6	5 – 7	99	96 – 102	56	53 – 58	76.6	76.3 – 76.9	80.6	80.3 – 81.0
84	7	6 – 8	6	6 – 7	110	107 – 113	53	52 – 56	76.0	75.6 – 76.3	82.4	82.0 – 82.7
85	17	14 – 20	14	11 – 17	169	147 – 180	127	110 – 140	72.8	72.0 – 74.7	76.6	75.3 – 78.3
86	5	5 – 6	4	4 – 5	98	96 – 99	44	42 – 45	77.5	77.4 – 77.7	84.7	84.4 – 85.1
87	25	21 – 29	22	17 – 25	199	178 – 217	144	128 – 148	68.5	67.4 – 70.0	72.5	72.1 – 73.8
88	80	75 – 80	60	56 – 64	366	350 – 375	201	182 – 215	58.0	57.6 – 58.9	68.4	67.2 – 70.0
89	107	99 – 114	98	90 – 105	578	533 – 617	529	486 – 568	48.2	46.2 – 50.3	49.6	47.5 – 51.8
90	93	79 – 104	74	61 – 85	269	210 – 319	208	172 – 259	60.4	57.8 – 64.0	64.5	61.2 – 67.3
91	13	11 – 17	12	9 – 15	100	93 – 107	68	62 – 74	74.2	73.5 – 75.0	76.8	76.0 – 77.6
92	70	62 – 78	58	50 – 67	335	306 – 364	175	152 – 200	60.0	58.5 – 61.7	68.8	66.8 – 70.8
93	152	130 – 189	134	120 – 169	355	323 – 422	299	271 – 339	52.2	47.4 – 54.9	56.1	52.0 – 58.3
94	20	12 – 25	14	11 – 16	328	315 – 355	122	112 – 134	64.2	62.8 – 64.9	75.5	74.5 – 76.5
95	22	17 – 27	18	14 – 22	192	168 – 215	136	121 – 151	69.1	67.7 – 70.7	73.3	72.2 – 74.7
96	159	143 – 172	150	134 – 164	667	572 – 742	630	536 – 706	42.0	38.8 – 45.7	42.2	38.6 – 47.3
97	205	173 – 233	187	161 – 211	448	367 – 521	385	312 – 452	46.6	43.3 – 51.3	49.1	45.7 – 53.9
98	31	25 – 37	29	23 – 34	210	192 – 228	157	143 – 171	67.5	66.4 – 68.7	71.0	70.0 – 72.2
99	15	11 – 17	12	9 – 14	286	270 – 300	106	98 – 110	66.9	66.1 – 67.8	77.2	76.7 – 78.2
100	5	4 – 7	5	4 – 6	135	122 – 148	64	57 – 72	73.9	73.0 – 74.8	80.8	79.8 – 82.1
101	156	147 – 162	142	134 – 149	385	348 – 417	322	290 – 350	51.7	50.3 – 53.7	54.6	53.2 – 56.6
102	229	206 – 251	211	190 – 234	701	604 – 779	653	557 – 733	37.1	33.6 – 41.1	37.8	34.0 – 42.2
103	15	13 – 18	12	10 – 15	202	186 – 218	113	100 – 125	68.3	67.4 – 69.4	74.1	73.1 – 75.3
104	62	45 – 80	66	45 – 85	228	209 – 248	226	199 – 248	64.6	62.9 – 66.2	64.4	62.4 – 66.7
105	231	216 – 241	220	206 – 230	518	452 – 578	446	387 – 501	42.7	40.3 – 45.2	44.6	42.2 – 47.3
106	10	8 – 11	6	4 – 7	111	103 – 119	46	41 – 55	75.4	74.7 – 76.2	80.7	79.3 – 82.0
107	48	41 – 56	39	32 – 47	302	275 – 324	230	213 – 248	62.8	61.4 – 64.3	67.8	66.6 – 69.0
108	175	161 – 186	168	154 – 179	357	304 – 410	302	256 – 347	51.7	49.2 – 54.2	53.5	51.1 – 56.2
109	21	20 – 25	16	16 – 20	228	220 – 240	109	106 – 116	67.6	67.0 – 68.1	74.6	74.1 – 75.0
110	31	27 – 35	25	22 – 28	180	167 – 187	101	96 – 106	71.0	70.4 – 72.0	76.2	75.7 – 76.8

Annex Table 1 Basic indicators for all Member States

	Member State	POPULATION ESTIMATES							
		Total population (000)	Annual growth rate (%)	Dependency ratio (per 100)		Percentage of population aged 60+ years		Total fertility rate	
		2000	1990–2000	1990	2000	1990	2000	1990	2000
111	Micronesia, Federated States of	123	2.6	69	76	6.0	6.8	4.8	5.1
112	Monaco	33	1.1	52	53	19.1	20.5	1.8	1.7
113	Mongolia	2 533	1.3	84	64	5.8	5.6	4.1	2.5
114	Morocco	29 878	2.0	77	63	6.0	6.4	4.3	3.2
115	Mozambique	18 292	3.0	89	89	5.1	5.1	6.5	6.1
116	Myanmar	47 749	1.7	71	61	6.8	6.8	4.0	3.1
117	Namibia	1 757	2.5	88	90	5.5	5.6	6.0	5.1
118	Nauru	12	2.6	69	76	6.0	6.8	4.3	4.6
119	Nepal	23 043	2.4	81	81	5.8	5.9	5.2	4.7
120	Netherlands	15 864	0.6	45	47	17.3	18.3	1.6	1.5
121	New Zealand	3 778	1.2	53	53	15.3	15.6	2.1	2.0
122	Nicaragua	5 071	2.9	97	84	4.4	4.6	4.9	4.1
123	Niger	10 832	3.5	109	108	3.5	3.3	8.1	8.0
124	Nigeria	113 862	2.9	97	93	4.7	4.8	6.5	5.7
125	Niue	2	−1.4	70	65	5.7	6.8	3.3	2.6
126	Norway	4 469	0.5	54	54	21.0	19.6	1.8	1.8
127	Oman	2 538	3.6	95	87	3.8	4.2	7.0	5.7
128	Pakistan	141 256	2.6	83	83	5.5	5.8	6.0	5.3
129	Palau	19	2.3	69	76	6.0	6.8	2.6	2.8
130	Panama	2 856	1.8	67	58	7.3	8.1	3.0	2.5
131	Papua New Guinea	4 809	2.5	79	74	4.2	4.1	5.1	4.5
132	Paraguay	5 496	2.7	84	75	5.4	5.3	4.7	4.0
133	Peru	25 662	1.8	73	62	6.1	7.2	3.7	2.8
134	Philippines	75 653	2.2	79	70	4.9	5.5	4.3	3.4
135	Poland	38 605	0.1	54	46	14.9	16.6	2.0	1.4
136	Portugal	10 016	0.1	51	48	19.0	20.8	1.6	1.5
137	Qatar	565	2.2	42	39	2.1	3.1	4.4	3.5
138	Republic of Korea	46 740	0.9	45	39	7.7	11.0	1.6	1.5
139	Republic of Moldova	4 295	−0.2	57	48	12.8	13.7	2.4	1.5
140	Romania	22 438	−0.3	51	46	15.7	18.8	1.9	1.3
141	Russian Federation	145 491	−0.2	49	44	16.0	18.5	1.8	1.2
142	Rwanda	7 609	1.2	99	88	4.1	4.2	6.9	6.0
143	Saint Kitts and Nevis	38	−0.8	64	57	9.1	9.9	2.8	2.4
144	Saint Lucia	148	1.2	78	61	8.8	7.8	3.4	2.6
145	Saint Vincent and the Grenadines	113	0.7	64	57	9.1	9.9	2.3	1.9
146	Samoa	159	−0.1	80	84	6.1	6.8	4.8	4.4
147	San Marino	27	1.4	45	48	21.1	24.1	1.7	1.5
148	Sao Tome and Principe	138	1.9	93	78	7.0	6.5	6.3	6.1
149	Saudi Arabia	20 346	2.8	84	85	4.1	4.8	6.9	5.8
150	Senegal	9 421	2.5	94	88	4.7	4.2	6.3	5.3
151	Seychelles	80	1.5	54	47	8.3	9.0	2.2	1.9
152	Sierra Leone	4 405	0.8	87	89	5.0	4.8	6.5	6.5
153	Singapore	4 018	2.9	37	41	8.4	10.6	1.7	1.5
154	Slovakia	5 399	0.3	55	45	14.8	15.4	2.0	1.3
155	Slovenia	1 988	0.4	45	42	17.1	19.2	1.5	1.2
156	Solomon Islands	447	3.5	95	90	4.6	4.2	5.9	5.4
157	Somalia	8 778	2.1	102	101	4.3	3.9	7.3	7.3
158	South Africa	43 309	1.8	71	60	5.0	5.7	3.6	3.0
159	Spain	39 910	0.2	50	46	19.2	21.8	1.4	1.1
160	Sri Lanka	18 924	1.1	59	48	8.0	9.3	2.6	2.1
161	Sudan	31 095	2.3	83	77	5.0	5.5	5.5	4.7
162	Suriname	417	0.4	68	56	6.8	8.1	2.7	2.1
163	Swaziland	925	1.9	90	82	4.9	5.3	5.6	4.6
164	Sweden	8 842	0.3	56	55	22.8	22.4	2.0	1.4
165	Switzerland	7 170	0.5	45	48	19.1	21.3	1.5	1.4

	PROBABILITY OF DYING (per 1000)								LIFE EXPECTANCY AT BIRTH (years)			
	Under age 5 years				Between ages 15 and 59 years							
	Males		Females		Males		Females		Males		Females	
	2000	Uncertainty interval	2000	Uncertainty interval	2000	Uncertainty interval	2000	Uncertainty interval	2000	Uncertainty interval	2000	Uncertainty interval
	61	45 – 79	48	35 – 64	243	211 – 270	188	160 – 209	63.7	61.6 – 66.1	67.7	65.8 – 69.9
	7	3 – 10	5	3 – 10	123	93 – 140	54	45 – 75	76.8	75.2 – 79.8	84.4	81.6 – 86.4
	92	75 – 109	76	60 – 90	280	265 – 305	199	184 – 214	61.2	59.1 – 62.6	66.9	65.4 – 68.4
	68	60 – 75	59	52 – 66	174	159 – 183	113	105 – 130	66.1	65.2 – 67.4	70.4	68.7 – 71.4
	227	217 – 232	208	199 – 214	674	634 – 712	612	573 – 646	37.9	36.7 – 39.5	39.5	38.2 – 41.2
	111	96 – 136	97	84 – 122	343	320 – 380	245	225 – 285	56.2	53.5 – 58.0	61.1	57.6 – 62.8
	125	109 – 139	119	106 – 131	695	585 – 777	661	568 – 735	42.8	39.2 – 48.1	42.6	39.2 – 47.6
	16	14 – 21	11	9 – 15	480	374 – 567	310	225 – 399	58.8	55.3 – 62.9	66.6	62.5 – 71.3
	101	90 – 110	116	108 – 124	314	288 – 337	314	292 – 337	58.5	56.8 – 60.5	58.0	56.5 – 59.7
	7	6 – 8	5	5 – 6	95	92 – 100	64	61 – 67	75.4	74.9 – 76.0	81.0	80.4 – 81.5
	7	6 – 8	6	4 – 6	108	100 – 114	69	63 – 78	75.9	75.2 – 76.7	80.9	79.8 – 81.9
	49	44 – 52	39	35 – 44	225	211 – 241	161	151 – 171	66.4	65.4 – 67.5	71.1	70.2 – 72.0
	257	231 – 264	252	234 – 259	473	402 – 537	408	351 – 461	42.7	40.5 – 46.1	43.9	42.1 – 46.7
	158	149 – 164	151	142 – 157	443	402 – 478	393	356 – 426	49.8	48.3 – 51.9	51.4	49.8 – 53.6
	34	24 – 46	28	18 – 39	181	151 – 219	144	100 – 159	69.5	66.7 – 71.9	72.8	71.4 – 77.3
	5	5 – 6	4	4 – 5	105	100 – 108	60	56 – 62	75.7	75.5 – 76.0	81.4	80.9 – 82.0
	20	15 – 25	17	14 – 22	187	171 – 204	135	123 – 147	69.5	68.4 – 70.6	73.5	72.6 – 74.5
	120	104 – 134	132	109 – 139	221	192 – 237	198	179 – 227	60.1	58.6 – 62.5	60.7	58.6 – 63.1
	26	18 – 32	22	16 – 30	264	255 – 285	183	163 – 200	64.7	63.6 – 65.2	69.3	68.4 – 70.3
	28	24 – 31	22	21 – 27	145	136 – 155	93	90 – 98	71.5	70.7 – 72.2	76.3	75.8 – 76.7
	118	85 – 134	109	74 – 124	359	336 – 395	329	310 – 370	55.1	52.8 – 57.7	57.5	54.8 – 60.0
	35	28 – 38	31	25 – 35	173	157 – 189	129	115 – 147	70.2	69.0 – 71.5	74.2	72.4 – 75.7
	53	48 – 56	48	44 – 52	190	178 – 201	139	128 – 151	66.7	65.9 – 67.6	71.6	70.4 – 72.7
	44	40 – 47	37	33 – 40	249	235 – 267	142	126 – 155	64.6	63.6 – 65.5	71.1	70.0 – 72.7
	12	11 – 13	11	9 – 12	226	222 – 232	88	84 – 92	69.2	68.9 – 69.5	77.7	77.2 – 78.2
	10	9 – 11	7	6 – 8	164	161 – 169	66	64 – 70	71.7	71.4 – 72.0	79.3	78.8 – 79.8
	20	17 – 23	13	11 – 15	173	170 – 177	121	117 – 124	70.4	70.1 – 70.7	75.0	74.6 – 75.4
	10	7 – 14	9	7 – 13	186	160 – 210	71	60 – 85	70.5	69.1 – 72.2	78.3	76.8 – 79.8
	26	23 – 29	21	18 – 24	325	310 – 340	165	152 – 178	63.1	62.4 – 63.8	70.5	69.6 – 71.4
	25	22 – 27	21	18 – 23	260	245 – 275	117	105 – 125	66.2	65.5 – 67.0	73.5	72.7 – 74.6
	23	22 – 25	17	16 – 19	428	394 – 453	156	143 – 161	59.4	58.4 – 60.8	72.0	71.6 – 73.0
	219	202 – 227	199	182 – 207	667	604 – 722	599	537 – 653	38.5	36.8 – 41.1	40.5	38.6 – 43.3
	25	22 – 28	22	18 – 25	243	219 – 258	148	133 – 162	66.1	65.3 – 67.3	72.0	70.8 – 73.3
	20	17 – 24	14	13 – 19	210	200 – 225	135	125 – 150	69.2	68.2 – 69.9	74.2	73.1 – 75.2
	20	17 – 25	17	15 – 22	246	230 – 269	165	149 – 181	67.7	66.5 – 68.7	73.3	72.2 – 74.8
	37	32 – 44	30	22 – 36	242	226 – 261	151	140 – 164	66.7	65.5 – 67.7	72.9	71.8 – 74.0
	8	7 – 11	9	7 – 10	81	75 – 89	38	35 – 43	76.1	75.1 – 77.2	83.8	82.8 – 84.7
	94	66 – 110	97	65 – 114	269	250 – 308	226	211 – 246	60.3	57.8 – 62.5	61.9	60.0 – 64.2
	40	35 – 45	26	22 – 30	181	166 – 195	116	105 – 126	68.1	67.1 – 69.1	73.5	72.7 – 74.5
	141	133 – 148	133	125 – 140	355	321 – 384	303	272 – 328	54.0	52.6 – 56.0	56.1	54.7 – 58.1
	16	14 – 18	12	10 – 14	268	240 – 296	122	105 – 145	66.5	65.2 – 67.9	74.2	72.4 – 76.2
	292	237 – 324	265	213 – 286	587	482 – 683	531	436 – 625	37.0	32.9 – 43.3	38.8	35.3 – 44.7
	5	4 – 6	4	4 – 5	114	110 – 120	61	57 – 66	75.4	74.7 – 76.0	80.2	79.5 – 81.1
	11	9 – 12	8	8 – 10	216	211 – 222	83	81 – 87	69.2	68.8 – 69.6	77.5	77.2 – 77.9
	6	6 – 8	5	4 – 6	170	164 – 174	76	72 – 81	71.9	71.5 – 72.3	79.4	78.9 – 80.2
	37	31 – 43	27	21 – 33	221	176 – 259	154	112 – 193	66.6	64.4 – 69.6	71.4	68.5 – 75.3
	221	211 – 225	199	191 – 205	516	480 – 548	452	420 – 482	43.8	42.6 – 45.4	45.9	44.7 – 47.6
	90	86 – 92	78	74 – 82	567	545 – 585	502	487 – 521	49.6	48.8 – 50.6	52.1	51.0 – 53.0
	6	6 – 7	5	5 – 6	122	118 – 128	49	47 – 51	75.4	74.7 – 75.8	82.3	82.0 – 82.6
	24	21 – 28	17	14 – 20	244	224 – 284	124	119 – 140	67.6	65.1 – 68.9	75.3	73.8 – 76.0
	124	108 – 138	117	102 – 131	341	277 – 399	291	235 – 340	55.4	52.9 – 59.1	57.8	55.1 – 61.5
	29	25 – 35	21	18 – 26	230	204 – 255	138	118 – 160	68.0	66.6 – 69.6	73.5	71.8 – 75.3
	135	99 – 169	123	93 – 153	627	513 – 718	587	473 – 678	44.7	39.4 – 50.7	45.6	40.8 – 52.0
	5	4 – 5	3	3 – 4	87	85 – 91	56	52 – 57	77.3	77.0 – 77.6	82.0	81.7 – 82.4
	6	6 – 7	6	5 – 6	99	97 – 104	58	56 – 61	76.7	76.3 – 77.0	82.5	82.1 – 82.9

Annex Table 1 Basic indicators for all Member States

	Member State	POPULATION ESTIMATES							
		Total population (000)	Annual growth rate (%)	Dependency ratio (per 100)		Percentage of population aged 60+ years		Total fertility rate	
		2000	1990–2000	1990	2000	1990	2000	1990	2000
166	Syrian Arab Republic	16 189	2.7	102	78	4.4	4.7	5.7	3.8
167	Tajikistan	6 087	1.4	89	78	6.2	6.8	4.9	3.3
168	Thailand	62 806	1.4	56	47	6.2	8.1	2.3	2.1
169	The former Yugoslav Republic of Macedonia	2 034	0.6	51	48	11.5	14.4	2.0	1.7
170	Togo	4 527	2.7	95	90	4.8	4.9	6.3	5.6
171	Tonga	99	0.3	70	65	5.7	6.8	4.8	3.8
172	Trinidad and Tobago	1 294	0.6	66	46	8.7	9.6	2.4	1.6
173	Tunisia	9 459	1.5	72	55	6.6	8.4	3.6	2.2
174	Turkey	66 668	1.7	65	56	7.1	8.4	3.4	2.5
175	Turkmenistan	4 737	2.6	79	72	6.2	6.5	4.3	3.4
176	Tuvalu	10	1.5	70	65	5.7	6.8	3.5	2.8
177	Uganda	23 300	3.1	103	107	4.1	3.8	7.1	7.1
178	Ukraine	49 568	−0.5	51	46	18.5	20.5	1.8	1.2
179	United Arab Emirates	2 606	2.6	45	40	2.5	5.1	4.2	3.0
180	United Kingdom	59 415	0.3	54	53	20.9	20.6	1.8	1.7
181	United Republic of Tanzania	35 119	3.0	96	90	3.7	4.0	6.1	5.3
182	United States of America	283 230	1.1	52	52	16.6	16.1	2.0	2.0
183	Uruguay	3 337	0.7	60	60	16.4	17.2	2.5	2.3
184	Uzbekistan	24 881	1.9	82	69	6.5	7.1	4.0	2.6
185	Vanuatu	197	2.8	91	83	5.3	5.0	4.9	4.4
186	Venezuela, Bolivarian Republic of	24 170	2.2	72	63	5.7	6.6	3.5	2.9
187	Viet Nam	78 137	1.7	78	63	7.3	7.5	3.7	2.4
188	Yemen	18 349	4.7	106	110	4.1	3.6	7.6	7.6
189	Yugoslavia	10 552	0.4	49	50	15.2	18.3	2.1	1.7
190	Zambia	10 421	2.6	95	98	4.4	4.5	6.3	5.9
191	Zimbabwe	12 627	2.1	95	94	4.6	4.7	5.8	4.8

	PROBABILITY OF DYING (per 1000)								LIFE EXPECTANCY AT BIRTH (years)			
	Under age 5 years				Between ages 15 and 59 years							
	Males		Females		Males		Females		Males		Females	
	2000	Uncertainty interval	2000	Uncertainty interval	2000	Uncertainty interval	2000	Uncertainty interval	2000	Uncertainty interval	2000	Uncertainty interval
166	32	30 – 38	28	25 – 32	170	160 – 184	132	125 – 144	69.3	68.4 – 69.9	72.4	71.6 – 73.0
167	85	76 – 96	82	75 – 97	293	264 – 313	204	176 – 224	60.4	59.0 – 62.3	64.7	63.0 – 66.9
168	35	31 – 38	32	28 – 35	245	230 – 260	150	130 – 164	66.0	65.0 – 67.1	72.4	71.1 – 74.2
169	16	14 – 20	15	13 – 18	160	153 – 167	89	85 – 92	70.2	69.8 – 70.8	74.8	74.5 – 75.3
170	138	124 – 149	121	108 – 133	460	392 – 519	406	344 – 460	50.5	48.1 – 54.0	53.0	50.5 – 56.6
171	29	24 – 33	19	15 – 23	226	211 – 236	159	145 – 160	67.4	66.8 – 68.3	72.9	72.6 – 73.9
172	16	13 – 22	13	10 – 18	209	176 – 229	133	124 – 144	68.5	67.4 – 70.5	73.8	72.8 – 74.7
173	29	24 – 32	34	31 – 40	169	158 – 182	99	91 – 113	69.2	68.3 – 70.0	73.4	71.9 – 74.3
174	49	45 – 52	45	41 – 48	218	201 – 220	120	107 – 126	66.8	66.6 – 68.0	72.5	71.9 – 74.0
175	59	54 – 66	52	49 – 60	343	328 – 353	217	201 – 224	60.0	59.3 – 60.8	64.9	64.3 – 66.0
176	43	30 – 55	40	30 – 50	262	242 – 287	198	182 – 227	63.6	62.0 – 64.8	67.6	65.7 – 68.7
177	165	148 – 178	151	138 – 165	617	531 – 686	567	486 – 637	43.5	40.8 – 47.3	44.6	41.7 – 48.7
178	18	17 – 19	13	12 – 14	365	353 – 378	135	129 – 140	62.6	62.0 – 63.1	73.3	72.9 – 73.8
179	16	13 – 19	14	11 – 16	143	128 – 157	93	84 – 102	72.3	71.2 – 73.5	76.4	75.4 – 77.7
180	7	7 – 8	6	5 – 6	109	108 – 112	67	65 – 68	74.8	74.6 – 75.0	79.9	79.7 – 80.2
181	150	143 – 153	140	135 – 145	569	554 – 583	520	508 – 531	45.8	45.1 – 46.7	47.2	46.4 – 47.9
182	9	9 – 10	8	7 – 8	147	143 – 149	84	83 – 85	73.9	73.7 – 74.2	79.5	79.3 – 79.6
183	19	18 – 21	14	13 – 16	185	182 – 188	89	86 – 92	70.0	69.8 – 70.3	77.9	77.5 – 78.2
184	69	64 – 72	57	52 – 60	282	270 – 290	176	165 – 185	62.1	61.6 – 62.9	68.0	67.3 – 68.9
185	57	42 – 72	45	32 – 57	240	169 – 303	185	134 – 243	64.2	60.5 – 69.1	68.1	64.2 – 72.3
186	26	22 – 30	21	18 – 26	178	170 – 185	99	96 – 105	70.6	70.0 – 71.2	76.5	75.8 – 77.0
187	38	35 – 41	30	27 – 33	203	188 – 217	139	128 – 151	66.7	65.7 – 67.8	71.0	69.9 – 72.0
188	104	96 – 111	96	89 – 101	278	251 – 305	226	205 – 242	59.3	57.6 – 60.9	62.0	60.9 – 63.5
189	18	16 – 20	15	14 – 17	180	175 – 181	100	98 – 102	69.8	69.6 – 70.1	74.7	74.5 – 75.0
190	170	150 – 185	156	143 – 170	725	630 – 798	687	600 – 754	39.2	36.1 – 43.8	39.5	36.5 – 43.7
191	108	101 – 111	98	91 – 101	650	628 – 662	612	596 – 631	45.4	44.7 – 46.5	46.0	44.9 – 47.1

Annex Table 2 Deaths by cause, sex and mortality stratum in WHO Regions,[a] estimates for 2000

Cause[b]	SEX						AFRICA		THE AMERICAS		
							Mortality stratum		Mortality stratum		
	Both sexes		Males		Females		High child, high adult	High child, very high adult	Very low child, very low adult	Low child, low adult	High child, high adult
Population (000)	6 045 172		3 045 372		2 999 800		294 099	345 533	325 186	430 951	71 235
	(000)	% total	(000)	% total	(000)	% total	(000)	(000)	(000)	(000)	(000)
TOTAL DEATHS	55 694	100	29 696	100	25 998	100	4 245	6 327	2 778	2 587	510
I. Communicable diseases, maternal and perinatal conditions and nutritional deficiencies	17 777	31.9	9 282	31.3	8 495	32.7	2 893	4 597	203	475	185
Infectious and parasitic diseases	10 457	18.8	5 637	19.0	4 819	18.5	1 969	3 467	60	213	93
Tuberculosis	1 660	3.0	1 048	3.5	613	2.4	146	235	2	33	22
STDs excluding HIV	217	0.4	119	0.4	97	0.4	43	58	0	1	0
Syphilis	197	0.4	118	0.4	79	0.3	42	56	0	0	0
Chlamydia	7	0.0	0	0.0	7	0.0	1	1	0	0	0
Gonorrhoea	4	0.0	0	0.0	4	0.0	1	1	0	0	0
HIV/AIDS	2 943	5.3	1 500	5.0	1 443	5.6	517	1 875	15	34	23
Diarrhoeal diseases	2 124	3.8	1 178	4.0	946	3.6	272	433	2	49	27
Childhood diseases	1 385	2.5	693	2.3	692	2.7	432	308	0	2	6
Pertussis	296	0.5	148	0.5	148	0.6	92	74	0	1	6
Poliomyelitis	1	0.0	0	0.0	0	0.0	0	0	0	0	0
Diphtheria	3	0.0	2	0.0	2	0.0	1	1	0	0	0
Measles	777	1.4	388	1.3	388	1.5	264	188	0	0	0
Tetanus	309	0.6	154	0.5	154	0.6	75	45	0	1	1
Meningitis	156	0.3	87	0.3	69	0.3	19	23	1	9	1
Hepatitis[c]	128	0.2	70	0.2	57	0.2	15	18	5	3	1
Malaria	1 080	1.9	522	1.8	558	2.1	489	477	0	1	1
Tropical diseases	124	0.2	76	0.3	48	0.2	33	30	0	20	3
Trypanosomiasis	50	0.1	32	0.1	18	0.1	25	24	0	0	0
Chagas disease	21	0.0	12	0.0	9	0.0	0	0	0	18	3
Schistosomiasis	11	0.0	8	0.0	3	0.0	3	2	0	1	0
Leishmaniasis	41	0.1	23	0.1	18	0.1	5	4	0	0	0
Lymphatic filariasis	0	0.0	0	0.0	0	0.0	0	0	0	0	0
Onchocerciasis	0	0.0	0	0.0	0	0.0	0	0	0	0	0
Leprosy	2	0.0	2	0.0	1	0.0	0	0	0	0	0
Dengue	12	0.0	8	0.0	4	0.0	0	0	0	0	0
Japanese encephalitis	4	0.0	1	0.0	2	0.0	0	0	0	0	0
Trachoma	0	0.0	0	0.0	0	0.0	0	0	0	0	0
Intestinal nematode infections	17	0.0	9	0.0	8	0.0	1	2	0	2	1
Ascariasis	6	0.0	3	0.0	3	0.0	0	1	0	1	0
Trichuriasis	2	0.0	1	0.0	1	0.0	0	0	0	0	0
Hookworm disease	6	0.0	4	0.0	2	0.0	1	1	0	0	0
Respiratory infections	3 941	7.1	2 121	7.1	1 821	7.0	460	622	115	104	43
Lower respiratory infections	3 866	6.9	2 084	7.0	1 782	6.9	454	614	115	102	42
Upper respiratory infections	69	0.1	34	0.1	35	0.1	4	5	0	1	1
Otitis media	6	0.0	3	0.0	3	0.0	1	2	0	0	0
Maternal conditions	495	0.9	0	0.0	495	1.9	97	146	0	13	7
Perinatal conditions	2 439	4.4	1 307	4.4	1 133	4.4	296	281	17	106	28
Nutritional deficiencies	445	0.8	218	0.7	227	0.9	70	81	10	39	13
Protein–energy malnutrition	271	0.5	137	0.5	134	0.5	49	52	5	28	8
Iodine deficiency	9	0.0	5	0.0	5	0.0	1	2	0	0	0
Vitamin A deficiency	41	0.1	17	0.1	24	0.1	11	13	0	0	0
Iron-deficiency anaemia	103	0.2	49	0.2	53	0.2	8	13	6	11	2

Cause[b]	EASTERN MEDITERRANEAN		EUROPE			SOUTH-EAST ASIA		WESTERN PACIFIC	
	Mortality stratum		Mortality stratum			Mortality stratum		Mortality stratum	
	Low child, Low adult	High child, high adult	Very low child, very low adult	Low child, low adult	Low child, high adult	Low child, low adult	High child, high adult	Very low child, very low adult	Low child, low adult
Population (000)	139 071	342 584	411 910	218 473	243 192	293 821	1 241 813	154 358	1 532 946
	(000)	(000)	(000)	(000)	(000)	(000)	(000)	(000)	(000)
TOTAL DEATHS	690	3 346	4 076	1 952	3 636	2 142	12 015	1 152	10 238
I. Communicable diseases, maternal and perinatal conditions and nutritional deficiencies	153	1 556	240	221	152	604	4 913	131	1 454
Infectious and parasitic diseases	84	836	49	85	86	332	2 540	25	618
Tuberculosis	7	129	6	19	49	157	517	6	336
STDs excluding HIV	0	12	0	2	1	1	95	0	3
Syphilis	0	10	0	1	0	1	85	0	2
Chlamydia	0	0	0	0	0	0	4	0	0
Gonorrhoea	0	0	0	0	0	0	2	0	0
HIV/AIDS	0	54	10	1	10	37	334	0	32
Diarrhoeal diseases	24	262	2	27	4	30	921	1	71
Childhood diseases	1	196	0	8	0	43	337	0	52
Pertussis	0	57	0	0	0	1	62	0	2
Poliomyelitis	0	0	0	0	0	0	0	0	0
Diphtheria	0	0	0	0	0	0	1	0	0
Measles	0	81	0	7	0	34	168	0	34
Tetanus	0	57	0	0	0	8	105	0	17
Meningitis	2	22	2	7	5	12	42	1	11
Hepatitis[c]	3	7	4	5	2	5	32	5	22
Malaria	0	47	0	0	0	8	43	0	13
Tropical diseases	1	5	0	0	0	0	30	0	2
Trypanosomiasis	0	1	0	0	0	0	0	0	0
Chagas disease	0	0	0	0	0	0	0	0	0
Schistosomiasis	1	2	0	0	0	0	0	0	2
Leishmaniasis	0	2	0	0	0	0	30	0	0
Lymphatic filariasis	0	0	0	0	0	0	0	0	0
Onchocerciasis	0	0	0	0	0	0	0	0	0
Leprosy	0	0	0	0	0	0	1	0	0
Dengue	0	1	0	0	0	1	10	0	1
Japanese encephalitis	0	0	0	0	0	0	0	0	3
Trachoma	0	0	0	0	0	0	0	0	0
Intestinal nematode infections	0	2	0	0	0	1	5	0	3
Ascariasis	0	1	0	0	0	0	1	0	1
Trichuriasis	0	0	0	0	0	0	0	0	1
Hookworm disease	0	0	0	0	0	0	3	0	0
Respiratory infections	40	330	168	86	44	142	1 221	102	463
Lower respiratory infections	39	327	165	85	42	141	1 199	101	439
Upper respiratory infections	1	3	3	1	1	1	22	1	24
Otitis media	0	0	0	0	0	0	1	0	0
Maternal conditions	3	62	0	2	1	21	122	0	19
Perinatal conditions	20	284	11	42	19	90	919	2	321
Nutritional deficiencies	5	43	11	6	2	19	110	1	32
Protein–energy malnutrition	2	23	3	2	1	8	66	1	22
Iodine deficiency	0	2	0	0	0	0	3	0	0
Vitamin A deficiency	0	6	0	0	0	0	10	0	0
Iron-deficiency anaemia	1	8	8	3	2	6	27	0	7

Annex Table 2 Deaths by cause, sex and mortality stratum in WHO Regions,[a] estimates for 2000

Cause[b]	SEX						AFRICA		THE AMERICAS		
							Mortality stratum		Mortality stratum		
	Both sexes		Males		Females		High child, high adult	High child, very high adult	Very low child, very low adult	Low child, low adult	High child, high adult
Population (000)	6 045 172		3 045 372		2 999 800		294 099	345 533	325 186	430 951	71 235
	(000)	% total	(000)	% total	(000)	% total	(000)	(000)	(000)	(000)	(000)
II. Noncommunicable conditions	**32 855**	**59.0**	**16 998**	**57.2**	**15 856**	**61.0**	**1 043**	**1 286**	**2 397**	**1 779**	**276**
Malignant neoplasms	6 930	12.4	3 918	13.2	3 011	11.6	228	305	652	371	50
Mouth and oropharynx cancers	340	0.6	242	0.8	98	0.4	11	22	11	10	2
Oesophagus cancer	413	0.7	274	0.9	139	0.5	5	21	16	14	1
Stomach cancer	744	1.3	464	1.6	280	1.1	18	18	19	42	10
Colon/rectum cancer	579	1.0	303	1.0	276	1.1	11	15	77	26	3
Liver cancer	626	1.1	433	1.5	193	0.7	28	35	15	14	3
Pancreas cancer	214	0.4	114	0.4	100	0.4	3	5	34	13	1
Trachea/bronchus/lung cancers	1 213	2.2	895	3.0	318	1.2	9	14	182	47	3
Melanoma and other skin cancers	65	0.1	35	0.1	30	0.1	4	5	13	5	0
Breast cancer	459	0.8	0	0.0	458	1.8	14	24	56	28	3
Cervix uteri cancer	288	0.5	0	0.0	288	1.1	21	38	6	17	6
Corpus uteri cancer	76	0.1	0	0.0	76	0.3	1	2	9	10	1
Ovary cancer	128	0.2	0	0.0	128	0.5	3	7	16	6	1
Prostate cancer	258	0.5	258	0.9	0	0.0	24	19	45	26	3
Bladder cancer	157	0.3	117	0.4	40	0.2	8	6	16	6	1
Lymphomas, multiple myeloma	291	0.5	173	0.6	118	0.5	18	19	47	16	3
Leukaemia	265	0.5	145	0.5	119	0.5	8	12	27	18	3
Other neoplasms	115	0.2	59	0.2	56	0.2	1	2	10	9	2
Diabetes mellitus	810	1.5	345	1.2	465	1.8	19	35	76	120	23
Nutritional/endocrine disorders	224	0.4	103	0.3	121	0.5	17	20	29	24	6
Neuropsychiatric disorders	948	1.7	477	1.6	472	1.8	31	44	135	51	13
Unipolar depressive disorders	0	0.0	0	0.0	0	0.0	0	0	0	0	0
Bipolar affective disorder	4	0.0	1	0.0	3	0.0	0	0	0	0	0
Schizophrenia	17	0.0	8	0.0	9	0.0	0	0	1	0	0
Epilepsy	98	0.2	59	0.2	38	0.1	9	15	2	6	2
Alcohol use disorders	84	0.2	73	0.2	12	0.0	2	5	8	13	4
Alzheimer's and other dementias	276	0.5	93	0.3	183	0.7	2	3	61	7	1
Parkinson disease	90	0.2	44	0.1	45	0.2	2	2	16	2	0
Multiple sclerosis	17	0.0	6	0.0	10	0.0	0	0	3	1	0
Drug use disorders	15	0.0	14	0.0	2	0.0	0	0	2	1	0
Post-traumatic stress disorder	0	0.0	0	0.0	0	0.0	0	0	0	0	0
Obsessive–compulsive disorder	0	0.0	0	0.0	0	0.0	0	0	0	0	0
Panic disorder	0	0.0	0	0.0	0	0.0	0	0	0	0	0
Insomnia (primary)	0	0.0	0	0.0	0	0.0	0	0	0	0	0
Migraine	0	0.0	0	0.0	0	0.0	0	0	0	0	0
Sense organ disorders	7	0.0	3	0.0	4	0.0	0	0	0	0	0
Glaucoma	1	0.0	0	0.0	0	0.0	0	0	0	0	0
Cataracts	1	0.0	0	0.0	1	0.0	0	0	0	0	0
Hearing loss, adult onset	0	0.0	0	0.0	0	0.0	0	0	0	0	0
Cardiovascular diseases	16 701	30.0	8 195	27.6	8 506	32.7	460	514	1 138	786	98
Rheumatic heart disease	332	0.6	137	0.5	195	0.7	13	16	6	6	3
Ischaemic heart disease	6 894	12.4	3 625	12.2	3 269	12.6	162	167	581	306	29
Cerebrovascular disease	5 101	9.2	2 406	8.1	2 695	10.4	137	166	197	229	24
Inflammatory heart disease	395	0.7	216	0.7	180	0.7	15	19	34	27	3

Cause[b]	EASTERN MEDITERRANEAN Mortality stratum		EUROPE Mortality stratum			SOUTH-EAST ASIA Mortality stratum		WESTERN PACIFIC Mortality stratum	
	Low child, Low adult	High child, high adult	Very low child, very low adult	Low child, low adult	Low child, high adult	Low child, low adult	High child, high adult	Very low child, very low adult	Low child, low adult
Population (000)	139 071	342 584	411 910	218 473	243 192	293 821	1 241 813	154 358	1 532 946
	(000)	(000)	(000)	(000)	(000)	(000)	(000)	(000)	(000)
II. Noncommunicable conditions	459	1 530	3 637	1 588	3 009	1 307	5 961	942	7 640
Malignant neoplasms	78	164	1 056	290	536	226	877	341	1 756
Mouth and oropharynx cancers	2	20	25	9	18	18	152	6	34
Oesophagus cancer	4	10	28	11	15	3	68	12	205
Stomach cancer	10	7	70	33	83	9	55	56	313
Colon/rectum cancer	5	7	141	29	67	23	32	44	100
Liver cancer	4	7	38	9	20	26	26	35	365
Pancreas cancer	2	1	52	12	30	4	11	20	26
Trachea/bronchus/lung cancers	11	20	206	59	109	35	118	62	339
Melanoma and other skin cancers	1	1	15	4	9	1	2	3	2
Breast cancer	5	12	91	21	43	26	78	12	46
Cervix uteri cancer	5	14	8	8	13	15	102	3	33
Corpus uteri cancer	1	1	16	6	13	2	2	3	9
Ovary cancer	1	3	26	5	17	7	17	5	15
Prostate cancer	3	4	71	9	14	6	15	11	9
Bladder cancer	3	9	37	9	18	5	15	6	18
Lymphomas, multiple myeloma	5	12	54	9	14	14	40	14	27
Leukaemia	7	9	37	9	15	12	38	9	62
Other neoplasms	1	4	27	3	5	26	5	10	10
Diabetes mellitus	11	52	86	26	25	50	146	17	123
Nutritional/endocrine disorders	3	25	24	2	2	15	16	8	33
Neuropsychiatric disorders	11	73	158	27	33	51	169	20	131
Unipolar depressive disorders	0	0	0	0	0	0	0	0	0
Bipolar affective disorder	0	0	0	0	0	0	3	0	0
Schizophrenia	1	1	1	0	0	2	6	0	5
Epilepsy	2	5	6	5	4	5	19	1	18
Alcohol use disorders	0	2	13	5	9	5	7	1	11
Alzheimer's and other dementias	1	5	76	4	7	20	37	7	48
Parkinson disease	1	4	21	1	1	2	10	4	24
Multiple sclerosis	0	0	4	1	2	0	3	0	1
Drug use disorders	0	0	4	0	0	1	3	1	3
Post-traumatic stress disorder	0	0	0	0	0	0	0	0	0
Obsessive–compulsive disorder	0	0	0	0	0	0	0	0	0
Panic disorder	0	0	0	0	0	0	0	0	0
Insomnia (primary)	0	0	0	0	0	0	0	0	0
Migraine	0	0	0	0	0	0	0	0	0
Sense organ disorders	0	0	0	0	0	0	1	0	3
Glaucoma	0	0	0	0	0	0	0	0	0
Cataracts	0	0	0	0	0	0	0	0	1
Hearing loss, adult onset	0	0	0	0	0	0	0	0	0
Cardiovascular diseases	276	811	1 797	1 051	2 125	598	3 493	406	3 147
Rheumatic heart disease	4	17	12	10	16	11	106	3	110
Ischaemic heart disease	136	288	762	472	1 115	237	1 706	140	792
Cerebrovascular disease	58	158	470	276	741	181	625	173	1 667
Inflammatory heart disease	4	12	28	23	26	13	111	8	74

Annex Table 2 Deaths by cause, sex and mortality stratum in WHO Regions,[a] estimates for 2000

Cause[b]	SEX						AFRICA		THE AMERICAS		
							Mortality stratum		Mortality stratum		
	Both sexes		Males		Females		High child, high adult	High child, very high adult	Very low child, very low adult	Low child, low adult	High child, high adult
Population (000)	6 045 172		3 045 372		2 999 800		294 099	345 533	325 186	430 951	71 235
	(000)	% total	(000)	% total	(000)	% total	(000)	(000)	(000)	(000)	(000)
Respiratory diseases	3 542	6.4	1 891	6.4	1 651	6.3	101	131	172	170	16
Chronic obstructive pulmonary disease	2 523	4.5	1 367	4.6	1 156	4.4	51	63	124	76	6
Asthma	218	0.4	107	0.4	111	0.4	8	16	7	11	3
Digestive diseases	1 923	3.5	1 151	3.9	772	3.0	87	112	97	144	32
Peptic ulcer disease	237	0.4	140	0.5	96	0.4	6	10	6	11	4
Cirrhosis of the liver	797	1.4	531	1.8	266	1.0	31	38	30	58	17
Appendicitis	33	0.1	19	0.1	13	0.1	1	1	1	2	1
Diseases of the genitourinary system	825	1.5	447	1.5	378	1.5	54	67	57	49	14
Nephritis/nephrosis	620	1.1	327	1.1	293	1.1	35	44	31	38	12
Benign prostatic hypertrophy	35	0.1	35	0.1	0	0.0	3	4	1	2	1
Skin diseases	68	0.1	30	0.1	38	0.1	10	12	4	5	2
Musculoskeletal diseases	104	0.2	36	0.1	68	0.3	6	7	12	9	3
Rheumatoid arthritis	20	0.0	6	0.0	14	0.1	1	1	2	2	1
Osteoarthritis	4	0.0	1	0.0	3	0.0	0	0	1	1	0
Congenital abnormalities	657	1.2	341	1.1	315	1.2	30	36	15	40	16
Oral diseases	2	0.0	1	0.0	1	0.0	0	0	0	0	0
Dental caries	0	0.0	0	0.0	0	0.0	0	0	0	0	0
Periodontal disease	0	0.0	0	0.0	0	0.0	0	0	0	0	0
Edentulism	0	0.0	0	0.0	0	0.0	0	0	0	0	0
III. Injuries	5 062	9.1	3 415	11.5	1 647	6.3	308	445	178	333	50
Unintentional	3 403	6.1	2 262	7.6	1 141	4.4	196	245	119	185	29
Road traffic accidents	1 260	2.3	931	3.1	329	1.3	69	99	49	82	10
Poisoning	315	0.6	204	0.7	112	0.4	15	20	12	3	2
Falls	283	0.5	170	0.6	113	0.4	8	10	23	15	2
Fires	238	0.4	104	0.3	135	0.5	18	17	4	5	1
Drowning	450	0.8	301	1.0	148	0.6	44	40	5	20	2
Other unintentional injuries	857	1.5	553	1.9	304	1.2	42	60	26	60	12
Intentional	1 659	3.0	1 153	3.9	506	1.9	112	199	59	148	21
Self-inflicted	815	1.5	509	1.7	305	1.2	10	17	39	23	4
Violence	520	0.9	401	1.4	119	0.5	40	76	20	123	17
War	310	0.6	233	0.8	77	0.3	62	106	0	2	0

[a] See list of Member States by WHO Region and mortality stratum (pp. 168–169).

[b] Estimates for specific causes may not sum to broader cause groupings due to omission of residual categories.

[c] Does not include liver cancer and cirrhosis deaths resulting from chronic hepatitis virus infection.

Cause[b]	EASTERN MEDITERRANEAN		EUROPE			SOUTH-EAST ASIA		WESTERN PACIFIC	
	Mortality stratum		Mortality stratum			Mortality stratum		Mortality stratum	
	Low child, Low adult	High child, high adult	Very low child, very low adult	Low child, low adult	Low child, high adult	Low child, low adult	High child, high adult	Very low child, very low adult	Low child, low adult
Population (000)	139 071	342 584	411 910	218 473	243 192	293 821	1 241 813	154 358	1 532 946
	(000)	(000)	(000)	(000)	(000)	(000)	(000)	(000)	(000)
Respiratory diseases	26	126	205	65	127	135	482	57	1 728
Chronic obstructive pulmonary disease	13	43	136	42	93	52	255	23	1 545
Asthma	5	17	14	9	11	22	35	7	55
Digestive diseases	23	123	185	81	112	115	367	46	399
Peptic ulcer disease	3	6	18	7	14	21	53	5	74
Cirrhosis of the liver	7	28	68	47	55	42	181	15	180
Appendicitis	0	1	1	1	1	1	18	0	6
Diseases of the genitourinary system	17	69	60	26	28	56	140	27	162
Nephritis/nephrosis	11	58	40	18	11	45	122	24	131
Benign prostatic hypertrophy	1	1	1	2	3	1	8	0	8
Skin diseases	0	5	8	1	2	5	6	1	8
Musculoskeletal diseases	1	3	18	2	4	10	3	5	20
Rheumatoid arthritis	0	0	4	1	1	2	1	2	2
Osteoarthritis	0	0	1	0	0	0	0	0	0
Congenital abnormalities	12	76	13	12	10	20	254	4	119
Oral diseases	0	0	0	0	0	0	1	0	0
Dental caries	0	0	0	0	0	0	0	0	0
Periodontal disease	0	0	0	0	0	0	0	0	0
Edentulism	0	0	0	0	0	0	0	0	0
III. Injuries	79	259	199	143	475	231	1 141	78	1 144
Unintentional	61	181	140	88	285	155	900	49	769
Road traffic accidents	40	51	46	20	55	115	320	16	288
Poisoning	2	16	6	14	89	4	78	1	53
Falls	4	17	48	11	17	8	31	8	81
Fires	4	20	3	4	15	7	121	2	19
Drowning	3	16	4	10	33	12	85	6	169
Other unintentional injuries	8	61	34	29	76	8	266	16	158
Intentional	17	78	59	55	190	76	241	30	376
Self-inflicted	7	16	54	25	107	19	150	28	315
Violence	7	24	4	11	62	11	66	1	58
War	3	36	0	17	20	45	18	0	2

Annex Table 3 Burden of disease in disability-adjusted life years (DALYs) by cause, sex and mortality stratum in WHO Regions,[a] estimates for 2000

Cause[b]	Both sexes (000)	Both sexes % total	Males (000)	Males % total	Females (000)	Females % total	AFRICA High child, high adult (000)	AFRICA High child, very high adult (000)	THE AMERICAS Very low child, very low adult (000)	THE AMERICAS Low child, low adult (000)	THE AMERICAS High child, high adult (000)
Population (000)	6 045 172		3 045 372		2 999 800		294 099	345 533	325 186	430 951	71 235
TOTAL DALYs	1 472 392	100	765 774	100	706 619	100	143 671	209 616	45 991	79 562	16 803
I. Communicable diseases, maternal and perinatal conditions and nutritional deficiencies	610 353	41.5	294 708	38.5	315 645	44.7	102 806	155 682	3 181	17 565	6 213
Infectious and parasitic diseases	340 176	23.1	173 704	22.7	166 473	23.6	68 459	114 085	1 478	7 820	3 058
Tuberculosis	35 792	2.4	21 829	2.9	13 962	2.0	3 754	6 034	20	633	482
STDs excluding HIV	15 839	1.1	5 808	0.8	10 031	1.4	2 837	3 351	110	601	98
Syphilis	5 574	0.4	3 095	0.4	2 479	0.4	1 353	1 817	1	23	4
Chlamydia	6 128	0.4	902	0.1	5 226	0.7	829	837	91	389	63
Gonorrhoea	3 919	0.3	1 758	0.2	2 161	0.3	655	693	16	186	31
HIV/AIDS	90 392	6.1	44 366	5.8	46 026	6.5	15 605	57 046	504	1 145	714
Diarrhoeal diseases	62 227	4.2	32 399	4.2	29 828	4.2	8 070	13 424	108	1 838	882
Childhood diseases	50 380	3.4	25 151	3.3	25 229	3.6	15 396	11 043	50	202	256
Pertussis	12 768	0.9	6 369	0.8	6 398	0.9	3 612	2 922	50	178	236
Poliomyelitis	184	0.0	95	0.0	89	0.0	16	7	0	6	1
Diphtheria	114	0.0	61	0.0	53	0.0	24	23	0	2	0
Measles	27 549	1.9	13 755	1.8	13 793	2.0	9 344	6 646	0	2	3
Tetanus	9 766	0.7	4 870	0.6	4 895	0.7	2 400	1 446	0	14	17
Meningitis	5 751	0.4	3 011	0.4	2 740	0.4	698	817	47	437	46
Hepatitis[c]	2 739	0.2	1 400	0.2	1 339	0.2	334	444	82	59	35
Malaria	40 213	2.7	19 237	2.5	20 976	3.0	17 916	17 832	1	83	27
Tropical diseases	12 289	0.8	8 271	1.1	4 018	0.6	3 051	3 012	9	701	109
Trypanosomiasis	1 585	0.1	1 013	0.1	572	0.1	804	754	0	0	0
Chagas disease	680	0.0	360	0.0	320	0.0	0	0	7	582	91
Schistosomiasis	1 713	0.1	1 037	0.1	676	0.1	648	724	1	70	9
Leishmaniasis	1 810	0.1	1 067	0.1	744	0.1	222	173	1	41	5
Lymphatic filariasis	5 549	0.4	4 245	0.6	1 304	0.2	894	966	0	8	1
Onchocerciasis	951	0.1	549	0.1	402	0.1	484	395	0	1	2
Leprosy	141	0.0	76	0.0	65	0.0	8	8	0	15	0
Dengue	433	0.0	286	0.0	147	0.0	2	4	0	3	7
Japanese encephalitis	426	0.0	207	0.0	219	0.0	0	0	0	0	0
Trachoma	1 181	0.1	319	0.0	862	0.1	212	232	0	0	0
Intestinal nematode infections	4 811	0.3	2 461	0.3	2 350	0.3	289	364	11	549	123
Ascariasis	1 252	0.1	636	0.1	616	0.1	48	70	3	168	27
Trichuriasis	1 640	0.1	836	0.1	803	0.1	50	70	5	239	46
Hookworm disease	1 829	0.1	939	0.1	890	0.1	191	222	3	125	20
Respiratory infections	97 658	6.6	50 452	6.6	47 206	6.7	13 210	17 823	561	2 400	1 144
Lower respiratory infections	94 222	6.4	48 786	6.4	45 436	6.4	12 933	17 467	509	2 233	1 095
Upper respiratory infections	1 963	0.1	916	0.1	1 047	0.1	149	188	15	56	27
Otitis media	1 472	0.1	750	0.1	722	0.1	128	168	37	110	22
Maternal conditions	34 480	2.3	0	0.0	34 480	4.9	5 166	7 710	182	1 321	431
Perinatal conditions	91 797	6.2	49 072	6.4	42 726	6.0	11 390	10 845	613	3 905	1 034
Nutritional deficiencies	46 242	3.1	21 480	2.8	24 761	3.5	4 580	5 219	347	2 119	547
Protein–energy malnutrition	16 483	1.1	8 298	1.1	8 185	1.2	2 578	2 904	34	763	239
Iodine deficiency	1 218	0.1	572	0.1	646	0.1	140	193	3	7	2
Vitamin A deficiency	1 392	0.1	587	0.1	805	0.1	382	440	0	3	1
Iron-deficiency anaemia	26 650	1.8	11 807	1.5	14 843	2.1	1 468	1 680	306	1 341	237

Cause[b]	EASTERN MEDITERRANEAN Mortality stratum		EUROPE Mortality stratum			SOUTH-EAST ASIA Mortality stratum		WESTERN PACIFIC Mortality stratum	
	Low child, Low adult	High child, high adult	Very low child, very low adult	Low child, low adult	Low child, high adult	Low child, low adult	High child, high adult	Very low child, very low adult	Low child, low adult
Population (000)	*139 071*	*342 584*	*411 910*	*218 473*	*243 192*	*293 821*	*1 241 813*	*154 358*	*1 532 946*
	(000)	(000)	(000)	(000)	(000)	(000)	(000)	(000)	(000)
TOTAL DALYs	22 400	110 959	52 862	40 278	59 972	60 423	364 581	16 393	248 883
I. Communicable diseases, maternal and perinatal conditions and nutritional deficiencies	6 592	56 529	2 800	8 608	5 164	20 700	163 137	1 110	60 266
Infectious and parasitic diseases	2 965	28 474	1 097	3 118	2 608	9 745	76 637	397	20 234
Tuberculosis	176	2 775	63	444	1 096	3 063	11 929	53	5 272
STDs excluding HIV	79	1 150	122	201	194	541	5 981	51	521
Syphilis	3	316	1	24	4	33	1 932	1	62
Chlamydia	51	463	105	120	140	291	2 442	41	266
Gonorrhoea	20	313	15	35	38	215	1 505	8	189
HIV/AIDS	2	1 784	307	36	421	1 198	10 279	11	1 340
Diarrhoeal diseases	815	8 358	109	963	166	976	22 387	45	4 084
Childhood diseases	63	6 934	66	332	34	1 599	12 128	37	2 240
Pertussis	42	2 204	63	63	29	133	2 737	36	462
Poliomyelitis	5	16	1	5	1	11	62	0	52
Diphtheria	0	16	0	6	1	4	35	0	4
Measles	10	2 882	1	252	2	1 212	5 989	1	1 206
Tetanus	7	1 816	1	6	1	239	3 306	0	516
Meningitis	71	800	66	206	125	442	1 429	14	555
Hepatitis[c]	73	181	45	142	46	98	756	56	389
Malaria	47	1 898	2	19	0	292	1 582	2	514
Tropical diseases	62	846	0	7	0	242	3 772	4	472
Trypanosomiasis	0	26	0	0	0	0	0	0	0
Chagas disease	0	0	0	0	0	0	0	0	0
Schistosomiasis	43	154	0	0	0	3	1	0	60
Leishmaniasis	16	124	0	6	0	6	1 210	0	9
Lymphatic filariasis	4	473	0	1	0	233	2 562	4	403
Onchocerciasis	0	69	0	0	0	0	0	0	0
Leprosy	0	12	0	0	0	7	83	0	6
Dengue	0	19	0	0	0	25	346	0	26
Japanese encephalitis	0	6	0	0	0	22	61	0	336
Trachoma	71	108	0	0	0	24	50	0	484
Intestinal nematode infections	47	248	0	8	1	469	1 044	6	1 651
Ascariasis	20	83	0	7	0	114	123	1	588
Trichuriasis	1	31	0	0	0	194	202	2	799
Hookworm disease	26	134	0	0	0	160	703	2	242
Respiratory infections	1 279	10 120	676	2 264	951	3 456	29 005	381	14 387
Lower respiratory infections	1 212	9 929	612	2 182	894	3 350	28 134	358	13 316
Upper respiratory infections	28	77	28	48	31	38	528	10	741
Otitis media	40	115	37	34	27	69	343	13	330
Maternal conditions	693	3 502	206	908	448	1 992	9 132	76	2 713
Perinatal conditions	819	10 424	435	1 669	771	3 224	34 473	94	12 101
Nutritional deficiencies	836	4 009	386	649	385	2 283	13 890	161	10 830
Protein–energy malnutrition	176	1 647	25	151	61	567	4 907	21	2 409
Iodine deficiency	31	173	5	27	32	32	486	2	85
Vitamin A deficiency	3	161	0	1	0	6	373	0	23
Iron-deficiency anaemia	588	1 890	352	445	266	1 624	8 053	137	8 264

Annex Table 3 Burden of disease in disability-adjusted life years (DALYs) by cause, sex and mortality stratum in WHO Regions,[a] estimates for 200(

Cause[b]	SEX						AFRICA		THE AMERICAS		
	Both sexes		Males		Females		Mortality stratum		Mortality stratum		
							High child, high adult	High child, very high adult	Very low child, very low adult	Low child, low adult	High child, high adult
Population (000)	6 045 172		3 045 372		2 999 800		294 099	345 533	325 186	430 951	71 235
	(000)	% total	(000)	% total	(000)	% total	(000)	(000)	(000)	(000)	(000)
II. Noncommunicable conditions	679 484	46.1	352 434	46.0	327 050	46.3	28 701	36 552	38 260	49 550	8 658
Malignant neoplasms	78 508	5.3	42 208	5.5	36 300	5.1	2 741	3 942	5 624	4 320	628
Mouth and oropharynx cancers	4 379	0.3	3 152	0.4	1 227	0.2	124	297	110	119	16
Oesophagus cancer	4 096	0.3	2 721	0.4	1 375	0.2	56	237	133	127	7
Stomach cancer	7 326	0.5	4 565	0.6	2 761	0.4	198	211	143	386	96
Colon/rectum cancer	5 659	0.4	3 074	0.4	2 585	0.4	132	171	617	260	26
Liver cancer	7 948	0.5	5 600	0.7	2 348	0.3	402	519	126	140	35
Pancreas cancer	1 867	0.1	1 064	0.1	803	0.1	31	53	242	114	11
Trachea/bronchus/lung cancers	11 418	0.8	8 303	1.1	3 115	0.4	98	157	1 443	481	27
Melanoma and other skin cancers	690	0.0	387	0.1	303	0.0	35	60	133	54	5
Breast cancer	6 386	0.4	4	0.0	6 382	0.9	182	315	686	392	41
Cervix uteri cancer	4 649	0.3	0	0.0	4 649	0.7	273	515	98	273	83
Corpus uteri cancer	993	0.1	0	0.0	993	0.1	13	21	93	174	27
Ovary cancer	1 651	0.1	0	0.0	1 651	0.2	44	95	149	85	13
Prostate cancer	1 526	0.1	1 526	0.2	0	0.0	144	124	255	147	19
Bladder cancer	1 329	0.1	998	0.1	331	0.0	69	64	116	50	5
Lymphomas, multiple myeloma	3 994	0.3	2 569	0.3	1 424	0.2	317	366	396	224	41
Leukaemia	5 147	0.3	2 835	0.4	2 312	0.3	131	234	254	382	87
Other neoplasms	1 394	0.1	728	0.1	666	0.1	28	46	81	130	31
Diabetes mellitus	14 943	1.0	7 002	0.9	7 941	1.1	289	433	1 290	1 901	292
Nutritional/endocrine disorders	8 061	0.5	3 728	0.5	4 332	0.6	751	867	768	1 205	307
Neuropsychiatric disorders	181 755	12.3	88 423	11.5	93 332	13.2	6 920	8 539	14 076	16 711	2 841
Unipolar depressive disorders	64 963	4.4	25 901	3.4	39 063	5.5	1 906	2 154	5 031	5 589	867
Bipolar affective disorder	13 645	0.9	6 897	0.9	6 747	1.0	743	852	504	1 026	172
Schizophrenia	15 686	1.1	8 013	1.0	7 672	1.1	732	827	509	1 221	204
Epilepsy	7 067	0.5	3 832	0.5	3 235	0.5	423	690	262	848	190
Alcohol use disorders	18 469	1.3	15 844	2.1	2 624	0.4	368	858	3 032	2 848	446
Alzheimer's and other dementias	12 464	0.8	5 381	0.7	7 083	1.0	280	300	1 415	750	64
Parkinson disease	1 473	0.1	723	0.1	750	0.1	30	37	227	43	6
Multiple sclerosis	1 475	0.1	630	0.1	845	0.1	51	40	110	100	15
Drug use disorders	5 830	0.4	4 535	0.6	1 295	0.2	526	601	697	788	227
Post-traumatic stress disorder	3 230	0.2	896	0.1	2 335	0.3	141	158	176	200	31
Obsessive–compulsive disorder	4 761	0.3	2 048	0.3	2 713	0.4	370	428	218	535	85
Panic disorder	6 591	0.4	2 239	0.3	4 352	0.6	336	386	262	494	83
Insomnia (primary)	3 361	0.2	1 447	0.2	1 914	0.3	134	150	258	310	47
Migraine	7 539	0.5	2 045	0.3	5 494	0.8	182	236	490	729	146
Sense organ disorders	37 673	2.6	19 253	2.5	18 420	2.6	2 537	3 187	1 278	2 676	483
Glaucoma	1 744	0.1	628	0.1	1 115	0.2	220	369	21	122	8
Cataracts	10 585	0.7	4 981	0.7	5 604	0.8	1 190	1 114	45	363	141
Hearing loss, adult onset	25 276	1.7	13 610	1.8	11 665	1.7	1 122	1 698	1 212	2 188	332
Cardiovascular diseases	150 975	10.3	80 325	10.5	70 651	10.0	5 049	6 445	7 240	7 753	1 064
Rheumatic heart disease	6 528	0.4	2 773	0.4	3 755	0.5	320	446	53	113	78
Ischaemic heart disease	55 682	3.8	31 997	4.2	23 685	3.4	1 526	1 721	3 288	2 673	255
Cerebrovascular disease	45 677	3.1	23 072	3.0	22 606	3.2	1 439	2 058	1 594	2 735	317
Inflammatory heart disease	6 631	0.5	3 860	0.5	2 771	0.4	334	435	390	409	48

Cause[b]	EASTERN MEDITERRANEAN Mortality stratum		EUROPE Mortality stratum			SOUTH-EAST ASIA Mortality stratum		WESTERN PACIFIC Mortality stratum	
	Low child, Low adult	High child, high adult	Very low child, very low adult	Low child, low adult	Low child, high adult	Low child, low adult	High child, high adult	Very low child, very low adult	Low child, low adult
Population (000)	*139 071*	*342 584*	*411 910*	*218 473*	*243 192*	*293 821*	*1 241 813*	*154 358*	*1 532 946*
	(000)	(000)	(000)	(000)	(000)	(000)	(000)	(000)	(000)
II. Noncommunicable conditions	12 654	43 155	45 608	26 860	41 365	31 624	155 306	13 643	147 547
Malignant neoplasms	1 086	2 514	8 659	3 278	5 706	3 160	12 398	2 820	21 633
Mouth and oropharynx cancers	30	277	291	107	217	259	1 978	59	495
Oesophagus cancer	36	114	233	107	150	34	804	96	1 960
Stomach cancer	108	103	475	323	800	99	669	452	3 264
Colon/rectum cancer	60	115	1 082	283	606	287	442	397	1 181
Liver cancer	48	91	772	87	187	333	369	291	5 048
Pancreas cancer	16	19	365	113	289	53	134	143	282
Trachea/bronchus/lung cancers	121	211	1 665	604	1 093	369	1 223	430	3 495
Melanoma and other skin cancers	10	19	146	43	92	11	29	27	27
Breast cancer	80	191	1 013	297	558	454	1 220	194	763
Cervix uteri cancer	70	235	106	124	169	262	1 888	34	519
Corpus uteri cancer	14	12	144	89	160	29	35	33	149
Ovary cancer	9	61	234	70	200	118	281	58	233
Prostate cancer	15	28	376	61	106	40	94	63	54
Bladder cancer	22	100	273	87	166	48	134	41	152
Lymphomas, multiple myeloma	94	271	445	136	186	230	720	115	454
Leukaemia	154	246	334	163	197	265	1 004	97	1 600
Other neoplasms	25	72	175	37	66	387	98	68	151
Diabetes mellitus	366	963	1 008	667	841	764	3 294	457	2 378
Nutritional/endocrine disorders	178	912	618	183	162	381	498	220	1 008
Neuropsychiatric disorders	3 812	10 497	15 285	6 599	9 196	7 669	39 250	3 878	36 482
Unipolar depressive disorders	1 184	3 507	4 074	2 548	2 634	2 832	17 123	1 000	14 515
Bipolar affective disorder	354	809	621	466	450	702	2 990	243	3 713
Schizophrenia	453	956	595	559	437	1 055	3 530	235	4 365
Epilepsy	131	400	358	256	219	371	1 528	99	1 291
Alcohol use disorders	18	303	2 691	297	2 253	304	1 910	595	2 546
Alzheimer's and other dementias	170	458	3 101	450	994	428	1 873	505	1 678
Parkinson disease	20	58	281	62	77	49	231	105	248
Multiple sclerosis	34	72	155	63	81	63	318	29	346
Drug use disorders	391	214	717	156	295	120	511	250	335
Post-traumatic stress disorder	78	180	207	123	131	179	706	81	841
Obsessive–compulsive disorder	184	326	257	267	284	170	823	63	752
Panic disorder	174	397	323	241	237	361	1 479	128	1 691
Insomnia (primary)	33	151	345	116	159	114	839	129	576
Migraine	144	394	747	250	240	334	1 686	155	1 805
Sense organ disorders	1 032	2 644	1 348	1 158	1 644	2 425	10 795	474	5 991
Glaucoma	92	194	61	52	146	47	98	11	303
Cataracts	212	885	21	101	279	760	3 788	21	1 665
Hearing loss, adult onset	728	1 557	1 265	1 005	1 219	1 616	6 890	442	4 001
Cardiovascular diseases	2 852	10 287	9 533	8 262	15 586	6 771	39 658	2 584	27 892
Rheumatic heart disease	85	501	81	177	232	279	2 384	22	1 757
Ischaemic heart disease	1 321	2 795	4 066	3 536	7 887	2 327	16 435	797	7 055
Cerebrovascular disease	600	2 101	2 732	2 415	5 284	1 936	6 950	1 268	14 248
Inflammatory heart disease	58	248	280	381	503	272	2 322	82	869

Annex Table 3 Burden of disease in disability-adjusted life years (DALYs) by cause, sex and mortality stratum in WHO Regions,ª estimates for 200

Cause[b]	SEX						AFRICA		THE AMERICAS		
	Both sexes		Males		Females		Mortality stratum		Mortality stratum		
							High child, high adult	High child, very high adult	Very low child, very low adult	Low child, low adult	High child, high adult
Population (000)	*6 045 172*		*3 045 372*		*2 999 800*		*294 099*	*345 533*	*325 186*	*430 951*	*71 235*
	(000)	% total	(000)	% total	(000)	% total	(000)	(000)	(000)	(000)	(000)
Respiratory diseases	68 737	4.7	37 408	4.9	31 329	4.4	3 270	4 397	2 667	4 718	719
Chronic obstructive pulmonary disease	33 748	2.3	18 677	2.4	15 071	2.1	717	961	1 262	1 032	88
Asthma	13 858	0.9	7 509	1.0	6 350	0.9	892	1 278	769	1 574	301
Digestive diseases	48 874	3.3	29 367	3.8	19 507	2.8	2 764	3 501	1 677	3 676	779
Peptic ulcer disease	4 113	0.3	2 651	0.3	1 462	0.2	132	201	53	144	44
Cirrhosis of the liver	14 856	1.0	10 358	1.4	4 497	0.6	492	648	492	1 121	306
Appendicitis	887	0.1	542	0.1	345	0.0	22	33	14	40	17
Diseases of the genitourinary system	15 875	1.1	9 099	1.2	6 777	1.0	1 194	1 559	564	1 037	268
Nephritis/nephrosis	9 150	0.6	4 921	0.6	4 229	0.6	597	818	172	479	170
Benign prostatic hypertrophy	2 304	0.2	2 304	0.3	0	0.0	122	134	84	193	28
Skin diseases	1 859	0.1	1 033	0.1	827	0.1	272	376	51	124	36
Musculoskeletal diseases	29 938	2.0	12 919	1.7	17 019	2.4	903	952	1 883	2 194	314
Rheumatoid arthritis	5 099	0.3	1 434	0.2	3 665	0.5	55	45	331	604	92
Osteoarthritis	16 446	1.1	6 650	0.9	9 796	1.4	574	598	1 024	941	113
Congenital abnormalities	32 871	2.2	17 053	2.2	15 819	2.2	1 749	2 041	719	2 291	749
Oral diseases	8 021	0.5	3 890	0.5	4 131	0.6	235	268	343	813	146
Dental caries	4 626	0.3	2 344	0.3	2 282	0.3	174	202	176	693	128
Periodontal disease	293	0.0	148	0.0	144	0.0	14	16	13	20	3
Edentulism	2 979	0.2	1 359	0.2	1 620	0.2	42	44	152	92	12
III. Injuries	**182 555**	**12.4**	**118 631**	**15.5**	**63 924**	**9.0**	**12 164**	**17 382**	**4 550**	**12 447**	**1 931**
Unintentional	136 485	9.3	87 309	11.4	49 176	7.0	8 605	11 122	3 099	7 565	1 285
Road traffic accidents	41 234	2.8	30 333	4.0	10 902	1.5	2 289	3 473	1 512	2 781	326
Poisoning	8 235	0.6	5 057	0.7	3 178	0.4	493	705	283	97	44
Falls	19 518	1.3	11 760	1.5	7 758	1.1	802	990	414	994	193
Fires	9 989	0.7	3 929	0.5	6 060	0.9	851	839	139	175	25
Drowning	13 263	0.9	8 874	1.2	4 389	0.6	1 428	1 260	124	588	59
Other unintentional injuries	44 246	3.0	27 356	3.6	16 890	2.4	2 741	3 854	627	2 929	639
Intentional	46 070	3.1	31 323	4.1	14 748	2.1	3 559	6 260	1 451	4 882	646
Self-inflicted	19 257	1.3	11 145	1.5	8 112	1.1	245	432	799	604	117
Violence	16 122	1.1	12 438	1.6	3 683	0.5	1 246	2 420	641	4 208	515
War	10 324	0.7	7 486	1.0	2 838	0.4	2 068	3 408	0	55	14

ª See list of Member States by WHO Region and mortality stratum (pp. 168–169).

[b] Estimates for specific causes may not sum to broader cause groupings due to omission of residual categories.

[c] Does not include liver cancer and cirrhosis DALYs resulting from chronic hepatitis virus infection.

Cause[b]	EASTERN MEDITERRANEAN Mortality stratum		EUROPE Mortality stratum			SOUTH-EAST ASIA Mortality stratum		WESTERN PACIFIC Mortality stratum	
	Low child, Low adult	High child, high adult	Very low child, very low adult	Low child, low adult	Low child, high adult	Low child, low adult	High child, high adult	Very low child, very low adult	Low child, low adult
Population (000)	*139 071*	*342 584*	*411 910*	*218 473*	*243 192*	*293 821*	*1 241 813*	*154 358*	*1 532 946*
	(000)	(000)	(000)	(000)	(000)	(000)	(000)	(000)	(000)
Respiratory diseases	701	4 036	2 648	1 597	2 170	2 784	13 917	856	24 256
Chronic obstructive pulmonary disease	178	827	1 239	731	1 241	959	5 206	179	19 127
Asthma	308	918	717	346	237	678	2 718	380	2 743
Digestive diseases	577	3 996	2 457	2 086	2 544	2 964	12 057	733	9 063
Peptic ulcer disease	34	178	133	118	227	289	1 310	37	1 213
Cirrhosis of the liver	136	628	931	765	932	857	4 116	215	3 216
Appendicitis	6	19	16	14	19	33	538	5	111
Diseases of the genitourinary system	387	1 431	547	579	727	981	3 117	227	3 258
Nephritis/nephrosis	174	1 022	196	271	184	649	2 351	103	1 965
Benign prostatic hypertrophy	62	120	120	66	80	107	459	49	679
Skin diseases	11	156	68	33	89	164	296	14	167
Musculoskeletal diseases	480	1 395	2 289	1 328	1 688	1 465	6 542	936	7 571
Rheumatoid arthritis	79	300	283	295	367	133	1 507	113	894
Osteoarthritis	244	704	1 474	759	996	848	3 415	634	4 121
Congenital abnormalities	743	3 606	621	669	595	1 071	11 699	238	6 082
Oral diseases	405	645	352	384	350	638	1 687	140	1 615
Dental caries	197	356	200	189	167	241	1 053	76	775
Periodontal disease	5	18	16	11	13	15	97	6	46
Edentulism	201	255	133	182	169	377	503	58	759
III. Injuries	**3 153**	**11 275**	**4 454**	**4 810**	**13 443**	**8 098**	**46 138**	**1 639**	**41 070**
Unintentional	2 586	8 719	3 308	3 404	8 890	5 720	38 960	1 113	32 110
Road traffic accidents	1 400	1 935	1 407	635	1 721	3 913	10 120	359	9 363
Poisoning	52	524	128	348	1 799	106	2 293	20	1 342
Falls	467	1 474	742	577	956	697	4 388	198	6 624
Fires	118	1 010	58	134	334	233	5 397	30	646
Drowning	100	498	78	274	823	376	2 376	69	5 210
Other unintentional injuries	449	3 277	895	1 435	3 258	394	14 386	436	8 925
Intentional	567	2 556	1 147	1 406	4 553	2 379	7 178	526	8 960
Self-inflicted	221	506	1 015	574	2 315	509	4 396	485	7 042
Violence	234	735	129	322	1 643	450	1 791	40	1 751
War	112	1 254	1	472	570	1 388	822	0	154

Annex Table 4 Healthy life expectancy (HALE) in all Member States, estimates for 2000

	Member State	Total population At birth	Males At birth	Males Uncertainty interval	Males At age 60	Males Uncertainty interval	Females At birth	Females Uncertainty interval	Females At age 60	Females Uncertainty interval	Expectation of lost healthy years at birth (years) Males	Expectation of lost healthy years at birth (years) Females	Percentage of total life expectancy lost Males	Percentage of total life expectancy lost Females
1	Afghanistan	33.8	35.1	30.3 – 40.4	7.1	5.5 – 8.8	32.5	26.2 – 39.5	5.8	2.6 – 9.0	9.1	12.5	20.5	27.8
2	Albania	59.4	56.5	54.4 – 59.3	11.4	10.3 – 12.6	62.3	59.9 – 64.8	14.4	13.0 – 16.0	7.9	10.6	12.2	14.5
3	Algeria	58.4	58.4	55.8 – 61.9	11.1	9.4 – 13.1	58.3	54.5 – 62.2	11.0	8.9 – 12.9	9.7	12.9	14.3	18.1
4	Andorra	71.8	69.8	67.4 – 73.0	17.0	15.4 – 18.7	73.7	70.7 – 77.9	19.4	17.3 – 22.5	7.3	10.1	9.5	12.1
5	Angola	36.9	36.2	33.7 – 42.0	7.4	5.3 – 10.1	37.6	33.3 – 42.8	7.3	4.6 – 10.3	8.1	10.8	18.2	22.3
6	Antigua and Barbuda	61.9	61.7	58.4 – 64.8	14.8	13.5 – 16.3	62.1	59.0 – 65.2	15.4	14.1 – 16.9	10.1	14.5	14.1	18.9
7	Argentina	63.9	61.8	59.6 – 64.0	13.2	12.0 – 14.6	65.9	63.0 – 68.6	16.0	14.8 – 17.5	8.4	11.9	12.0	15.2
8	Armenia	59.0	56.9	55.0 – 58.6	9.7	8.8 – 10.6	61.1	58.1 – 64.1	12.0	10.9 – 13.1	7.5	10.1	11.7	14.2
9	Australia	71.5	69.6	67.8 – 71.5	17.0	16.1 – 18.1	73.3	69.8 – 75.4	19.5	18.7 – 20.6	6.9	8.8	9.1	10.7
10	Austria	70.3	68.1	66.9 – 69.4	15.2	14.5 – 16.0	72.5	70.3 – 74.3	18.4	17.8 – 19.2	6.8	8.9	9.0	10.9
11	Azerbaijan	55.4	53.3	50.6 – 56.3	12.2	10.8 – 14.0	57.5	54.3 – 60.8	14.6	12.9 – 16.5	8.4	11.4	13.6	16.5
12	Bahamas	58.1	57.2	54.0 – 60.5	12.4	10.2 – 14.7	59.1	54.2 – 64.0	12.6	10.1 – 15.2	10.8	15.7	15.9	21.0
13	Bahrain	62.7	63.0	61.0 – 65.2	11.3	9.8 – 12.8	62.3	59.1 – 65.1	11.4	10.2 – 12.6	9.7	12.4	13.3	16.6
14	Bangladesh	49.3	50.6	47.4 – 54.1	8.8	7.5 – 10.4	47.9	43.6 – 52.6	8.0	6.4 – 9.9	9.8	12.9	16.2	21.2
15	Barbados	63.3	62.3	59.7 – 65.0	13.4	12.1 – 14.9	64.3	60.9 – 67.7	16.1	14.1 – 18.4	9.3	13.4	13.0	17.2
16	Belarus	60.1	55.4	53.4 – 57.5	9.9	9.2 – 10.8	64.8	62.7 – 66.9	14.4	13.2 – 15.9	6.6	9.2	10.7	12.4
17	Belgium	69.4	67.7	66.2 – 69.2	15.3	14.5 – 16.2	71.0	69.0 – 73.0	18.0	17.2 – 18.7	6.9	9.9	9.2	12.2
18	Belize	59.2	58.0	55.2 – 61.0	12.7	11.2 – 14.1	60.4	55.6 – 64.9	13.6	11.0 – 16.4	11.1	14.3	16.1	19.2
19	Benin	42.5	43.1	39.8 – 46.5	8.4	6.7 – 10.1	41.9	37.5 – 46.5	7.4	3.9 – 10.5	8.5	11.9	16.5	22.0
20	Bhutan	49.2	50.1	44.8 – 55.1	9.3	7.5 – 11.1	48.2	43.5 – 53.7	8.8	6.1 – 11.7	10.3	14.3	17.0	22.9
21	Bolivia	51.4	51.4	47.4 – 55.5	9.8	8.3 – 11.5	51.4	47.1 – 55.9	10.0	8.0 – 11.8	9.5	12.1	15.6	19.1
22	Bosnia and Herzegovina	63.7	62.1	60.3 – 64.3	12.4	11.3 – 13.5	65.3	62.8 – 67.9	14.3	13.0 – 15.7	6.6	9.4	9.5	12.5
23	Botswana	37.3	38.1	34.3 – 42.0	8.3	6.4 – 10.1	36.5	33.2 – 40.0	8.9	6.3 – 11.5	6.5	7.9	14.6	17.7
24	Brazil[b]	57.1	54.9	51.4 – 58.1	10.7	9.2 – 12.0	59.2	54.8 – 64.1	12.6	9.8 – 15.2	9.5	12.7	14.8	17.6
25	Brunei Darussalam	64.9	63.8	61.5 – 66.0	13.3	12.0 – 14.6	65.9	62.4 – 69.6	15.1	13.8 – 16.5	9.6	12.7	13.1	16.2
26	Bulgaria	63.4	61.0	59.4 – 62.6	12.4	11.8 – 13.1	65.8	63.8 – 67.7	15.2	14.0 – 16.4	6.3	9.2	9.4	12.2
27	Burkina Faso	34.8	35.4	32.5 – 38.3	8.0	6.2 – 9.7	34.1	30.5 – 37.9	7.4	4.9 – 10.0	7.2	9.5	16.8	21.7
28	Burundi	33.4	33.9	30.4 – 37.5	7.6	6.0 – 9.1	32.9	29.3 – 36.9	7.7	5.4 – 10.3	6.7	8.5	16.5	20.5
29	Cambodia	47.1	45.6	43.1 – 48.0	9.0	7.8 – 10.3	48.7	45.4 – 52.4	10.1	8.0 – 12.2	7.8	9.8	14.7	16.8
30	Cameroon	40.4	40.9	37.6 – 44.0	8.4	6.2 – 10.6	39.9	36.7 – 43.2	8.0	5.7 – 10.5	8.1	10.5	16.5	20.8
31	Canada	70.0	68.3	66.9 – 69.7	15.4	14.6 – 16.3	71.7	70.0 – 73.5	17.8	17.0 – 18.6	7.7	9.8	10.2	12.0
32	Cape Verde	58.4	56.9	53.7 – 60.2	11.3	9.8 – 12.8	60.0	56.3 – 63.8	12.0	10.0 – 14.1	9.6	12.3	14.4	17.0
33	Central African Republic	34.1	34.7	31.6 – 38.2	8.2	6.6 – 9.8	33.6	30.3 – 37.3	7.9	5.9 – 9.8	6.9	8.9	16.7	20.9
34	Chad	39.3	38.6	35.3 – 43.7	7.4	5.5 – 9.4	39.9	36.1 – 44.5	7.5	4.6 – 10.5	8.7	11.2	18.4	22.0
35	Chile	65.5	63.5	61.5 – 66.0	13.1	11.8 – 14.5	67.4	64.5 – 70.3	15.7	14.4 – 17.1	9.0	12.1	12.4	15.2
36	China	62.1	60.9	59.5 – 62.5	11.8	11.0 – 12.8	63.3	59.1 – 65.8	14.3	13.6 – 15.1	8.0	9.7	11.6	13.2
37	Colombia	60.9	58.6	56.2 – 61.0	12.9	11.6 – 14.2	63.3	59.8 – 66.2	14.0	12.8 – 15.1	8.6	11.8	12.8	15.7
38	Comoros	46.0	46.2	42.8 – 49.6	8.0	6.6 – 9.5	45.8	41.4 – 50.3	7.7	5.4 – 9.9	9.1	12.3	16.4	21.1
39	Congo	42.6	42.5	39.3 – 47.0	8.7	7.0 – 11.0	42.8	39.1 – 47.2	8.9	6.1 – 11.7	7.7	10.1	15.3	19.1
40	Cook Islands	60.7	60.4	58.1 – 62.8	11.4	10.4 – 12.3	61.1	57.7 – 64.9	13.0	11.6 – 14.6	8.3	11.0	12.0	15.3
41	Costa Rica	65.3	64.2	61.9 – 66.9	14.0	12.4 – 15.6	66.4	63.1 – 69.2	15.6	14.2 – 17.1	9.2	12.4	12.6	15.7
42	Côte d'Ivoire	39.0	39.1	36.7 – 42.6	8.6	7.3 – 10.1	38.9	35.9 – 42.1	8.5	5.9 – 11.2	7.2	9.5	15.6	19.7
43	Croatia	64.0	60.8	59.5 – 62.0	11.4	10.8 – 12.1	67.1	64.7 – 69.2	15.2	14.6 – 15.8	9.0	10.6	12.9	13.6
44	Cuba	65.9	65.1	63.0 – 67.2	14.5	13.4 – 15.6	66.7	64.4 – 68.8	15.5	14.1 – 16.9	8.6	10.9	11.6	14.0
45	Cyprus	66.3	66.4	64.6 – 68.7	14.5	12.9 – 16.3	66.2	63.4 – 68.8	14.1	12.8 – 15.7	8.4	12.7	11.2	16.1
46	Czech Republic	65.6	62.9	61.3 – 64.4	13.0	12.2 – 13.8	68.3	65.7 – 70.5	15.8	15.2 – 16.4	8.6	9.9	12.0	12.6
47	Democratic People's Republic of Korea	55.4	54.9	51.5 – 58.4	11.1	10.0 – 12.4	56.0	52.2 – 59.8	12.1	10.6 – 13.8	9.6	11.2	14.8	16.7
48	Democratic Republic of the Congo	34.4	34.4	31.6 – 39.4	7.2	5.9 – 8.8	34.4	30.5 – 39.3	7.4	5.1 – 9.6	7.2	9.6	17.4	21.9
49	Denmark	69.5	68.9	67.5 – 70.3	15.7	14.9 – 16.6	70.1	68.2 – 72.0	16.5	15.8 – 17.3	5.3	8.4	7.2	10.7
50	Djibouti	35.1	35.6	31.3 – 40.4	7.4	5.5 – 9.5	34.6	30.1 – 39.6	7.0	4.6 – 9.6	7.8	10.1	18.0	22.5
51	Dominica	64.6	63.2	59.7 – 66.1	14.4	13.1 – 15.9	66.1	63.3 – 69.3	16.4	14.8 – 18.1	9.4	12.2	13.0	15.6
52	Dominican Republic	56.2	54.7	50.9 – 58.2	12.3	11.0 – 13.5	57.7	53.4 – 61.9	13.0	11.0 – 15.0	10.8	14.0	16.4	19.5
53	Ecuador	60.3	58.4	55.4 – 61.3	12.7	11.3 – 14.0	62.2	58.6 – 66.0	14.4	12.4 – 16.5	9.9	12.0	14.5	16.2
54	Egypt	57.1	57.1	55.4 – 58.8	9.9	8.6 – 11.2	57.0	54.1 – 59.3	10.0	8.9 – 11.2	8.3	12.0	12.6	17.4
55	El Salvador	57.3	55.3	52.0 – 58.7	11.9	10.5 – 13.5	59.4	55.3 – 63.3	13.3	10.7 – 15.9	11.0	13.9	16.6	19.0

	Member State	Total population At birth	Healthy life expectancy[a] (years)									Expectation of lost healthy years at birth (years)		Percentage of total life expectancy lost	
			Males				Females								
		At birth	At birth	Uncertainty interval	At age 60	Uncertainty interval	At birth	Uncertainty interval	At age 60	Uncertainty interval		Males	Females	Males	Females
56	Equatorial Guinea	44.8	44.9	40.6 − 48.7	8.7	7.1 − 10.3	44.8	40.2 − 49.4	8.3	5.8 − 10.9		8.7	11.4	16.2	20.2
57	Eritrea	41.0	41.4	38.1 − 45.0	8.3	6.5 − 10.0	40.5	36.5 − 45.0	8.1	5.6 − 10.7		7.7	10.4	15.7	20.4
58	Estonia	60.8	56.2	54.7 − 57.6	10.0	9.1 − 10.9	65.4	62.5 − 67.7	14.8	14.0 − 15.8		9.3	11.0	14.2	14.4
59	Ethiopia	35.4	35.7	32.2 − 40.9	7.7	5.8 − 9.7	35.1	30.4 − 40.9	7.5	4.9 − 10.3		7.1	9.6	16.6	21.4
60	Fiji	59.6	58.7	55.9 − 61.3	11.2	9.6 − 12.7	60.5	56.9 − 64.3	12.7	10.8 − 14.4		8.3	10.7	12.3	15.1
61	Finland	68.8	66.1	64.9 − 67.2	14.8	14.0 − 15.4	71.5	69.9 − 73.0	17.9	17.4 − 18.5		7.6	9.5	10.3	11.7
62	France	70.7	68.5	67.4 − 69.5	16.6	15.9 − 17.2	72.9	71.4 − 74.5	19.4	18.9 − 20.0		6.7	10.2	8.9	12.2
63	Gabon	46.6	46.8	42.9 − 50.0	9.2	7.7 − 10.8	46.5	42.6 − 49.9	9.3	7.6 − 11.2		7.8	10.4	14.2	18.4
64	Gambia	46.9	47.3	44.1 − 50.6	8.5	6.8 − 10.3	46.6	42.4 − 50.8	8.1	6.0 − 10.5		8.6	12.1	15.4	20.6
65	Georgia	58.2	56.1	54.1 − 58.3	9.5	8.5 − 10.5	60.2	57.3 − 62.8	11.1	10.3 − 11.9		9.6	11.6	14.6	16.1
66	Germany	69.4	67.4	66.0 − 68.7	14.8	14.0 − 15.6	71.5	69.4 − 73.3	17.6	16.9 − 18.2		6.9	9.2	9.3	11.4
67	Ghana	46.7	46.5	43.4 − 49.7	8.9	6.9 − 10.8	46.9	43.5 − 51.1	9.0	6.5 − 11.3		8.5	11.0	15.5	18.9
68	Greece	71.0	69.7	68.5 − 70.8	16.0	15.2 − 16.6	72.3	69.9 − 74.0	17.6	17.1 − 18.3		5.7	8.5	7.6	10.5
69	Grenada	61.9	62.1	59.5 − 65.1	14.0	12.6 − 15.4	61.8	57.8 − 65.7	14.1	12.0 − 16.4		8.8	11.5	12.4	15.7
70	Guatemala	54.7	53.5	49.9 − 57.2	11.3	9.1 − 13.6	56.0	52.3 − 59.7	11.7	10.0 − 13.5		10.1	12.6	15.8	18.3
71	Guinea	40.3	40.4	36.7 − 44.0	7.3	5.6 − 9.1	40.1	35.9 − 45.5	7.0	3.9 − 10.3		8.6	11.9	17.5	22.8
72	Guinea-Bissau	36.6	36.7	33.6 − 39.8	7.2	5.1 − 9.1	36.4	33.0 − 40.3	7.1	4.1 − 10.1		7.7	10.5	17.4	22.3
73	Guyana	52.1	51.4	48.3 − 54.6	10.3	9.1 − 11.6	52.8	47.7 − 58.4	11.1	8.9 − 13.6		10.1	14.2	16.4	21.2
74	Haiti	43.1	41.3	37.0 − 46.2	7.8	6.1 − 9.5	44.9	38.8 − 51.1	8.5	5.7 − 11.4		8.4	11.2	16.9	20.0
75	Honduras	56.8	55.8	52.5 − 59.6	11.7	10.0 − 13.3	57.8	53.6 − 62.0	12.7	10.9 − 14.7		10.6	13.2	16.0	18.6
76	Hungary	59.9	55.3	53.7 − 56.9	9.4	8.3 − 10.3	64.5	61.8 − 66.7	13.8	13.0 − 14.6		11.0	10.7	16.5	14.2
77	Iceland	71.2	69.8	68.1 − 71.5	16.2	15.1 − 17.4	72.6	70.3 − 74.9	18.6	17.6 − 19.6		7.3	9.3	9.5	11.3
78	India	52.0	52.2	50.2 − 54.2	9.9	8.7 − 11.0	51.7	48.5 − 54.8	10.9	9.6 − 12.1		7.6	11.0	12.7	17.5
79	Indonesia	57.4	56.5	55.7 − 58.2	11.6	10.8 − 12.5	58.4	55.8 − 61.0	12.5	11.8 − 13.3		6.9	9.1	10.9	13.5
80	Iran, Islamic Republic of	58.8	59.0	56.4 − 61.6	11.3	9.7 − 12.9	58.6	55.3 − 61.9	11.4	10.0 − 12.7		9.1	11.4	13.3	16.2
81	Iraq	52.6	52.6	48.6 − 57.0	9.3	6.7 − 12.0	52.5	48.6 − 57.3	9.5	7.5 − 11.9		9.2	12.1	14.8	18.7
82	Ireland	69.3	67.8	66.3 − 69.1	14.3	13.5 − 15.1	70.9	68.6 − 72.7	16.9	16.2 − 17.6		6.3	8.8	8.5	11.0
83	Israel	69.9	69.3	67.7 − 71.0	16.2	15.2 − 17.3	70.6	68.3 − 72.9	17.1	15.8 − 18.4		7.3	10.0	9.6	12.4
84	Italy	71.2	69.5	68.4 − 70.8	16.3	15.6 − 17.2	72.8	70.5 − 74.5	18.8	18.1 − 19.4		6.4	9.6	8.5	11.6
85	Jamaica	64.0	62.9	59.8 − 65.8	14.6	13.5 − 15.9	65.0	62.1 − 68.1	15.7	13.7 − 17.7		10.0	11.5	13.7	15.1
86	Japan	73.8	71.2	69.9 − 72.5	17.6	16.8 − 18.4	76.3	74.6 − 77.8	21.4	20.3 − 22.5		6.3	8.4	8.1	9.9
87	Jordan	58.5	58.2	56.4 − 60.3	10.3	9.0 − 11.7	58.8	56.0 − 61.4	11.3	10.1 − 12.6		10.3	13.6	15.0	18.8
88	Kazakhstan	54.3	50.5	48.0 − 53.1	10.9	9.9 − 11.9	58.1	55.6 − 60.6	14.6	13.1 − 16.0		7.5	10.3	13.0	15.0
89	Kenya	40.7	41.2	38.7 − 44.4	9.3	8.0 − 10.7	40.1	36.7 − 43.8	9.1	7.0 − 11.0		7.0	9.4	14.5	19.1
90	Kiribati	53.6	52.8	49.6 − 56.1	10.7	9.2 − 12.2	54.4	50.7 − 57.9	11.4	9.3 − 13.3		7.6	10.1	12.6	15.7
91	Kuwait	64.7	64.6	62.1 − 66.8	12.4	10.8 − 13.8	64.8	61.4 − 68.0	13.0	10.7 − 15.0		9.6	12.0	13.0	15.6
92	Kyrgyzstan	52.6	49.6	46.5 − 53.1	8.5	6.2 − 10.9	55.6	51.2 − 60.1	11.8	9.7 − 13.9		10.4	13.2	17.4	19.2
93	Lao People's Democratic Republic	44.7	43.7	39.1 − 47.5	9.6	8.1 − 11.2	45.7	40.6 − 49.6	10.6	8.4 − 12.7		8.6	10.4	16.4	18.5
94	Latvia	57.7	51.4	49.0 − 53.5	9.1	7.9 − 10.0	63.9	60.9 − 66.5	14.4	13.5 − 15.4		12.8	11.6	19.9	15.3
95	Lebanon	60.7	60.3	57.6 − 63.1	11.3	9.6 − 12.8	61.1	57.4 − 65.1	12.2	10.3 − 14.3		8.9	12.2	12.8	16.7
96	Lesotho	35.3	36.1	33.1 − 39.7	8.7	6.8 − 10.6	34.5	31.2 − 38.7	8.8	6.4 − 11.3		5.9	7.7	14.1	18.2
97	Liberia	37.8	38.2	34.0 − 42.4	7.3	6.1 − 8.5	37.4	33.5 − 41.5	6.9	4.3 − 9.5		8.4	11.7	18.1	23.9
98	Libyan Arab Jamahiriya	58.5	58.4	55.7 − 61.4	10.6	9.0 − 12.4	58.6	55.2 − 62.5	11.3	9.2 − 13.4		9.2	12.4	13.6	17.4
99	Lithuania	58.4	53.6	51.6 − 55.5	10.1	9.0 − 11.0	63.2	60.2 − 65.9	14.2	13.2 − 15.2		13.3	14.0	19.8	18.2
100	Luxembourg	69.8	67.6	66.2 − 69.2	14.9	14.1 − 15.8	72.0	69.5 − 74.0	18.4	17.6 − 19.1		6.3	8.7	8.5	10.8
101	Madagascar	42.9	43.2	40.6 − 46.1	8.0	6.4 − 9.5	42.6	38.0 − 47.3	7.5	4.6 − 10.9		8.5	12.0	16.5	22.1
102	Malawi	30.9	31.4	28.2 − 34.6	7.6	5.8 − 9.4	30.5	26.8 − 34.4	7.8	5.1 − 11.0		5.8	7.4	15.5	19.5
103	Malaysia	61.6	59.7	57.3 − 62.1	10.6	8.9 − 12.3	63.4	60.3 − 66.6	12.7	11.3 − 14.1		8.6	10.7	12.6	14.5
104	Maldives	52.4	54.2	50.3 − 58.2	10.1	8.4 − 11.9	50.6	46.4 − 55.9	8.6	6.1 − 10.8		10.4	13.8	16.1	21.5
105	Mali	34.5	34.8	31.5 − 39.3	7.1	5.9 − 8.9	34.1	29.5 − 38.9	7.2	4.3 − 10.1		7.9	10.5	18.5	23.5
106	Malta	70.4	68.7	67.3 − 70.2	15.6	14.7 − 16.5	72.1	69.7 − 74.1	17.7	16.9 − 18.5		6.7	8.6	8.9	10.7
107	Marshall Islands	56.1	54.8	51.9 − 57.9	10.4	8.8 − 12.2	57.4	54.3 − 60.3	12.3	10.6 − 14.2		7.9	10.4	12.7	15.3
108	Mauritania	41.5	42.1	37.7 − 46.3	7.8	5.7 − 10.0	40.8	35.5 − 46.0	7.1	3.7 − 10.3		9.6	12.7	18.5	23.8
109	Mauritius	60.5	58.6	55.6 − 61.3	10.1	8.6 − 11.5	62.5	58.4 − 66.3	12.3	10.1 − 14.6		9.1	12.2	13.4	16.3
110	Mexico	64.2	63.1	60.8 − 65.2	14.5	13.1 − 16.0	65.3	61.5 − 68.1	15.0	13.8 − 16.4		7.9	10.9	11.2	14.3

Annex Table 4 Healthy life expectancy (HALE) in all Member States, estimates for 2000

	Member State	Total population At birth	Males At birth	Males Uncertainty interval	Males At age 60	Males Uncertainty interval	Females At birth	Females Uncertainty interval	Females At age 60	Females Uncertainty interval	Expectation of lost healthy years at birth (years) Males	Females	Percentage of total life expectancy lost Males	Females
111	Micronesia, Federated States of	56.6	55.8	52.8 – 58.8	11.0	9.5 – 12.5	57.5	54.0 – 61.0	12.0	10.6 – 13.4	8.0	10.3	12.5	15.2
112	Monaco	71.7	69.4	67.5 – 72.1	17.2	16.0 – 18.8	73.9	71.1 – 76.7	20.2	18.4 – 22.4	7.4	10.5	9.6	12.4
113	Mongolia	52.4	50.3	46.3 – 54.3	10.8	9.0 – 12.6	54.5	50.8 – 58.2	12.7	10.4 – 15.1	10.9	12.4	17.8	18.5
114	Morocco	54.9	55.3	53.4 – 57.3	9.9	8.4 – 11.4	54.5	51.3 – 57.2	10.0	8.7 – 11.2	10.8	16.0	16.3	22.7
115	Mozambique	31.3	31.5	28.9 – 34.9	7.3	5.4 – 9.6	31.1	28.1 – 34.7	7.3	5.4 – 9.7	6.4	8.4	17.0	21.3
116	Myanmar	49.1	47.7	43.8 – 51.6	9.2	7.6 – 10.9	50.5	45.7 – 54.3	10.1	7.8 – 12.1	8.5	10.7	15.1	17.4
117	Namibia	35.6	36.5	32.5 – 41.2	9.2	7.4 – 11.0	34.7	31.4 – 38.8	9.1	6.6 – 11.7	6.3	7.9	14.8	18.6
118	Nauru	52.9	50.4	47.0 – 54.4	7.9	6.6 – 9.5	55.4	51.0 – 60.2	10.5	8.2 – 13.2	8.3	11.1	14.1	16.7
119	Nepal	45.8	47.5	44.4 – 51.1	10.2	8.3 – 12.0	44.2	39.1 – 49.8	9.6	6.3 – 12.7	11.0	13.8	18.8	23.9
120	Netherlands[b]	69.7	68.2	67.1 – 69.3	15.2	14.6 – 15.9	71.2	69.7 – 72.7	17.8	17.2 – 18.4	7.3	9.7	9.6	12.0
121	New Zealand	70.8	69.5	68.0 – 71.0	16.7	15.8 – 17.7	72.1	69.8 – 74.0	18.8	17.9 – 19.6	6.4	8.9	8.5	11.0
122	Nicaragua	56.9	55.8	51.8 – 60.3	11.3	9.6 – 13.4	58.0	54.3 – 62.4	12.5	10.6 – 14.7	10.6	13.0	16.0	18.3
123	Niger	33.1	33.9	30.9 – 37.7	6.6	3.8 – 9.3	32.4	27.1 – 37.6	5.8	3.2 – 8.4	8.8	11.5	20.7	26.2
124	Nigeria	41.6	42.1	39.2 – 45.0	8.4	6.8 – 10.0	41.1	37.7 – 45.0	8.2	6.4 – 10.1	7.7	10.3	15.5	20.1
125	Niue	61.1	60.8	57.1 – 64.2	13.0	11.4 – 14.7	61.4	58.6 – 65.2	13.8	11.9 – 16.2	8.7	11.4	12.6	15.6
126	Norway	70.5	68.8	67.0 – 70.5	15.8	14.8 – 16.8	72.3	70.2 – 74.6	18.2	16.9 – 19.5	6.9	9.1	9.2	11.2
127	Oman	59.7	59.2	57.2 – 61.4	10.3	8.8 – 11.9	60.3	56.6 – 63.1	12.0	10.5 – 13.5	10.3	13.2	14.8	17.9
128	Pakistan[b]	48.1	50.2	46.6 – 54.2	9.8	8.7 – 11.2	46.1	41.5 – 51.1	8.7	5.6 – 11.8	10.0	14.7	16.6	24.1
129	Palau	57.7	56.5	54.3 – 58.6	9.5	8.4 – 10.3	58.9	55.7 – 62.4	10.7	9.2 – 12.2	8.2	10.4	12.6	15.0
130	Panama	63.9	62.6	60.1 – 65.1	13.7	12.4 – 14.9	65.3	62.6 – 68.0	15.3	13.8 – 16.8	8.9	11.0	12.5	14.4
131	Papua New Guinea	46.8	46.6	42.8 – 50.5	9.2	7.7 – 10.6	47.1	43.6 – 50.9	10.5	8.7 – 12.1	8.5	10.4	15.4	18.1
132	Paraguay	60.9	59.9	56.7 – 63.4	12.3	10.4 – 14.3	61.9	58.8 – 65.5	14.0	12.4 – 15.6	10.3	12.3	14.7	16.6
133	Peru	58.8	57.8	55.2 – 60.6	12.0	10.5 – 13.6	59.8	56.2 – 63.6	13.6	11.6 – 15.8	8.9	11.8	13.4	16.4
134	Philippines	59.0	57.0	54.3 – 59.4	11.5	10.3 – 12.6	60.9	57.7 – 64.3	13.6	11.9 – 15.5	7.7	10.2	11.9	14.3
135	Poland	61.8	59.3	57.9 – 60.5	10.9	10.1 – 11.7	64.3	61.2 – 66.7	13.8	12.9 – 14.6	10.0	13.4	14.4	17.2
136	Portugal	66.3	63.9	62.5 – 65.4	13.6	12.7 – 14.4	68.6	66.2 – 70.5	16.0	15.3 – 16.7	7.8	10.7	10.9	13.5
137	Qatar	60.6	59.3	56.5 – 62.6	9.2	7.0 – 11.4	61.8	58.4 – 65.4	11.6	9.8 – 13.6	11.1	13.2	15.7	17.6
138	Republic of Korea	66.0	63.2	60.8 – 65.3	12.3	11.1 – 13.4	68.8	64.0 – 71.4	16.0	15.1 – 17.0	7.3	9.5	10.3	12.1
139	Republic of Moldova	58.4	55.4	52.4 – 57.9	10.2	8.8 – 11.4	61.5	59.1 – 64.3	12.5	11.1 – 13.9	7.7	8.9	12.3	12.7
140	Romania	61.7	59.5	57.4 – 61.4	12.1	11.0 – 12.9	64.0	61.6 – 66.8	14.4	13.1 – 15.7	6.8	9.5	10.2	12.9
141	Russian Federation	55.5	50.3	48.6 – 52.4	8.2	7.3 – 8.9	60.6	57.0 – 63.3	12.2	11.5 – 13.0	9.1	11.4	15.3	15.8
142	Rwanda	31.9	32.0	29.6 – 36.5	7.0	4.8 – 9.4	31.8	28.3 – 36.2	7.2	5.3 – 9.2	6.5	8.7	17.0	21.5
143	Saint Kitts and Nevis	59.6	57.6	54.7 – 60.7	10.3	9.4 – 11.3	61.5	57.8 – 65.6	12.6	10.8 – 14.5	8.4	10.5	12.8	14.5
144	Saint Lucia	62.0	60.7	58.1 – 63.0	12.5	11.3 – 13.8	63.3	60.0 – 66.5	13.9	12.1 – 15.6	8.5	10.9	12.2	14.7
145	Saint Vincent and the Grenadines	60.9	59.7	57.1 – 62.2	12.1	11.0 – 13.3	62.1	59.1 – 65.0	14.1	12.5 – 15.7	8.0	11.3	11.9	15.4
146	Samoa	59.9	58.2	55.6 – 60.6	12.3	10.9 – 13.7	61.6	59.0 – 64.4	14.3	12.7 – 16.0	8.5	11.3	12.7	15.6
147	San Marino	72.0	69.7	68.0 – 71.8	15.9	14.8 – 17.0	74.3	72.2 – 76.4	19.9	18.4 – 21.5	6.5	9.5	8.5	11.4
148	Sao Tome and Principe	50.0	50.3	46.8 – 53.6	9.6	8.0 – 11.0	49.7	44.8 – 54.7	9.2	7.5 – 10.6	10.0	12.2	16.6	19.8
149	Saudi Arabia	59.5	58.3	55.0 – 61.1	10.5	8.4 – 12.3	60.7	56.5 – 64.9	12.1	9.8 – 14.2	9.7	12.8	14.3	17.4
150	Senegal	44.9	45.2	42.1 – 48.0	8.4	6.8 – 9.8	44.5	40.9 – 48.4	8.0	5.0 – 11.1	8.8	11.6	16.3	20.7
151	Seychelles	58.7	57.0	54.1 – 59.7	9.4	7.2 – 11.5	60.4	57.1 – 64.0	10.7	8.8 – 13.1	9.5	13.8	14.3	18.6
152	Sierra Leone	29.5	29.7	26.4 – 36.0	6.5	4.7 – 8.8	29.3	25.2 – 35.1	6.0	2.9 – 9.5	7.3	9.6	19.6	24.6
153	Singapore	67.8	66.8	64.3 – 69.0	14.5	13.1 – 15.8	68.9	65.8 – 71.7	16.2	14.6 – 18.0	8.6	11.3	11.4	14.1
154	Slovakia	62.4	59.6	58.1 – 60.9	10.7	9.9 – 11.6	65.2	62.3 – 67.5	14.0	13.2 – 14.9	9.7	12.3	14.0	15.9
155	Slovenia	66.9	64.5	62.1 – 66.7	13.6	12.8 – 14.3	69.3	66.5 – 71.9	16.7	15.4 – 18.0	7.4	10.2	10.3	12.8
156	Solomon Islands	59.0	58.0	55.1 – 61.5	11.2	9.4 – 13.3	60.1	56.6 – 63.8	12.4	10.7 – 14.1	8.6	11.3	12.9	15.9
157	Somalia	35.1	35.5	32.5 – 38.9	7.3	5.2 – 9.5	34.7	30.6 – 38.8	6.4	2.6 – 9.7	8.3	11.2	18.9	24.4
158	South Africa	43.2	43.0	41.1 – 45.0	9.1	7.9 – 10.5	43.5	40.5 – 46.4	10.4	8.7 – 12.1	6.6	8.6	13.3	16.5
159	Spain	70.6	68.7	67.3 – 70.3	15.8	14.9 – 16.8	72.5	70.3 – 74.2	18.3	17.5 – 19.1	6.6	9.8	8.8	11.9
160	Sri Lanka	61.1	58.6	55.7 – 61.5	12.5	10.9 – 14.1	63.6	61.0 – 67.0	14.6	12.8 – 16.6	9.0	11.7	13.4	15.6
161	Sudan	45.1	45.7	42.2 – 49.3	8.3	6.5 – 10.1	44.4	39.2 – 50.2	7.8	5.8 – 9.6	9.8	13.4	17.6	23.1
162	Suriname	60.6	59.5	57.0 – 61.9	12.2	11.0 – 13.6	61.7	58.5 – 64.6	13.3	11.5 – 15.1	8.5	11.9	12.5	16.1
163	Swaziland	38.2	38.8	34.1 – 44.2	9.3	7.0 – 11.5	37.6	32.6 – 42.7	9.6	7.5 – 12.0	6.0	8.0	13.3	17.4
164	Sweden	71.4	70.1	68.7 – 71.6	16.8	15.9 – 17.7	72.7	70.6 – 74.6	18.7	18.0 – 19.4	7.2	9.2	9.3	11.3
165	Switzerland	72.1	70.4	68.7 – 72.1	17.0	16.1 – 17.9	73.7	71.3 – 75.7	19.7	19.0 – 20.4	6.2	8.8	8.1	10.7

	Member State	Total population At birth	Healthy life expectancy[a] (years) Males				Females				Expectation of lost healthy years at birth (years)		Percentage of total life expectancy lost	
			At birth	Uncertainty interval	At age 60	Uncertainty interval	At birth	Uncertainty interval	At age 60	Uncertainty interval	Males	Females	Males	Females
166	Syrian Arab Republic	59.6	59.6	56.6 – 62.3	11.2	9.1 – 13.2	59.5	55.7 – 63.0	11.6	9.3 – 13.7	9.7	12.9	14.0	17.9
167	Tajikistan	50.8	49.6	46.2 – 53.2	9.0	7.1 – 11.0	52.0	47.8 – 56.1	10.3	7.7 – 12.8	10.8	12.7	17.9	19.7
168	Thailand	59.7	57.7	55.7 – 59.7	13.2	12.1 – 14.3	61.8	57.9 – 64.9	14.4	13.4 – 15.5	8.4	10.5	12.6	14.6
169	The former Yugoslav Republic of Macedonia	64.9	63.9	62.0 – 65.6	12.5	11.7 – 13.4	65.9	64.1 – 67.6	14.3	13.3 – 15.2	6.3	8.9	9.0	12.0
170	Togo	42.7	42.7	39.3 – 46.5	8.6	6.7 – 10.7	42.7	39.3 – 46.8	8.6	6.5 – 10.9	7.9	10.3	15.5	19.4
171	Tonga	60.7	59.3	57.0 – 61.9	11.6	10.3 – 13.0	62.0	58.4 – 65.2	13.6	12.3 – 15.0	8.1	10.8	12.0	14.9
172	Trinidad and Tobago	61.7	60.3	57.9 – 63.1	11.6	10.2 – 13.1	63.0	59.0 – 65.8	13.3	12.1 – 14.5	8.2	10.7	12.0	14.5
173	Tunisia	61.4	61.0	59.2 – 62.9	11.4	10.6 – 12.2	61.7	58.0 – 65.4	12.6	10.6 – 14.7	8.2	11.7	11.8	15.9
174	Turkey	58.7	56.8	55.4 – 58.2	11.2	10.3 – 12.1	60.5	57.4 – 63.2	13.4	12.7 – 14.2	10.0	12.0	14.9	16.5
175	Turkmenistan	52.1	51.2	48.3 – 54.3	8.8	7.5 – 10.3	53.0	50.1 – 56.7	9.5	7.9 – 11.1	8.8	11.9	14.7	18.3
176	Tuvalu	57.0	56.4	54.0 – 58.9	9.9	8.8 – 11.0	57.6	54.0 – 61.0	11.5	8.8 – 13.7	7.2	10.0	11.3	14.8
177	Uganda	35.7	36.2	33.4 – 39.8	7.7	6.2 – 9.3	35.2	31.1 – 39.6	7.4	4.9 – 10.0	7.2	9.4	16.7	21.1
178	Ukraine	56.8	52.3	51.0 – 53.7	8.1	7.3 – 8.9	61.3	58.0 – 63.5	11.8	11.3 – 12.5	10.3	12.0	16.4	16.4
179	United Arab Emirates	63.1	62.3	60.0 – 64.5	11.5	9.8 – 13.2	63.9	59.9 – 66.9	13.3	11.8 – 14.7	10.0	12.5	13.8	16.4
180	United Kingdom	69.9	68.3	66.8 – 69.7	15.3	14.4 – 16.1	71.4	69.2 – 73.1	17.4	16.7 – 18.1	6.5	8.5	8.7	10.6
181	United Republic of Tanzania	38.1	38.6	35.4 – 42.7	7.8	5.9 – 9.8	37.5	34.0 – 41.1	7.7	5.2 – 10.2	7.2	9.6	15.7	20.4
182	United States of America[b]	67.2	65.7	63.8 – 67.5	15.0	14.0 – 16.0	68.8	66.5 – 71.0	16.8	15.8 – 17.9	8.2	10.7	11.1	13.4
183	Uruguay	64.1	61.7	59.0 – 64.6	12.6	11.6 – 13.6	66.5	63.5 – 69.4	15.8	14.0 – 17.7	8.4	11.4	11.9	14.6
184	Uzbekistan	54.3	52.7	49.2 – 56.3	9.9	7.9 – 11.9	55.8	51.5 – 60.2	11.6	9.6 – 13.7	9.4	12.2	15.1	17.9
185	Vanuatu	56.7	56.0	52.6 – 59.7	10.9	9.4 – 12.6	57.4	53.6 – 61.8	11.7	9.9 – 13.8	8.2	10.8	12.8	15.8
186	Venezuela, Bolivarian Republic of	62.3	60.4	57.7 – 63.2	13.0	11.1 – 14.7	64.2	59.9 – 67.2	14.7	13.2 – 16.1	10.1	12.3	14.4	16.1
187	Viet Nam	58.9	58.2	55.6 – 60.7	11.4	10.3 – 12.6	59.7	56.5 – 62.8	12.3	10.3 – 14.2	8.5	11.3	12.7	15.9
188	Yemen	49.1	48.9	45.7 – 51.9	8.5	6.8 – 10.4	49.3	44.4 – 53.9	8.8	6.7 – 10.8	10.4	12.7	17.5	20.5
189	Yugoslavia	64.3	63.3	62.1 – 64.7	13.0	12.2 – 13.7	65.4	63.2 – 67.3	14.6	13.4 – 15.7	6.5	9.3	9.3	12.5
190	Zambia	33.0	33.7	30.6 – 37.0	8.2	6.8 – 9.6	32.3	28.9 – 36.1	8.5	5.5 – 11.5	5.5	7.2	14.1	18.3
191	Zimbabwe	38.8	39.6	37.4 – 41.9	9.3	7.7 – 10.8	38.1	34.7 – 41.3	9.7	8.0 – 11.4	5.8	7.9	12.8	17.1

Healthy life expectancy estimates published here are not directly comparable to those published in the *World Health Report 2000*, due to improvements in survey methodology and the use of new epidemiological data for some diseases. See Statistical Annex notes (pp.130–135). The figures reported in this Table along with the data collection and estimation methods have been largely developed by WHO and do not necessarily reflect official statistics of Member States. Further development in collaboration with Member States is underway for improved data collection and estimation methods.

Figures not yet endorsed by Member States as official statistics.

Annex Table 5 Selected National Health Accounts indicators for all Member States, estimates for 1997 and 1998

	Member State	Total expenditure on health as % of GDP		Public expenditure on health as % of total expenditure on health		Private expenditure on health as % of total expenditure on health		Public expenditure on health as % of general government expenditure		Social security expenditure on health as % of public expenditure on health		Tax funded expenditure on health as % of public expenditure on health		External resources for health as % of public expenditure on health		Private insurance on health as % of private expenditure on health		Out-of-pocket disbursement for health as % of private expenditure on health	
		1997	1998	1997	1998	1997	1998	1997	1998	1997	1998	1997	1998	1997	1998	1997	1998	1997	199
1	Afghanistan	1.4	1.6	52.6	57.7	47.4	42.3	3.6	4.2	0.0	0.0	92.5	96.2	7.5	3.8	0.0	0.0	100	100
2	Albania	3.8	3.7	71.5	70.2	28.5	29.8	9.5	8.7	17.5	19.8	81.6	77.9	0.9	2.3	45.9	45.1	54.1	54
3	Algeria	4.0	4.1	79.8	80.2	20.2	19.8	11.3	12.4	66.7	66.7	33.3	33.3	...	...	0.0	0.0	100	100
4	Andorra	9.3	10.6	86.6	89.0	13.4	11.0	22.1	24.8	84.8	66.6	15.3	33.4	0.0	0.0	...	...	100	100
5	Angola	4.1	4.6	47.9	53.8	52.1	46.2	6.1	6.4	0.0	0.0	89.1	87.5	10.9	12.5	0.0	0.0	100	100
6	Antigua and Barbuda	5.5	5.3	62.9	63.3	37.1	36.7	15.0	15.0	0.0	0.0	91.7	91.1	8.3	8.9	...	...	100	100
7	Argentina	8.0	8.1	55.2	55.0	44.8	45.0	20.1	20.0	60.2	59.5	39.7	40.4	0.2	0.2	24.8	24.8	75.2	75
8	Armenia	7.8	7.4	41.5	42.9	58.5	57.1	12.2	13.0	0.0	0.0	92.1	88.8	7.9	11.2	0.0	0.0	100	100
9	Australia	8.4	8.6	69.3	69.9	30.7	30.1	16.6	16.8	0.0	0.0	100	100	0.0	0.0	29.2	24.8	49.5	53
10	Austria	7.9	8.0	71.4	71.8	28.6	28.2	11.1	11.2	59.5	59.6	40.5	40.4	0.0	0.0	27.0	25.9	58.8	58
11	Azerbaijan	2.3	2.5	73.4	73.1	26.6	26.9	7.6	6.5	0.0	0.0	92.2	92.1	7.8	7.9	0.0	0.0	100	100
12	Bahamas	6.5	6.8	53.7	55.7	46.3	44.3	13.7	15.9	0.0	0.0	100	100	0.0	0.0	...	...	92.6	92
13	Bahrain	5.0	4.7	71.3	70.6	28.7	29.4	10.7	10.0	0.0	0.0	100	100	...	0.0	8.2	8.3	91.8	91
14	Bangladesh	3.8	3.8	34.7	36.5	65.3	63.5	5.8	6.9	0.0	0.0	87.4	89.0	12.6	11.0	0.0	0.0	95.0	93
15	Barbados	6.4	6.4	60.2	61.1	39.8	38.9	11.6	11.8	0.0	0.0	100	100	0.0	0.0	19.6	19.5	80.4	80
16	Belarus	6.2	6.1	87.2	86.1	12.8	13.9	11.6	11.9	0.0	0.0	99.9	99.1	0.1	0.9	0.0	0.0	100	100
17	Belgium	8.6	8.6	71.0	71.2	29.0	28.8	11.9	12.0	88.0	88.0	12.0	12.0	0.0	0.0	6.8	7.0	46.7	48
18	Belize	4.9	5.8	52.9	59.9	47.1	40.1	8.1	10.4	0.0	0.0	95.8	97.0	4.2	3.0	0.0	0.0	100	100
19	Benin	3.1	3.2	48.5	49.4	51.5	50.6	6.0	6.3	0.0	0.0	85.8	83.4	14.2	16.6	0.0	0.0	100	100
20	Bhutan	3.7	3.8	90.4	90.3	9.6	9.7	10.1	12.2	0.0	0.0	70.3	72.5	29.7	27.5	0.0	0.0	100	100
21	Bolivia	4.7	5.0	63.9	65.6	36.1	34.4	9.1	10.0	65.3	64.8	24.9	25.8	9.8	9.4	7.8	7.8	85.7	85
22	Bosnia and Herzegovina	4.0	3.9	55.4	57.1	44.6	42.9	6.2	6.4	0.0	0.0	69.1	71.3	30.9	28.7	0.0	0.0	100	100
23	Botswana	3.4	3.5	70.5	70.7	29.5	29.3	5.9	5.5	0.0	0.0	98.5	98.9	1.5	1.1	52.9	48.1	37.1	41
24	Brazil	6.5	6.9	40.3	48.2	59.7	51.8	9.7	9.0	0.0	0.0	100	100	0.0	0.0	48.0	53.2	52.0	46
25	Brunei Darussalam	5.4	5.7	40.6	43.5	59.4	56.5	4.5	5.0	0.0	0.0	100	100	0.0	0.0	0.0	0.0	100	100
26	Bulgaria	4.4	4.1	80.0	78.3	20.0	21.7	8.9	8.1	10.5	14.3	89.5	85.7	...	0.0	0.0	0.0	93.5	93
27	Burkina Faso	4.0	4.0	67.6	67.7	32.4	32.3	10.6	10.6	0.0	0.0	60.0	68.1	40	31.9	0.0	0.0	100	100
28	Burundi	2.1	2.3	42.2	41.2	57.8	58.8	4.0	3.9	0.0	0.0	69.4	66.3	30.6	33.7	0.0	0.0	100	100
29	Cambodia	7.2	7.2	9.4	8.4	90.6	91.6	7.0	6.1	0.0	0.0	49.0	34.1	51.0	65.9	0.0	0.0	100	100
30	Cameroon	2.8	2.7	29.4	30.9	70.6	69.1	5.7	5.6	0.0	0.0	63.8	57.4	36.2	42.6	...	...	81.6	80
31	Canada	9.0	9.3	69.9	70.1	30.1	29.9	14.2	14.7	1.6	1.7	98.4	98.3	0.0	0.0	36.1	37.5	56.9	55
32	Cape Verde	2.6	2.6	71.8	69.0	28.2	31.0	4.7	4.3	0.0	0.0	75.8	67.3	24.2	32.7	...	...	100	100
33	Central African Republic	2.4	2.4	51.4	48.9	48.6	51.1	4.0	3.8	0.0	0.0	75.7	72.9	24.3	27.1	0.0	0.0	77.3	78
34	Chad	3.1	2.9	79.3	78.6	20.7	21.4	13.2	12.6	0.0	0.0	78.0	65.7	22.0	34.3	0.0	0.0	100	100
35	Chile	7.2	7.5	37.9	39.6	62.1	60.4	12.1	12.4	83.6	75.7	16.0	23.9	0.4	0.4	33.7	33.8	66.3	66
36	China	4.2	4.5	39.4	38.8	60.6	61.2	13.6	12.8	87.0	80.1	12.6	19.3	0.4	0.6	0.0	0.0	78.9	80
37	Colombia	9.3	9.3	57.6	54.8	42.4	45.2	18.2	17.4	40.3	38.4	59.5	61.3	0.2	0.2	38.9	38.6	61.1	61
38	Comoros	4.5	4.9	68.2	71.8	31.8	28.2	8.7	9.4	0.0	0.0	75.8	76.0	24.2	24.0	0.0	0.0	100	100
39	Congo	2.8	3.0	64.6	67.2	35.4	32.8	4.8	4.3	0.0	0.0	84.5	80.3	15.5	19.7	0.0	0.0	100	100
40	Cook Islands	5.3	5.3	67.1	68.3	32.9	31.7	10.3	10.6	0.0	0.0	99.8	99.8	0.2	0.2	0.0	0.0	100	100
41	Costa Rica	7.0	6.8	78.3	77.4	21.7	22.6	21.6	20.7	84.9	89.5	14.5	9.9	0.6	0.6	3.0	3.0	97.0	97
42	Côte d'Ivoire	3.0	2.9	46.0	46.7	54.0	53.3	5.7	6.0	0.0	0.0	81.6	82.3	18.4	17.7	14.9	14.0	85.1	86
43	Croatia	8.2	8.8	80.5	81.7	19.5	18.3	13.2	13.7	92.6	86.1	7.4	13.9	...	0.0	0.0	0.0	100	100
44	Cuba	6.3	6.4	87.5	87.6	12.5	12.4	10.0	10.3	20.9	19.4	79.0	80.5	0.1	0.1	0.0	0.0	100	100
45	Cyprus	6.4	6.3	36.3	37.9	63.7	62.1	6.3	6.4	80.9	80.0	19.1	20.0	0.0	0.0	...	...	97.9	96
46	Czech Republic	7.1	7.1	91.7	91.9	8.3	8.1	14.2	15.0	89.5	90.2	10.5	9.8	...	0.0	...	...	100	100
47	Democratic People's Republic of Korea	3.0	3.0	83.5	83.5	16.5	16.5	5.5	5.5	0.0	0.0	99.0	99.0	1.0	1.0	0.0	0.0	100	100
48	Democratic Republic of the Congo	1.6	1.7	74.1	74.1	25.9	25.9	12.3	13.5	0.0	0.0	90.5	92.2	9.5	7.8	0.0	0.0	100	100
49	Denmark	8.2	8.3	82.3	81.9	17.7	18.1	12.1	12.5	0.0	0.0	100	100	0.0	0.0	7.9	8.2	92.1	91
50	Djibouti	4.6	4.9	44.4	46.3	55.6	53.7	5.7	5.9	0.0	0.0	96.7	95.7	3.3	4.3	0.0	0.0	29.8	29

	Per capita total expenditure on health at official exchange rate (US $)		Per capita public expenditure on health at official exchange rate (US $)		Per capita total expenditure on health in international dollars		Per capita public expenditure on health in international dollars	
	1997	1998	1997	1998	1997	1998	1997	1998
1	6	8	3	5	9	11	5	6
2	28	36	20	25	104	128	74	90
3	67	71	54	57	140	148	112	118
4	1 307	1 566	1 132	1 394	1 912	2 226	1 655	1 982
5	26	24	13	13	58	60	28	32
6	480	498	302	315	517	527	326	333
7	657	667	363	366	995	1 019	549	560
8	34	37	14	16	165	174	69	75
9	1 680	1 672	1 164	1 172	1 950	2 080	1 351	1 457
10	2 024	2 097	1 445	1 506	1 723	1 919	1 231	1 377
11	11	13	8	9	42	49	31	36
12	726	778	390	434	859	910	461	507
13	469	441	334	312	672	611	479	431
14	10	12	4	4	40	42	14	16
15	532	571	320	349	843	873	507	533
16	83	79	73	68	293	477	256	411
17	2 063	2 110	1 465	1 502	1 944	2 122	1 380	1 510
18	143	170	76	102	246	293	130	176
19	11	12	6	6	23	24	11	12
20	23	23	21	21	68	71	62	64
21	48	53	31	35	109	119	70	78
22	13	15	7	9	178	205	99	117
23	119	120	84	85	196	207	138	147
24	316	320	127	154	454	470	183	227
25	956	872	389	379	992	985	403	428
26	54	61	43	48	156	161	125	126
27	9	9	6	6	30	32	20	21
28	3	3	1	1	10	11	4	5
29	18	16	2	1	54	54	5	5
30	17	17	5	5	32	33	9	10
31	1 876	1 847	1 311	1 296	2 183	2 363	1 525	1 657
32	34	35	24	24	76	83	54	57
33	7	7	3	3	19	21	10	10
34	7	7	5	5	19	19	15	15
35	371	369	141	146	642	664	243	263
36	31	34	12	13	127	143	50	55
37	247	226	142	124	433	413	249	227
38	13	15	9	11	36	40	25	28
39	24	20	15	14	45	48	29	33
40	276	241	185	165	423	419	284	286
41	239	245	187	189	448	460	351	356
42	21	22	10	10	47	50	22	23
43	354	408	285	334	549	623	442	509
44	131	138	114	121	282	303	247	266
45	714	728	259	276	904	966	328	367
46	363	392	333	360	870	946	798	869
47	14	14	12	11	30	30	25	25
48	26	27	19	20	35	46	26	34
49	2 637	2 737	2 170	2 241	1 953	2 138	1 607	1 751
50	39	41	18	19	84	88	37	41

Annex Table 5 Selected National Health Accounts indicators for all Member States, estimates for 1997 and 1998

	Member State	Total expenditure on health as % of GDP		Public expenditure on health as % of total expenditure on health		Private expenditure on health as % of total expenditure on health		Public expenditure on health as % of general government expenditure		Social security expenditure on health as % of public expenditure on health		Tax funded expenditure on health as % of public expenditure on health		External resources for health as % of public expenditure on health		Private insurance on health as % of private expenditure on health		Out-of-pocket disbursement for health as % of private expenditure on health	
		1997	1998	1997	1998	1997	1998	1997	1998	1997	1998	1997	1998	1997	1998	1997	1998	1997	1998
51	Dominica	5.9	5.8	69.6	68.4	30.4	31.6	10.9	10.9	0.0	0.0	97.5	97.5	2.5	2.5	17.6	17.0	82.4	83.
52	Dominican Republic	6.4	6.5	29.1	28.3	70.9	71.7	10.5	10.2	22.3	21.9	75.4	74.3	2.3	3.7	13.1	14.2	77.1	76.
53	Ecuador	3.7	3.6	50.8	45.9	49.2	54.1	7.0	6.8	48.8	44.1	49.1	53.5	2.1	2.4	10.5	10.3	65.4	63.
54	Egypt	4.3	4.6	31.8	30.8	68.2	69.2	4.5	4.4	39.6	39.5	56.1	55.2	4.3	5.3	0.4	0.4	93.2	93.
55	El Salvador	8.1	8.3	38.7	42.5	61.3	57.5	21.1	22.0	43.3	41.7	47.8	51.5	8.9	6.8	2.7	3.3	97.1	96.
56	Equatorial Guinea	3.6	4.2	56.0	59.4	44.0	40.6	7.9	8.3	0.0	0.0	85.9	81.3	14.1	18.7	0.0	0.0	100	100
57	Eritrea	4.4	5.4	65.8	66.1	34.2	33.9	5.3	4.5	0.0	0.0	83.1	82.6	16.9	17.4	0.0	0.0	100	100
58	Estonia	6.3	6.0	88.5	86.3	11.5	13.7	15.2	13.3	72.2	77.2	26.7	21.2	1.1	1.7	...	...	97.9	96.
59	Ethiopia	4.7	5.2	41.4	46.6	58.6	53.4	8.1	9.5	0.0	0.0	85.9	85.9	14.1	14.1	0.0	0.0	87.6	86.
60	Fiji	4.0	4.1	66.7	65.4	33.3	34.6	7.4	6.9	0.0	0.0	99.2	86.9	0.8	13.1	0.0	0.0	100	100
61	Finland	7.3	6.9	76.1	76.3	23.9	23.7	10.3	10.5	19.6	19.8	80.4	80.2	0.0	0.0	10.4	10.5	83.0	82.
62	France	9.4	9.3	76.1	76.1	23.9	23.9	13.5	13.6	96.8	96.8	3.2	3.2	0.0	0.0	51.7	52.7	44.0	43.
63	Gabon	3.1	3.0	66.5	66.7	33.5	33.3	6.2	6.4	0.0	0.0	92.6	92.9	7.4	7.1	0.0	0.0	100	100
64	Gambia	3.0	3.2	78.7	78.2	21.3	21.8	11.5	11.9	0.0	0.0	86.2	82.9	13.8	17.1	0.0	0.0	100	100
65	Georgia	4.4	4.8	8.6	7.1	91.4	92.9	2.6	2.3	0.0	0.0	91.6	81.8	8.4	18.2	...	...	100	100
66	Germany	10.5	10.3	76.6	75.8	23.4	24.2	16.7	16.4	90.7	91.6	9.3	8.3	0.0	0.0	29.5	29.5	52.2	52.
67	Ghana	3.6	4.3	55.1	54.0	44.9	46	9.6	9.0	0.0	0.0	72.1	77.3	27.9	22.7	0.0	0.0	100	100
68	Greece	8.7	8.4	55.2	56.3	44.8	43.7	9.4	9.3	28.0	39.0	72.0	61.0	0.0	0.0	4.9	5.2	82.5	87.
69	Grenada	4.6	4.5	65.7	64.0	34.3	36.0	10.4	10.4	0.0	0.0	98.2	98.8	1.8	1.2	...	...	100	100
70	Guatemala	4.3	4.4	44.9	47.5	55.1	52.5	15.5	14.0	57.7	55.3	36.3	37.9	6.1	6.9	3.8	4.5	92.3	93.
71	Guinea	3.6	3.6	57.2	60.4	42.8	39.6	9.7	12.9	0.0	0.0	73.9	73.2	26.1	26.8	0.0	0.0	100	100
72	Guinea-Bissau	3.9	4.0	64.0	65.1	36.0	34.9	2.2	1.9	0.0	0.0	79.2	76.9	20.8	23.1	0.0	0.0	100	100
73	Guyana	4.6	4.5	81.5	82.4	18.5	17.6	8.6	8.6	0.0	0.0	99.4	99.4	0.6	0.6	...	...	93.9	100
74	Haiti	3.6	3.6	33.5	28.5	66.5	71.5	10.8	9.7	0.0	0.0	63.4	66.7	36.6	33.3	...	...	43.2	40.
75	Honduras	6.4	6.4	55.4	60.8	44.6	39.2	17.0	18.9	9.7	9.8	84.9	84.6	5.3	5.6	0.1	0.1	91.4	91.
76	Hungary	6.8	6.8	75.3	76.5	24.7	23.5	10.4	9.7	35.5	38.0	64.5	62.0	...	0.0	...	...	46.9	50.
77	Iceland	8.0	8.4	83.7	83.9	16.3	16.1	18.9	21.0	31.5	29.8	68.5	70.2	0.0	0.0	0.0	0.0	100	100
78	India	5.5	5.1	15.3	18.0	84.7	82.0	4.7	5.6	0.0	0.0	96.0	96.4	4.0	3.6	0.0	0.0	97.3	97.
79	Indonesia	2.4	2.7	23.8	25.5	76.2	74.5	2.8	3.3	14.1	20.8	70.9	60.3	15.0	18.9	4.4	3.9	95.6	96.
80	Iran, Islamic Republic of	5.9	5.7	46.4	48.6	53.6	51.4	10.4	9.9	36.5	37.9	63.4	62.1	0.0	0.0	0.0	0.0	100	100
81	Iraq	4.2	4.2	58.9	59.1	41.1	40.9	12.5	13.5	0.0	0.0	100	100	0.0	0.0	0.0	0.0	100	100
82	Ireland	6.9	6.8	75.6	76.8	24.4	23.2	14.8	15.7	8.3	9.0	91.7	91.0	0.0	0.0	32.9	35.7	54.6	49.
83	Israel	8.8	8.8	68.1	66.8	31.9	33.2	12.5	12.0	0.0	0.0	100	100	...	...	0.0	0.0	81.7	84.
84	Italy	7.7	7.7	72.2	71.9	27.8	28.1	11.2	11.4	0.4	0.1	99.6	99.9	0.0	0.0	4.8	4.7	90.4	87.
85	Jamaica	5.4	5.5	53.5	53.0	46.5	47.0	8.7	8.1	0.0	0.0	97.3	96.4	2.7	3.6	7.6	7.3	50.6	48.
86	Japan[a]	7.4	7.5	79.5	78.1	20.5	21.9	16.5	13.6	89.0	89.2	11.0	10.8	0.0	0.0	...	1.3	78.9	77.
87	Jordan	8.8	8.5	62.6	62.1	37.4	37.9	14.7	14.4	0.0	0.0	98.0	97.2	2.0	2.8	0.0	0.0	83.1	82.
88	Kazakhstan	4.9	5.7	76.4	70.6	23.6	29.4	17.6	13.4	26.9	28.3	72.8	70.7	0.3	1.1	...	...	100	100
89	Kenya	7.6	7.6	28.2	28.1	71.8	71.9	7.9	7.8	13.5	13.6	60.1	59.9	26.3	26.5	4.7	4.5	73.9	74.
90	Kiribati	8.9	8.4	99.1	99.2	0.9	0.8	12.9	11.8	0.0	0.0	98.5	98.3	1.5	1.7	0.0	0.0	100	100
91	Kuwait	3.3	4.0	87.4	87.1	12.6	12.9	8.4	8.0	0.0	0.0	100	100	0.0	0.0	0.0	0.0	100	100
92	Kyrgyzstan	3.9	4.5	69.4	63.9	30.6	36.1	10.4	10.1	0.8	4.6	94.0	85.8	5.2	9.6	...	...	100	100
93	Lao People's Democratic Republic	4.3	4.1	36.8	37.1	63.2	62.9	6.0	5.7	0.6	0.6	86.3	87.2	13.1	12.1	0.0	0.0	100	100
94	Latvia	6.0	6.7	60.6	61.8	39.4	38.2	9.6	9.6	52.5	49.0	47.4	50.3	0.1	0.7	...	...	100	100
95	Lebanon	11.3	11.6	20.6	18.0	79.4	82.0	5.4	6.4	5.9	14.7	84.9	76.9	9.2	8.4	1.5	13.6	95.2	85.
96	Lesotho	5.3	6.0	76.0	78.3	24.0	21.7	12.4	10.8	0.0	0.0	79.5	82.0	20.5	18.0	0.0	0.0	100	100
97	Liberia	2.5	2.4	66.7	66.0	33.3	34.0	6.7	7.7	0.0	0.0	88.8	83.1	11.2	16.9	0.0	0.0	100	100
98	Libyan Arab Jamahiriya	3.7	3.9	47.6	47.6	52.4	52.4	2.6	2.7	0.0	0.0	100	100	...	...	0.0	0.0	90.9	90.
99	Lithuania	6.6	6.6	73.9	73.0	26.1	27.0	14.4	14.8	68.6	89.9	31.4	10.1	...	...	...	...	90.9	90.
100	Luxembourg	5.9	6.0	92.5	92.4	7.5	7.6	12.5	12.7	86.0	82.7	14.0	17.3	0.0	0.0	19.5	21.5	59.2	58.
101	Madagascar	2.3	2.3	57.2	57.8	42.8	42.2	7.6	7.7	0.0	0.0	87.1	83.2	12.9	16.8	...	...	100	100
102	Malawi	7.3	7.2	50.6	50.3	49.4	49.7	14.6	14.5	0.0	0.0	61.3	67.5	38.7	32.5	1.6	2.2	35.4	34.

	Per capita total expenditure on health at official exchange rate (US $)		Per capita public expenditure on health at official exchange rate (US $)		Per capita total expenditure on health in international dollars		Per capita public expenditure on health in international dollars	
	1997	1998	1997	1998	1997	1998	1997	1998
51	204	212	142	145	293	303	204	208
52	122	126	35	36	229	240	66	68
53	62	59	31	27	124	119	63	55
54	51	56	16	17	132	144	42	44
55	153	164	59	70	328	343	127	146
56	42	44	24	26	101	121	57	72
57	9	10	6	7	37	47	25	31
58	203	217	179	188	503	516	445	445
59	5	6	2	3	25	28	11	13
60	106	82	70	54	184	170	123	111
61	1 739	1 735	1 323	1 323	1 495	1 570	1 137	1 198
62	2 251	2 297	1 712	1 747	1 905	2 074	1 449	1 578
63	138	122	92	81	182	181	121	121
64	11	11	8	9	44	48	35	38
65	43	47	4	3	163	173	14	12
66	2 708	2 697	2 074	2 044	2 225	2 382	1 703	1 806
67	14	18	8	10	77	96	42	52
68	1 002	960	553	541	1 211	1 220	668	687
69	157	172	103	110	264	286	174	183
70	73	78	33	37	160	168	72	80
71	18	17	10	11	53	55	30	33
72	9	10	6	6	27	27	17	18
73	45	45	37	37	113	115	92	94
74	14	16	5	5	37	38	12	11
75	50	56	28	34	132	133	73	81
76	309	320	233	244	696	742	525	568
77	2 162	2 476	1 810	2 078	1 998	2 277	1 673	1 911
78	24	22	4	4	111	110	17	20
79	25	12	6	3	78	54	18	14
80	139	155	64	75	406	397	188	193
81	125	149	74	88	195	209	115	124
82	1 512	1 567	1 144	1 203	1 498	1 583	1 133	1 216
83	1 561	1 501	1 064	1 003	1 630	1 607	1 111	1 074
84	1 568	1 603	1 132	1 153	1 603	1 712	1 157	1 231
85	154	159	83	84	269	265	144	141
86	2 467	2 244	1 961	1 752	1 783	1 763	1 417	1 377
87	147	147	92	91	355	348	222	216
88	81	66	62	47	231	214	176	151
89	28	30	8	8	104	104	29	29
90	54	47	54	47	140	138	138	137
91	580	565	507	492	554	536	485	467
92	15	15	10	10	92	105	64	67
93	15	11	6	4	55	50	20	19
94	138	167	84	103	359	419	218	259
95	503	534	104	96	608	594	125	107
96	28	27	21	21	77	77	58	60
97	1	1	1	1	25	24	17	16
98	345	344	164	164	286	290	136	138
99	171	192	126	140	448	462	331	337
00	2 461	2 574	2 276	2 379	1 998	2 214	1 848	2 046
01	6	6	3	3	19	20	11	12
02	18	12	9	6	35	33	18	17

Annex Table 5 Selected National Health Accounts indicators for all Member States, estimates for 1997 and 1998

	Member State	Total expenditure on health as % of GDP		Public expenditure on health as % of total expenditure on health		Private expenditure on health as % of total expenditure on health		Public expenditure on health as % of general government expenditure		Social security expenditure on health as % of public expenditure on health		Tax funded expenditure on health as % of public expenditure on health		External resources for health as % of public expenditure on health		Private insurance on health as % of private expenditure on health		Out-of-pocket disbursement for health as % of private expenditure on health	
		1997	1998	1997	1998	1997	1998	1997	1998	1997	1998	1997	1998	1997	1998	1997	1998	1997	1998
103	Malaysia	2.3	2.5	57.6	57.7	42.4	42.3	5.6	6.0	0.0	0.0	98.8	98.5	1.2	1.5	0.0	0.0	100	100
104	Maldives	7.1	7.2	74.5	72.3	25.5	27.7	10.9	10.0	0.0	0.0	91.6	91.9	8.4	8.1	0.0	0.0	100	100
105	Mali	4.2	4.4	45.8	46.5	54.2	53.5	7.8	8.3	0.0	0.0	74.9	75.6	25.1	24.4	...	...	89.8	87.
106	Malta	8.2	8.4	70.9	69.3	29.1	30.7	14.0	14.1	62.7	62.4	37.3	37.6	0.0	0.0	...	...	100	100
107	Marshall Islands	9.2	9.5	61.9	61.6	38.1	38.4	14.1	13.9	0.0	0.0	61.5	62.3	38.5	37.7	0.0	0.0	100	100
108	Mauritania	2.9	3.3	69.7	69.1	30.3	30.9	7.7	10.5	0.0	0.0	84.8	79.4	15.2	20.6	0.0	0.0	100	100
109	Mauritius	3.4	3.4	51.1	51.8	48.9	48.2	7.1	7.1	0.0	0.0	79.1	80.2	20.9	19.8	...	...	100	100
110	Mexico	5.4	5.3	43.6	48.0	56.4	52.0	6.0	7.2	72.7	70.4	27.3	29.5	0.0	0.0	2.7	4.0	93.7	92.
111	Micronesia, Federated States of	10.7	10.5	56.7	55.3	43.3	44.7	11.3	11.2	0.0	0.0	63.0	61.5	37.0	38.5	0.0	0.0	33.3	33.
112	Monaco	7.0	7.2	50.0	49.3	50.0	50.7	17.8	17.9	93.8	94.1	6.3	5.9	0.0	0.0	...	...	100	100
113	Mongolia	5.0	6.2	62.7	65.4	37.3	34.6	13.4	14.7	36.8	39.9	51.8	55.3	11.4	4.8	0.0	0.0	73.3	74.
114	Morocco	4.6	4.4	28.6	30.0	71.4	70.0	3.9	3.9	8.4	8.5	89.8	89.8	1.8	1.7	23.1	23.2	76.8	76.
115	Mozambique	3.9	3.8	56.2	57.7	43.8	42.3	11.2	11.1	0.0	0.0	39.8	38.7	60.2	61.3	0.0	0.0	41.2	41.
116	Myanmar	1.6	1.5	20.3	15.1	79.7	84.9	3.6	3.9	3.4	2.8	93.1	93.7	3.4	3.5	...	...	100	100
117	Namibia	7.9	8.2	54.3	54.3	45.7	45.7	11.1	12.0	0.0	0.0	91.6	93.2	8.4	6.8	91.3	91.3	3.0	2.
118	Nauru	4.9	4.9	97.4	97.4	2.6	2.6	9.6	9.7	0.0	0.0	100	100	...	...	0.0	0.0	100	100
119	Nepal	4.7	5.4	20.6	23.5	79.4	76.5	5.3	6.2	0.0	0.0	67.1	66.2	32.9	33.8	0.0	0.0	73.5	72.
120	Netherlands	8.7	8.7	68.9	68.6	31.1	31.4	12.7	12.9	93.8	94.0	6.2	6.0	0.0	0.0	57.5	55.7	23.2	25.
121	New Zealand	7.6	8.1	77.3	77.0	22.7	23.0	12.7	13.5	0.0	0.0	100	100	0.0	0.0	29.8	27.7	70.2	72.
122	Nicaragua	5.9	5.7	61.3	62.8	38.7	37.2	22.1	22.3	18.7	17.6	61.2	66.5	20.1	15.9	...	...	100	100
123	Niger	3.0	3.0	51.1	48.6	48.9	51.4	6.0	5.5	0.0	0.0	61.0	63.8	39.0	36.2	0.0	0.0	81.4	80.
124	Nigeria	1.9	2.1	27.0	39.4	73.0	60.6	3.5	5.1	0.0	0.0	53.8	60.5	46.2	39.5	...	...	100	100
125	Niue	7.6	6.7	97.3	96.7	2.7	3.3	13.0	12.6	0.0	0.0	100	100	...	...	0.0	0.0	100	100
126	Norway	8.0	8.6	83.0	82.8	17.0	17.2	14.7	14.8	0.0	0.0	100	100	0.0	0.0	...	...	88.9	90.
127	Oman	3.2	3.6	82.1	81.6	17.9	18.4	6.9	7.3	0.0	0.0	100	100	0.0	0.0	0.0	0.0	49.9	51.
128	Pakistan	4.0	4.0	22.9	23.6	77.1	76.4	2.9	3.1	55.1	55.2	42.0	41.4	2.9	3.4	0.0	0.0	100	100
129	Palau	6.1	6.4	87.5	88.0	12.5	12.0	8.9	9.1	0.0	0.0	78.6	83.6	21.4	16.4	0.0	0.0	100	100
130	Panama	7.6	7.5	66.7	68.9	33.3	31.1	18.7	18.5	60.6	61.8	38.8	37.5	0.6	0.6	16.8	16.9	76.8	76.
131	Papua New Guinea	3.3	3.9	89.4	91.4	10.6	8.6	9.6	12.3	0.0	0.0	83.5	77.8	16.5	22.2	2.1	5.1	88.2	91.
132	Paraguay	7.5	7.3	33.1	37.7	66.9	62.3	13.6	14.9	47.8	44.9	48.7	38.1	3.5	17.0	20.8	12.0	69.2	77.
133	Peru	4.0	4.4	55.5	57.2	44.5	42.8	10.2	11.0	43.7	43.8	53.7	52.7	2.6	3.4	6.6	6.9	80.4	80.
134	Philippines	3.6	3.6	43.4	42.4	56.6	57.6	6.7	6.6	11.8	8.8	83.5	84.7	4.7	6.4	3.4	3.4	82.9	83.
135	Poland	6.1	6.4	72.0	65.4	28.0	34.6	9.5	9.4	0.0	0.0	100	100	...	0.0	0.0	0.0	100	100
136	Portugal	7.5	7.7	67.1	66.9	32.9	33.1	12.0	12.2	7.4	8.5	91.8	92.0	0.0	0.0	5.2	5.3	67.8	68.
137	Qatar	4.0	4.4	76.3	76.6	23.7	23.4	7.6	7.8	0.0	0.0	100	100	0.0	0.0	0.0	0.0	24.7	24.
138	Republic of Korea	5.0	5.1	41.0	46.2	59.0	53.8	9.4	9.6	71.9	74.5	28.1	25.5	0.0	0.0	11.3	12.9	78.2	77.
139	Republic of Moldova	8.0	6.5	75.4	68.1	24.6	31.9	11.9	11.9	0.0	0.0	97.6	96.2	2.4	3.8	0.0	0.0	100	100
140	Romania	4.1	3.8	62.9	56.9	37.1	43.1	7.5	7.9	18.7	21.6	80.3	77.4	1.0	0.9	...	...	100	100
141	Russian Federation	5.7	5.6	70.5	70.7	29.5	29.3	10.6	12.3	83.8	81.8	15.7	16.5	0.5	1.7	...	...	72.4	73.
142	Rwanda	5.2	5.0	34.1	37.2	65.9	62.8	8.7	9.8	0.9	0.9	28.5	24.3	70.6	74.9	0.2	0.2	62.4	52.
143	Saint Kitts and Nevis	4.7	4.7	68.4	67.6	31.6	32.4	10.9	10.9	0.0	0.0	92.5	92.6	7.5	7.4	...	...	100	100
144	Saint Lucia	4.1	4.4	62.3	65.6	37.7	34.4	9.0	8.8	...	...	97.0	97.4	3.0	2.6	...	...	100	100
145	Saint Vincent and the Grenadines	6.3	5.9	63.8	62.5	36.2	37.5	9.8	9.7	0.0	0.0	99.9	99.8	0.1	0.2	...	...	100	100
146	Samoa	3.5	3.5	71.4	68.9	28.6	31.1	12.5	12.4	0.0	0.0	97.8	93.0	2.2	7.0	0.0	0.0	100	100
147	San Marino	7.6	7.7	85.2	85.7	14.8	14.3	9.9	10.1	93.6	94.6	6.4	5.4	0.0	0.0	...	...	100	100
148	Sao Tome and Principe	3.0	2.9	66.7	67.9	33.3	32.1	2.9	3.6	0.0	0.0	78.8	80.9	21.3	19.1	0.0	0.0	100	100
149	Saudi Arabia	4.0	4.1	80.2	77.5	19.8	22.5	9.4	10.9	0.0	0.0	100	100	...	0.0	10.5	9.5	31.9	38.
150	Senegal	4.5	4.5	55.7	58.4	44.3	41.6	13.1	13.1	0.0	0.0	83.6	86.9	16.4	13.1	0.0	0.0	100	100
151	Seychelles	6.8	6.9	72.3	69.4	27.7	30.6	8.8	7.9	0.0	0.0	78.0	73.1	22.0	26.9	0.0	0.0	77.8	75.
152	Sierra Leone	3.0	2.8	41.4	40.4	58.6	59.6	7.2	7.3	0.0	0.0	73.2	78.6	26.8	21.4	0.0	0.0	100	100
153	Singapore	3.3	3.6	34.4	35.4	65.6	64.6	2.6	2.6	23.2	20.7	76.8	79.3	0.0	0.0	...	...	100	100

	Per capita total expenditure on health at official exchange rate (US $)		Per capita public expenditure on health at official exchange rate (US $)		Per capita total expenditure on health in international dollars		Per capita public expenditure on health in international dollars	
	1997	1998	1997	1998	1997	1998	1997	1998
03	110	84	63	48	194	168	112	97
04	91	96	68	69	198	211	147	152
05	10	11	5	5	23	26	11	12
06	715	761	507	527	1 011	1 135	717	786
07	144	143	89	88	187	184	116	113
08	13	13	9	9	32	38	22	26
09	122	117	62	61	264	280	135	145
10	228	234	99	112	443	443	193	212
11	213	206	121	114	383	364	217	202
12	1 661	1 772	831	873	1 435	1 628	718	802
13	22	24	14	16	79	88	49	58
14	54	54	16	16	137	145	39	43
15	8	8	4	5	23	25	13	14
16	65	86	13	13	24	32	5	5
17	155	145	84	79	330	337	179	183
18	168	141	164	138	523	507	510	493
19	11	11	2	3	51	58	11	14
20	2 086	2 166	1 436	1 487	1 856	2 056	1 278	1 411
21	1 339	1 159	1 035	893	1 374	1 469	1 062	1 132
22	51	53	31	33	132	139	81	87
23	5	5	3	3	16	17	8	8
24	20	24	5	10	17	18	5	7
25	411	328	399	317	411	328	400	317
26	2 831	2 848	2 348	2 359	2 148	2 246	1 782	1 860
27	303	294	249	240	327	353	268	288
28	18	18	4	4	66	67	15	16
29	442	449	387	395	444	437	388	384
30	241	255	161	175	412	427	275	294
31	35	32	31	29	67	79	60	73
32	142	120	47	45	307	282	102	106
33	98	100	54	57	188	197	104	112
34	41	32	18	14	162	144	70	61
35	228	264	164	173	465	535	334	350
36	801	859	537	575	1 081	1 217	725	814
37	836	842	638	645	919	919	701	705
38	523	354	215	164	716	580	294	268
39	36	25	27	17	181	125	137	85
40	63	65	40	37	258	238	162	135
41	173	109	122	77	418	317	295	225
42	17	16	6	6	41	39	14	14
43	320	349	219	236	501	530	343	358
44	169	186	105	122	231	255	144	167
45	163	170	104	106	313	319	200	199
46	52	48	37	33	107	106	77	73
47	2 288	2 404	1 949	2 060	1 606	1 674	1 369	1 435
48	10	8	6	6	26	25	17	17
49	310	316	248	245	461	459	370	356
50	23	23	13	14	47	50	26	29
51	500	509	362	353	765	806	553	559
52	6	5	3	2	23	22	10	9
53	846	792	291	280	679	744	233	263

Annex Table 5 Selected National Health Accounts indicators for all Member States, estimates for 1997 and 1998

	Member State	Total expenditure on health as % of GDP		Public expenditure on health as % of total expenditure on health		Private expenditure on health as % of total expenditure on health		Public expenditure on health as % of general government expenditure		Social security expenditure on health as % of public expenditure on health		Tax funded expenditure on health as % of public expenditure on health		External resources for health as % of public expenditure on health		Private insurance on health as % of private expenditure on health		Out-of-pocket disbursement for health as % of private expenditure on health	
		1997	1998	1997	1998	1997	1998	1997	1998	1997	1998	1997	1998	1997	1998	1997	1998	1997	1998
154	Slovakia	7.1	6.3	91.4	90.7	8.6	9.3	13.7	12.5	66.2	73.4	33.8	26.6	...	0.1	...	...	83.3	85.2
155	Slovenia	8.9	8.7	79.3	78.7	20.7	21.3	16.3	15.6	96.3	98.6	3.7	1.4	0.0	0.0	48.1	49.1	51.9	50.9
156	Solomon Islands	3.5	4.4	95.3	95.8	4.7	4.2	11.4	11.4	0.0	0.0	85.2	82.2	14.8	17.8	0.0	0.0	6.7	6.2
157	Somalia	2.4	2.0	62.5	62.4	37.5	37.6	5.6	4.5	0.0	0.0	92.6	81.5	7.4	18.5	0.0	0.0	100	100
158	South Africa	10.3	8.7	47.3	43.6	52.7	56.4	12.7	11.6	0.0	0.0	99.8	99.7	0.2	0.3	77.8	75.8	20.2	22.4
159	Spain	7.1	7.0	76.6	76.8	23.4	23.2	13.5	14.3	13.6	11.7	86.4	88.3	0.0	0.0	23.4	23.6	76.6	76.4
160	Sri Lanka	3.2	3.4	49.5	51.3	50.5	48.7	6.0	5.8	0.0	0.0	95.8	96.0	4.2	4.0	1.0	1.0	99.0	99.0
161	Sudan	4.4	4.2	20.9	24.1	79.1	75.9	3.4	4.4	0.0	0.0	99.7	99.2	0.3	0.8	0.0	0.0	100	100
162	Suriname	6.7	7.1	60.2	62.2	39.8	37.8	19.9	14.1	44.7	42.1	22.8	22.7	32.4	35.2	...	...	100	100
163	Swaziland	3.4	3.7	72.3	72.0	27.7	28.0	8.2	8.0	0.0	0.0	79.3	76.7	20.7	23.3	0.0	0.0	100	100
164	Sweden	8.1	7.9	84.3	83.8	15.7	16.2	11.3	11.4	0.0	0.0	100	100	0.0	0.0	...	...	100	100
165	Switzerland	10.4	10.6	55.2	54.9	44.8	45.1	10.9	10.4	71.6	72.3	28.4	27.7	0.0	0.0	25.7	23.8	72.0	72.0
166	Syrian Arab Republic	4.0	4.0	51.7	51.5	48.3	48.5	7.1	7.1	0.0	0.0	99.8	99.9	0.2	0.1	0.0	0.0	100	100
167	Tajikistan	3.0	2.3	66.0	61.5	34.0	38.5	9.4	8.2	0.0	0.0	96.5	97.5	3.5	2.5	0.0	0.0	100	100
168	Thailand	3.7	3.9	57.2	61.4	42.8	38.6	10.9	13.3	8.3	8.3	91.5	91.6	0.1	0.1	13.6	15	86.1	84.4
169	The former Yugoslav Republic of Macedonia	6.5	8.0	84.8	87.6	15.2	12.4	15.6	19.9	89.6	92.5	9.9	7.2	0.5	0.4	0.0	0.0	100	100
170	Togo	2.8	2.4	42.8	50.0	57.2	50.0	4.3	4.3	0.0	0.0	84.7	83.2	15.3	16.8	0.0	0.0	100	100
171	Tonga	7.9	7.7	46.8	46.1	53.2	53.9	13.1	14.2	0.0	0.0	90.7	90.8	9.3	9.2	0.0	0.0	100	100
172	Trinidad and Tobago	5.0	5.2	43.4	44.2	56.6	55.8	7.6	6.9	0.0	0.0	100	100	0.0	0.0	5.8	5.6	87.5	87.4
173	Tunisia	5.3	5.3	40.4	41.3	59.6	58.7	6.7	7.0	42.7	40.0	57.2	59.9	0.1	0.1	0.0	0.0	90.9	91.5
174	Turkey	4.2	4.9	71.5	71.9	28.5	28.1	10.7	11.5	39.0	43.8	61.0	56.2	0.0	0.0	0.2	0.2	99.6	99.6
175	Turkmenistan	3.9	5.5	74.5	79.2	25.5	20.8	11.7	16.7	9.9	5.3	87.7	93.2	2.4	1.6	0.0	0.0	100	100
176	Tuvalu	8.9	9.0	71.4	72.2	28.6	27.8	7.6	7.1	0.0	0.0	94.2	94.6	5.8	5.4	0.0	0.0	100	100
177	Uganda	3.7	3.5	50.7	38.2	49.3	61.8	11.5	9.3	0.0	0.0	38.2	51.2	61.8	48.8	0.6	0.5	59.1	54.4
178	Ukraine	5.4	5.0	75.0	71.1	25.0	28.9	9.3	8.0	0.0	0.0	99.2	99.5	0.8	0.5	0.0	0.0	100	100
179	United Arab Emirates	3.7	4.1	79.3	79.7	20.7	20.3	7.9	7.4	0.0	0.0	100	100	0.0	0.0	19	19.9	65.9	64.7
180	United Kingdom	6.7	6.8	83.7	83.3	16.3	16.7	13.7	14.3	11.6	11.8	88.4	88.2	0.0	0.0	21.3	20.8	67.1	66.8
181	United Republic of Tanzania	5.1	4.9	47.1	48.5	52.9	51.5	14.8	14.9	0.0	0.0	63.3	56.1	36.7	43.9	0.0	0.0	85.9	86.5
182	United States of America	13.0	12.9	45.5	44.8	54.5	55.2	17.3	16.9	31.9	33.2	68.1	66.8	0.0	0.0	60.6	60.7	28.2	28.5
183	Uruguay	10.0	10.2	45.9	46.4	54.1	53.6	13.7	14.2	51.7	53.0	47.7	46.4	0.6	0.6	63.3	63.7	36.7	36.3
184	Uzbekistan	4.6	4.1	82.9	82.9	17.1	17.1	11.6	10.3	0.0	0.0	99.4	99.2	0.6	0.8	0.0	0.0	100	100
185	Vanuatu	3.3	3.3	64.2	63.6	35.8	36.4	9.6	9.6	0.0	0.0	51.6	51.7	48.4	48.3	0.0	0.0	100	100
186	Venezuela, Bolivarian Republic of	4.6	4.9	50.6	53.1	49.4	46.9	9.4	10.9	27.7	28.6	72.3	71.4	0.0	0.0	4.7	5.2	86.8	94.5
187	Viet Nam	4.5	5.2	20.3	23.9	79.7	76.1	4.0	6.3	0.0	0.0	93.3	94.7	6.7	5.3	0.0	0.0	100	100
188	Yemen	2.9	3.9	37.9	39.1	62.1	60.9	3.3	3.9	0.0	0.0	90.1	89.2	9.9	10.8	0.0	0.0	100	100
189	Yugoslavia	6.7	5.6	58.6	50.9	41.4	49.1	13.8	10.5	0.0	0.0	100	99.9	...	0.1	0.0	0.0	100	100
190	Zambia	6.0	5.6	56.5	57.3	43.5	42.7	13.4	12.6	0.0	0.0	60.7	57.0	39.3	43.0	0.0	0.0	73.3	74.7
191	Zimbabwe	9.2	10.8	59.1	55.9	40.9	44.1	15.4	17.0	0.0	0.0	61.9	69.2	38.1	30.8	21.0	16.4	67.0	75.7

[a] Japan data for 1998 are preliminary. They are based on new Japanese national health accounts, estimated as pilot implementation of the OECD manual "A System of Health Accounts". Consequently, the comparability of data over time is limited and there are several breaks in series.

... Data not available or not applicable.

	Per capita total expenditure on health at official exchange rate (US $)		Per capita public expenditure on health at official exchange rate (US $)		Per capita total expenditure on health in international dollars		Per capita public expenditure on health in international dollars	
	1997	1998	1997	1998	1997	1998	1997	1998
154	270	251	247	228	695	652	635	592
155	811	852	643	671	1 240	1 340	984	1 055
156	43	38	41	36	100	92	95	88
157	5	4	3	3	13	11	8	7
158	321	275	152	120	628	530	297	231
159	995	1 026	762	788	1 104	1 215	846	933
160	26	29	13	15	89	99	44	51
161	120	121	25	29	60	60	13	14
162	148	140	89	87	276	225	166	140
163	52	51	37	37	160	167	116	120
164	2 272	2 144	1 914	1 797	1 709	1 731	1 440	1 450
165	3 720	3 877	2 052	2 127	2 532	2 861	1 396	1 570
166	42	46	22	24	106	109	55	56
167	5	5	3	3	40	37	26	23
168	93	71	53	44	221	197	126	121
169	121	140	103	123	268	355	227	311
170	10	9	4	4	34	31	15	16
171	143	123	67	57	276	266	129	123
172	228	248	99	109	358	398	155	176
173	109	115	44	47	282	310	114	128
174	125	150	90	108	273	326	195	234
175	23	32	17	25	117	172	87	136
176	125	110	90	79	300	293	214	212
177	12	11	6	4	32	30	16	11
178	53	42	40	30	189	158	142	112
179	729	752	578	600	743	739	589	589
180	1 499	1 628	1 254	1 357	1 457	1 512	1 220	1 260
181	10	10	5	5	21	20	10	10
182	3 915	4 055	1 780	1 817	3 915	4 055	1 780	1 817
183	662	697	304	324	884	943	406	438
184	26	26	22	21	98	97	81	80
185	46	41	29	26	96	95	62	61
186	179	200	91	106	289	286	146	152
187	15	19	3	4	90	112	18	27
188	12	13	5	5	37	49	14	19
189	125	87	73	45	284	233	167	119
190	24	20	14	12	51	45	29	26
191	67	60	40	33	222	242	131	135

LIST OF MEMBER STATES BY
WHO REGION AND MORTALITY STRATUM

African Region (AFR)

Algeria – High child, high adult
Angola – High child, high adult
Benin – High child, high adult
Botswana – High child, very high adult
Burkina Faso – High child, high adult
Burundi – High child, very high adult
Cameroon – High child, high adult
Cape Verde – High child, high adult
Central African Republic – High child, very high adult
Chad – High child, high adult
Comoros – High child, high adult
Congo – High child, very high adult
Côte d'Ivoire – High child, very high adult
Democratic Republic of the Congo – High child, very high adult
Equatorial Guinea – High child, high adult
Eritrea – High child, very high adult
Ethiopia – High child, very high adult
Gabon – High child, high adult
Gambia – High child, high adult
Ghana – High child, high adult
Guinea – High child, high adult
Guinea-Bissau – High child, high adult
Kenya – High child, very high adult
Lesotho – High child, very high adult
Liberia – High child, high adult
Madagascar – High child, high adult
Malawi – High child, very high adult
Mali – High child, high adult
Mauritania – High child, high adult
Mauritius – High child, high adult
Mozambique – High child, very high adult
Namibia – High child, very high adult
Niger – High child, high adult
Nigeria – High child, high adult
Rwanda – High child, very high adult
Sao Tome and Principe – High child, high adult
Senegal – High child, high adult
Seychelles – High child, high adult
Sierra Leone – High child, high adult
South Africa – High child, very high adult
Swaziland – High child, very high adult
Togo – High child, high adult
Uganda – High child, very high adult
United Republic of Tanzania – High child, very high adult
Zambia – High child, very high adult
Zimbabwe – High child, very high adult

Region of the Americas (AMR)

Antigua and Barbuda – Low child, low adult
Argentina – Low child, low adult
Bahamas – Low child, low adult
Barbados – Low child, low adult
Belize – Low child, low adult
Bolivia – High child, high adult
Brazil – Low child, low adult
Canada – Very low child, very low adult
Chile – Low child, low adult
Colombia – Low child, low adult
Costa Rica – Low child, low adult
Cuba – Very low child, very low adult
Dominica – Low child, low adult
Dominican Republic – Low child, low adult
Ecuador – High child, high adult
El Salvador – Low child, low adult
Grenada – Low child, low adult
Guatemala – High child, high adult
Guyana – Low child, low adult
Haiti – High child, high adult
Honduras – Low child, low adult
Jamaica – Low child, low adult
Mexico – Low child, low adult
Nicaragua – High child, high adult
Panama – Low child, low adult
Paraguay – Low child, low adult
Peru – High child, high adult
Saint Kitts and Nevis – Low child, low adult
Saint Lucia – Low child, low adult
Saint Vincent and the Grenadines – Low child, low adult
Suriname – Low child, low adult
Trinidad and Tobago – Low child, low adult
United States of America – Very low child, very low adult
Uruguay – Low child, low adult
Venezuela, Bolivarian Republic of – Low child, low adult

Eastern Mediterranean Region (EMR)

Afghanistan – High child, high adult
Bahrain – Low child, low adult
Cyprus – Low child, low adult
Djibouti – High child, high adult
Egypt – High child, high adult
Iran, Islamic Republic of – Low child, low adult
Iraq – High child, high adult
Jordan – Low child, low adult
Kuwait – Low child, low adult
Lebanon – Low child, low adult
Libyan Arab Jamahiriya – Low child, low adult
Morocco – High child, high adult
Oman – Low child, low adult

Pakistan – High child, high adult
Qatar – Low child, low adult
Saudi Arabia – Low child, low adult
Somalia – High child, high adult
Sudan – High child, high adult
Syrian Arab Republic – Low child, low adult
Tunisia – Low child, low adult
United Arab Emirates – Low child, low adult
Yemen – High child, high adult

European Region (EUR)

Albania – Low child, low adult
Andorra – Very low child, very low adult
Armenia – Low child, low adult
Austria – Very low child, very low adult
Azerbaijan – Low child, low adult
Belarus – Low child, high adult
Belgium – Very low child, very low adult
Bosnia and Herzegovina – Low child, low adult
Bulgaria – Low child, low adult
Croatia – Very low child, very low adult
Czech Republic – Very low child, very low adult
Denmark – Very low child, very low adult
Estonia – Low child, high adult
Finland – Very low child, very low adult
France – Very low child, very low adult
Georgia – Low child, low adult
Germany – Very low child, very low adult
Greece – Very low child, very low adult
Hungary – Low child, high adult
Iceland – Very low child, very low adult
Ireland – Very low child, very low adult
Israel – Very low child, very low adult
Italy – Very low child, very low adult
Kazakhstan – Low child, high adult

Kyrgyzstan – Low child, low adult
Latvia – Low child, high adult
Lithuania – Low child, high adult
Luxembourg – Very low child, very low adult
Malta – Very low child, very low adult
Monaco – Very low child, very low adult
Netherlands – Very low child, very low adult
Norway – Very low child, very low adult
Poland – Low child, low adult
Portugal – Very low child, very low adult
Republic of Moldova – Low child, high adult
Romania – Low child, low adult
Russian Federation – Low child, high adult
San Marino – Very low child, very low adult
Slovakia – Low child, low adult
Slovenia – Very low child, very low adult
Spain – Very low child, very low adult
Sweden – Very low child, very low adult
Switzerland – Very low child, very low adult
Tajikistan – Low child, low adult
The former Yugoslav Republic of Macedonia – Low child, low adult
Turkey – Low child, low adult
Turkmenistan – Low child, low adult
Ukraine – Low child, high adult
United Kingdom – Very low child, very low adult
Uzbekistan – Low child, low adult
Yugoslavia – Low child, low adult

South-East Asia Region (SEAR)

Bangladesh – High child, high adult
Bhutan – High child, high adult
Democratic People's Republic of Korea – High child, high adult
India – High child, high adult
Indonesia – Low child, low adult

Maldives – High child, high adult
Myanmar – High child, high adult
Nepal – High child, high adult
Sri Lanka – Low child, low adult
Thailand – Low child, low adult

Western Pacific Region (WPR)

Australia – Very low child, very low adult
Brunei Darussalam – Very low child, very low adult
Cambodia – Low child, low adult
China – Low child, low adult
Cook Islands – Low child, low adult
Fiji – Low child, low adult
Japan   Very low child, very low adult
Kiribati – Low child, low adult
Lao People's Democratic Republic – Low child, low adult
Malaysia – Low child, low adult
Marshall Islands – Low child, low adult
Micronesia, Federated States of – Low child, low adult
Mongolia – Low child, low adult
Nauru – Low child, low adult
New Zealand – Very low child, very low adult
Niue – Low child, low adult
Palau – Low child, low adult
Papua New Guinea – Low child, low adult
Philippines – Low child, low adult
Republic of Korea – Low child, low adult
Samoa – Low child, low adult
Singapore – Very low child, very low adult
Solomon Islands – Low child, low adult
Tonga – Low child, low adult
Tuvalu – Low child, low adult
Vanuatu – Low child, low adult
Viet Nam – Low child, low adult

Acknowledgements

Headquarters Advisory Group
Anarfi Asamoa-Baah
Ruth Bonita
Jane Ferguson
Bill Kean
Lorenzo Savioli
Mark Szczeniowski
Bedirhan Üstün
Eva Wallstam

Regional Advisory Groups:

AFRO
Jo Asare (Ghana)
Florence Baingana (World Bank)
Mariamo Barry (Guinea)
Mohammed Belhocine (AFRO)
Tecla Butau (AFRO)
Fidelis Chikara (Zimbabwe)
Joseph Delafosse (Côte d'Ivoire)
Fatoumata Diallo (AFRO)
Melvin Freeman (South Africa)
Geeneswar Gaya (Mauritius)
Eric Grunitzky (Togo)
Momar Gueye (Senegal)
Mohammed Hacen (AFRO)
Dia Houssenou (Mauritania)
Baba Koumare (Mali)
Itzack Levav (Israel)
Mapunza-ma-Mamiezi (Democratic
    Republic of the Congo)
Custodia Mandlhate (AFRO)
Elisabeth Matare (WFMH)
Ana Paula Mogne (Mozambique)
Patrick Msoni (Zambia)
Mercy Ngowenha (Zimbabwe)
Felicien N'tone Enime (Cameroon)
Olabisi Odejide (Nigeria)
David Okello (AFRO)
Michel Olatuwara (Nigeria)
Brian Robertson (South Africa)
Bokar Toure (AFRO)

AMRO
Jose Miguel Caldas De Almeida
    (AMRO-PAHO)
Rene Gonzales (Costa Rica)
Matilde Maddaleno (AMRO-PAHO)
Maria Elena Medina-Mora (Mexico)
Claudio Miranda (AMRO-PAHO)
Winnifred Mitchel-Frable (USA)
Grayson Norquist (USA)
Juan Ramos (USA)
Darrel Regier (USA)
Jorge Rodriguez (Guatemala)
Heather Stuart (Canada)
Charles Thesiger (Jamaica)
Benjamin Vincente (Chile)

EMRO
Youssef Adbdulghani (Saudi Arabia)
Ahmed Abdullatif (EMRO)
Fouad Antoun (Lebanon)
Ahmed Abou El Azayem (Egypt)
Mahmoud Abou Dannoun (Jordan)
Abdullah El Eryani (Yemen)
Zohier Hallaj (EMRO)
Ramez Mahaini (EMRO)
Abdel Masih Khalef (Syria)
Abdelhay Mechbal (EMRO)
Ahmed Mohit (EMRO)
Driss Moussaoui (Morocco)
Malik Mubbashar (Pakistan)
Mounira Nabli (Tunisia)
Ayad Nouri (Iraq)
Ahmad Okasha (Egypt)
Omar Shaheen (Egypt)
Davoud Shahmohammadi (Iran,
    Islamic Republic of)
Gihan Tawile (EMRO)

EURO
Fritz Henn (Germany)
Clemens Hosman (Netherlands)
Maria Kopp (Hungary)
Valery Krasnov (Russia)
Ulrik Malt (Norway)
Wolfgang Rutz (EURO)
Danuta Wasserman (Sweden)

SEARO
Nazmul Ahsan (Bangladesh)
Somchai Chakrabhand (Thailand)
Vijay Chandra (SEARO)
Chencho Dorji (Bhutan)
Kim Farley (WR-India)
Mohan Issac (India)
Nyoman Kumara Rai (SEARO)
Sao Sai Lon (Myanmar)
Rusdi Maslim (Indonesia)
Nalaka Mendis (Sri Lanka)
Imam Mochny (SEARO)
Davinder Mohan (India)
Sawat Ramaboot (SEARO)
Diyanath Samarasinghe (Sri Lanka)
Omaj Sutisnaputra (SEARO)
Than Sein (SEARO)
Kapil Dev Upadhyaya (Nepal)

WPRO
Abdul Aziz Abdullah (Malaysia)
Iokapeta Enoka (Samoa)
Gauden Galea (WPRO)
Helen Herrman (Australia)
Lourdes Ignacio (Philippines)
Linda Milan (WPRO)
Masato Nakauchi (WPRO)
Masahisa Nishizono (Japan)
Bou-Yong Rhi (Republic of Korea)
Shen Yucun (China)
Nguyen Viet (Viet Nam)

Additional inputs from:
Sarah Assamagan (USA)
José Ayuso-Mateos (WHO)
Meena Cabral de Mello (WHO)
Judy Chamberlain (USA)
Carlos Climent (Colombia)
John Cooper (UK)
Bhargavi Davar (India)
Vincent Dubois (Belgium)
Alexandra Fleischmann (WHO)
Alan Flisher (South Africa)
Hamid Godhse (INCB)
Zora Cazi Gotovac (Croatia)
Gopalakrishna Gururaj (India)
Rosanna de Guzman (Philippines)
Nick Hether (UK)
Rachel Jenkins (UK)
Sylvia Kaaya (Tanzania)
Martin Knapp (UK)
Robert Kohn (USA)
Julian Leff (UK)
Margaret Leggot (Canada)
Itzhak Levav (Israel)
Felice Lieh Mak (Hong Kong)
Ian Locjkhart (South Africa)
Jana Lojanova (Slovakia)
Crick Lund (UK)
Pallav Maulik (WHO)
Pat Mc Gorry (Australia)
Maria Elena Medina Mora (Mexico)
Brian Mishara (Denmark)
Protima Murthy (India)
Helen Nygren-Krugs (WHO)
Kathryn O'Connell (WHO)
Inge Peterson (South Africa)
Leonid Prilipko (WHO)
Lakshmi Ratnayeke (Sri Lanka)
Morton Silverman (USA)
Tirupathi Srinivasan (India)
Avdesh Sharma (India)
Michele Tansella (Italy)
Rangaswamy Thara (India)
Graham Thornicroft (UK)
Lakshmi Vijayakumar (India)
Frank Vocci (USA)
Erica Wheeler (WHO)
Harvey Whiteford (Australia)
Sik Jun Young (Korea, Republic of)

INDEX

Page numbers in **bold** type indicate main discussions.